Oral Radiology: Interpretation and Diagnostic Strategies

Editor

MEL MUPPARAPU

DENTAL CLINICS OF NORTH AMERICA

www.dental.theclinics.com

January 2016 • Volume 60 • Number 1

ELSEVIER

1600 John F. Kennedy Boulevard • Suite 1800 • Philadelphia, Pennsylvania, 19103-2899

http://www.dental.theclinics.com

DENTAL CLINICS OF NORTH AMERICA Volume 60, Number 1
January 2016 ISSN 0011-8532, ISBN: 978-0-323-41447-0

Editor: John Vassallo; j.vassallo@elsevier.com
Developmental Editor: Kristen Helm

Dental Clinics of North America (ISSN 0011-8532) is published quarterly by Elsevier Inc., 360 Park Avenue South, New York, NY 10010-1710. Months of issue are January, April, July, and October. Business and Editorial Offices: 1600 John F. Kennedy Boulevard, Suite 1800, Philadelphia, PA 19103-2899. Periodicals postage paid at New York, NY and additional mailing offices. Subscription prices are $280.00 per year (domestic individuals), $537.00 per year (domestic institutions), $100.00 per year (domestic students/residents), $340.00 per year (Canadian individuals), $695.00 per year (Canadian institutions), $410.00 per year (international individuals), $695.00 per year (international institutions), and $200.00 per year (international and Canadian students/residents). International air speed delivery is included in all *Clinics* subscription prices. All prices are subject to change without notice. **POSTMASTER:** Send address changes to *Dental Clinics of North America*, Elsevier Health Sciences Division, Subscription Customer Service, 3251 Riverport Lane, Maryland Heights, MO 63043. **Customer Service (orders, claims, online, change of address): Elsevier Health Sciences Division, Subscription Customer Service, 3251 Riverport Lane, Maryland Heights, MO 63043. Tel: 1-800-654-2452 (U.S. and Canada). Fax: 314-447-8029. E-mail: journalscustomer service-usa@elsevier.com (for print support); journalsonlinesupport-usa@elsevier.com (for online support).**

Reprints. For copies of 100 or more, of articles in this publication, please contact the Commercial Reprints Department, Elsevier Inc., 360 Park Avenue South, New York, NY 10010-1710. Tel.: 212-633-3874; Fax: 212-633-3820; E-mail: reprints@elsevier.com.

The *Dental Clinics of North America* is covered in *MEDLINE/PubMed (Index Medicus), Current Contents/Clinical Medicine, ISI/BIOMED* and *Clinahl.*

Contributors

EDITOR

MEL MUPPARAPU, DMD, MDS
Diplomate, American Board of Oral and Maxillofacial Radiology, Professor and Director of Radiology; Director, Fellowship program in Oral and Maxillofacial Radiology; Director of Faculty Advancement and Diversity, University of Pennsylvania School of Dental Medicine, Robert Schattner Center; Attending, Hospital of the University of Pennsylvania, Philadelphia, Pennsylvania

AUTHORS

KENNETH ABRAMOVITCH, DDS, MS
Professor and Chairman, Department of Radiologic and Imaging Sciences, School of Dentistry; Professor, Department of Radiology, School of Medicine, Loma Linda University, Loma Linda, California

MANSUR AHMAD, BDS, PhD
Associate Professor, University of Minnesota School of Dentistry, Minneapolis, Minnesota

SUNDAY O. AKINTOYE, BDS, DDS, MS
Associate Professor, Department of Oral Medicine, University of Pennsylvania School of Dental Medicine, Robert Schattner Center, Philadelphia, Pennsylvania

GHADA ALZAMEL, DDS
Staff Dentist, King Abdulaziz Medical City-Dental Center, Departmet of Dental Care Services, Division of Oral Medicine, Riyadh, Kingdom of Saudi Arabia

ALI ARATSU, DMD, MS
Instructor, Department of Periodontics, University of Pennsylvania School of Dental Medicine, Philadelphia, Pennsylvania

THOMAS R. BERARDI, DDS
Clinical Associate Professor, Oral Medicine, University of Pennsylvania School of Dental Medicine, Philadelphia, Pennsylvania

ADRIANA G. CREANGA, BDS, MS
Dipl. ABOMR; Assistant Professor, Division of Oral and Maxillofacial Radiology, Department of Diagnostic Sciences, Rutgers School of Dental Medicine, Newark, New Jersey

ANITA GOHEL, BDS, PhD
Oral and Maxillofacial Radiology, Department of General Dentistry, Henry M. Goldman School of Dental Medicine, Boston University, Boston, Massachusetts

BRIAN KASTEN, DMD
Post-Doctoral Fellow, Department of Periodontics, University of Pennsylvania School of Dental Medicine, Philadelphia, Pennsylvania

JONATHAN KOROSTOFF, DMD, PhD
Associate Professor-Clinician Educator, Department of Periodontics; Director, Master of Science in Oral Biology Program, University of Pennsylvania School of Dental Medicine, Philadelphia, Pennsylvania

ARTHUR S. KUPERSTEIN, DDS
Director, Oral Medicine Clinical Services; Assistant Professor, University of Pennsylvania School of Dental Medicine, Philadelphia, Pennsylvania

KIRAN K. KURUBA, BDS, MDS
Department of Oral and Maxillofacial Pathology, Sibar Institute of Dental Sciences, Guntur, India

MEL MUPPARAPU, DMD, MDS
Diplomate, American Board of Oral and Maxillofacial Radiology, Professor and Director of Radiology; Director, Fellowship program in Oral and Maxillofacial Radiology; Director of Faculty Advancement and Diversity, University of Pennsylvania School of Dental Medicine, Robert Schattner Center; Attending, Hospital of the University of Pennsylvania, Philadelphia, Pennsylvania

CHRISTINE NADEAU, DMD, MS
Professeur adjoint Médecinebuccale, Faculty of Dental Medicine, Université Laval, Québec, Québec, Canada

SCOTT ODELL, DMD
Clinical Assistant Professor, Department of Oral Medicine, University of Pennsylvania School of Dental Medicine, Philadelphia, Pennsylvania

TEMITOPE T. OMOLEHINWA, BDS
Department of Oral Medicine, University of Pennsylvania School of Dental Medicine, Robert Schattner Center, Philadelphia, Pennsylvania

BADDAM VENKAT RAMANA REDDY, BDS, MDS
Department of Oral and Maxillofacial Pathology, Sibar Institute of Dental Sciences, Guntur, India

DWIGHT D. RICE, DDS
Associate Professor, Department of Radiologic and Imaging Sciences, School of Dentistry, Loma Linda University, Loma Linda, California

OSAMU SAKAI, MD, PhD
Departments of Radiology, Otolaryngology – Head and Neck Surgery and Radiation Oncology, Boston Medical Center, Boston University School of Medicine, Boston, Massachusetts

ERIC L. SCHIFFMAN, DDS, MS
Professor, University of Minnesota School of Dentistry, Minneapolis, Minnesota

STEVEN R. SINGER, DDS
Professor and Chair, Division of Oral and Maxillofacial Radiology, Department of Diagnostic Sciences, Rutgers School of Dental Medicine, Newark, New Jersey

ALESSANDRO VILLA, DDS, PhD, MPH
Division of Oral Medicine and Dentistry, Department of Oral Medicine, Infection and Immunity, Dana Farber Cancer Institute, Brigham and Women's Hospital, Harvard School of Dental Medicine, Boston, Massachusetts

SAMATHA YALAMANCHILI, BDS, MDS
Department of Oral Medicine and Radiology, Sibar Institute of Dental Sciences, Guntur, India

Contents

Preface: Diagnostic Imaging in Dentistry   xi

Mel Mupparapu

Oral and Maxillofacial Imaging   1

Mel Mupparapu and Christine Nadeau

This article provides the reader with the knowledge and skills of identification and diagnostic interpretative skills using planar images, tomographic images, CBCT, MDCT, pertinent MR images, as well as bone scans and PET images. The goal is to provide sufficient in-depth knowledge of the technique, anatomy, and radiographic identifiers for the diagnosis of local and systemic pathoses. The information will train the reader to be an advocate of selection criteria as well as a follower of the "Image Gently" campaign and philosophy supported by the organized dentistry in the United States, especially in Diagnostic Radiology.

Developmental Disorders Affecting Jaws   39

Ghada AlZamel, Scott Odell, and Mel Mupparapu

Teeth are housed in mandible and maxilla and are known to undergo variations in clinical presentation depending on the degree of abnormality during growth and development. It is essential to identify these variations in normal anatomy so that appropriate treatment can be initiated. Some normal anatomic variations are harmless and best left alone, whereas others require intervention. Radiology plays a vital role in identification of such anomalies. This article focuses on the diagnostic radiographic interpretation and strategies including differential diagnosis. Also discussed is the importance of advanced imaging and its appropriateness in the diagnosis and interpretation.

Radiologic Assessment of the Periodontal Patient   91

Jonathan Korostoff, Ali Aratsu, Brian Kasten, and Mel Mupparapu

Periodontal examination involves evaluation of soft and hard tissue parameters to gauge gingival inflammatory changes and quantify attachment loss. Conventional radiographs are vital components of this process and can be used to assess the presence of calculus and other local factors to establish a diagnosis, prognosis, and periodontal treatment plan. The 2-dimensional nature of these images limits their utility. The advent of high-resolution cone beam computed tomography (CBCT) offers 3-dimensional images that might overcome these limitations. We discuss the use of conventional radiographic techniques as well as CBCT for evaluating, diagnosing, and treatment planning patients presenting for periodontal and/or implant therapy.

Temporomandibular Joint Disorders and Orofacial Pain   105

Mansur Ahmad and Eric L. Schiffman

> Temporomandibular disorders (TMD) affect 5% to 12% of the United
> States population. This article discusses common conditions related to
> temporomandibular joints, including disc displacements, inflammatory
> disturbances, loose joint bodies, traumatic disturbances, and develop-
> mental conditions. Also addressed are the appropriate imaging modalities
> and diagnostic criteria for TMD.

Benign Jaw Lesions   125

Anita Gohel, Alessandro Villa, and Osamu Sakai

> There are both odontogenic and nonodontogenic benign lesions in the
> maxilla and mandible. These lesions may have similar imaging features,
> and the key radiographic features are presented to help the clinician
> narrow the differential diagnosis and plan patient treatment. Both intraoral
> and panoramic radiographs and advanced imaging features are useful in
> assessing the benign lesions of the jaws. The location, margins, internal
> contents, and effects of the lesions on adjacent structures are important
> features in diagnosing the lesions.

Diagnostic Imaging of Malignant Tumors in the Orofacial Region   143

Steven R. Singer and Adriana G. Creanga

> Though rare, malignancies of the orofacial region often have serious con-
> sequences. Malignancies of the orofacial region are typically discovered
> during a clinical examination or from a patient complaint. Initial discovery
> from a radiograph is rare. Three-dimensional imaging using advanced im-
> aging techniques often provides adequate information about the aggres-
> sive nature of a lesion. Radiographically based imaging demonstrates
> mainly hard-tissue destruction and, rarely, bone deposition. MRI provides
> excellent visualization of soft-tissue densities without using ionizing radia-
> tion. Functional imaging is used to visualize increased metabolic activity
> associated with malignancies, and is excellent for determining the meta-
> static spread of a lesion.

Benign Fibro-Osseous Lesions of the Jaws   167

Kenneth Abramovitch and Dwight D. Rice

> Fibro-osseous lesions are grouped together because histologically they
> show similar cellular and mineralization patterns. Despite the histologic
> ubiquity, their behaviors vary significantly. Because of the histologic simi-
> larity and the broad range of morbidity among them, it is important to be
> able to differentiate between them in the preliminary diagnostic process.
> The radiographic presentations along with the location of the bony
> changes are often extremely critical diagnostic features to help render a
> differential or working diagnosis in lieu of an automatic biopsy procedure.
> Therefore the unique and specific radiographic presentations may be one
> of the main criteria for preliminary diagnosis.

Granulomatous Diseases Affecting Jaws 195

Baddam Venkat Ramana Reddy, Kiran K. Kuruba, Samatha Yalamanchili, and Mel Mupparapu

The common aspect of all granulomatous diseases is the typical form of chronic inflammatory response with distinct microscopic granulomas that are formed secondary to either definitive etiologic agents, like bacteria, fungal, or parasitic, or due to an unknown etiologic agent, such as trauma, autoimmune, or even neoplastic process. Although they can be histologically distinct, granulomatous diseases demonstrate a variety of clinical features that may not seem to be inflammatory. Two types of granulomas are typically encountered: foreign body granulomas and immune granulomas. The differences between the two types of granulomas lie in the pathogenesis.

Systemic Diseases and Conditions Affecting Jaws 235

Arthur S. Kuperstein, Thomas R. Berardi, and Mel Mupparapu

This article discusses the radiographic manifestation of jaw lesions whose etiology may be traced to underlying systemic disease. Some changes may be related to hematologic or metabolic disorders. A group of bone changes may be associated with disorders of the endocrine system. It is imperative for the clinician to compare the constantly changing and dynamic maxillofacial skeleton to the observed radiographic pathology as revealed on intraoral and extraoral imagery.

Chemical and Radiation-Associated Jaw Lesions 265

Temitope T. Omolehinwa and Sunday O. Akintoye

Osteonecrosis of the jaw is a major public health concern throughout the world. Use of radiotherapy for head and neck cancer and bone antiresorptives and antiangiogenic agents have increased its incidence. Medication-related osteonecrosis of the jaw is more common relative to other types of osteonecrosis. Osteoradionecrosis occurs despite better treatment planning and shielding to minimize collateral damage to bone. Other related necrotic lesions are secondary to usage of recreational drugs and steroids. This article provides comprehensive information about these different types of bone necrosis, and provides the readers with radiographic diagnostic criteria and updates on current theories on pathophysiology of osteonecrosis.

Index 279

DENTAL CLINICS OF NORTH AMERICA

FORTHCOMING ISSUES

April 2016
Clinical Pharmacology for Dentists
Harry Dym, *Editor*

July 2016
Special Care Dentistry
Burton S. Wasserman, *Editor*

October 2016
Impact of Oral Health on Interprofessional
Collaborative Practice
Linda M. Kaste and Leslie R. Halpern,
Editors

RECENT ISSUES

October 2015
Unanswered Questions in Periodontology
Frank A. Scannapieco, *Editor*

July 2015
Modern Concepts in Aesthetic Dentistry and
Multi-disciplined Reconstructive Grand
Rounds
John R. Calamia, Richard D. Trushkowsky,
Steven B. David, and Mark S. Wolff,
Editors

April 2015
Implant Procedures for the General Dentist
Harry Dym, *Editor*

ISSUE OF RELATED INTEREST

Oral and Maxillofacial Surgery Clinics of North America,
November 2015 (Vol. 27, No. 4)
Management of Medication-related Osteonecrosis of the Jaw
Salvatore L. Ruggiero, *Editor*
Available at: www.oralmaxsurgery.theclinics.com

THE CLINICS ARE AVAILABLE ONLINE!
Access your subscription at:
www.theclinics.com

Preface

Diagnostic Imaging in Dentistry

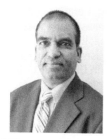

Mel Mupparapu, DMD, MDS
Editor

For every technological innovation in Oral and Maxillofacial Radiology, we have hailed the change as stunning and revolutionary. Better visualization of anatomy has led to better diagnosis. We are now able to image an anatomical region of interest with some sense of understanding thanks to the technological innovations in the field of radiology, including computed tomography (CT), MRI, and radionuclide imaging, followed by PET, PET/CT, and PET/MR, and cone-beam computed tomography (CBCT). CBCT is a game changer for all dental practitioners as they are able to finally look at teeth, their supporting structures, and jaws three-dimensionally. Since the discovery of radiographs in 1895 by Wilhelm Conrad Röntgen, what we have been able to accomplish in this short 120-year period is amazing. We have been able to better understand the effects of radiation on the human body at every level, selectively use radiation for diagnostic as well as therapeutic purposes, and recognize the concepts of radiation safety in order to introduce better radiation hygiene measures. We are certainly in a safer world than our predecessors; thanks to them, we are more prudent in our methods as we have learned the lessons of radiation injury from each and every amputation that the early radiologists went through. Father of modern dentistry and early radiology in the United States, Dr Charles Edmund Kells (1856-1928) of New Orleans, Louisiana, paid with his life trying to understand the biological effects of radiation. Selective and prescriptive radiology based on the selection criteria, guidelines, dose reduction strategies, and awareness campaigns like Image Gently changed radiology for the better.

Diagnostic radiology is both challenging and rewarding. When I approached the associate publisher for Elsevier Clinical Solutions, John Vassallo, I had only one concern in my mind: How can I make the topics in diagnostic dental radiology more interesting for students, residents, and practicing dentists? What insights can I provide the readers to make a topic more interesting? My mentor and former chair of Radiology at Penn Dental Medicine, the late Dr Bob Beideman, taught me the philosophy of being a good educator. His knowledge and love for radiology and his kindness always

Dent Clin N Am 60 (2016) xi–xiii
http://dx.doi.org/10.1016/j.cden.2015.10.001
0011-8532/16/$ – see front matter © 2016 Published by Elsevier Inc.

dental.theclinics.com

inspired me. For this issue, I knew that the study of diagnostic imaging should have an overview with current developments in the field of oral and maxillofacial imaging. I hope that my colleague, Dr Christine Nadeau from the Université Laval, and I were able to present a comprehensive treatise. The issue would not be complete without an article on the developmental disturbances. Dr Ghada AlZamel from the King Abdulaziz Medical City-Dental Center, Riyadh and Dr Scott Odell from Penn Dental Medicine aided me in authoring an extensive review on the anomalies related to teeth and jaws. We also hope that the tables come in handy for a quick look-up for syndromes of the head and neck. Learning radiology of periodontal diseases is an integral component in becoming an astute diagnostician. I teamed up with Drs Jon Korostoff, Ali Aratsu, and Brian Kasten from the Department of Periodontology at Penn Dental Medicine to present the readers with a comprehensive review of the radiology of periodontal diseases. I could not have gone to better experts than my colleagues, Drs Mansur Ahmad and Eric Schiffman from the University of Minnesota, for an article on temporomandibular disorders (TMD) and orofacial pain. They spearheaded and published the Research Diagnostic Criteria for TMD and the development of image analysis criteria that led to better understanding of TMD diagnosis. The article on benign lesions was written by my esteemed colleague from Boston University, Dr Anita Gohel, and her associates, Drs Osamu Sakai and Alessandro Villa. My colleagues from the Rutgers School of Dental Medicine, Drs Steven Singer and Adriana Creanga, undertook the arduous task of writing an article on cancerous lesions of jaws, a topic that is very difficult to condense due to the wealth of information available on the subject. They did a marvelous job in presenting the relevant material to the readers. There is one topic that most dental practitioners and specialists alike have a hard time understanding due to the ambiguous nature of the disease process and its variations—the benign fibro-osseous lesions of the jaws. My colleagues from Loma Linda University, Drs Ken Abramovitch and Dwight Rice, did a phenomenal job in comprehensively presenting the pathognomonic radiographic features to the audience by using pertinent radiographic images. My frequent trips to India as a visiting professor to the Sibar Institute of Dental Sciences fostered a valued friendship with my colleagues, Drs Baddam Venkat Ramana Reddy, Kiran Kuruba, and Samatha Yalamanchili, who helped me report the material on granulomatous lesions affecting the jaws. Drs Art Kuperstein and Tom Berardi from Penn Dental Medicine assisted me with writing the article on systemic diseases affecting jaws; a large majority of the lesions in this article were observed firsthand in the admissions clinic of Penn Dental Medicine. Finally, the issue would not be complete without the masterful writing skills of my colleagues from Penn Dental Medicine, Drs Sunday Akintoye and Temitope Omolehinwa, who presented the material on chemical and radiation-associated jaw lesions. I would like to thank the many contributors who readily shared their images for this publication, especially Dr Mansur Ahmad from Minnesota, Dr Elena Kurtz from Philadelphia, Dr Maano Milles from Newark, Drs Carl Bouchard and Joanne Ethier from Canada, and Dr Adrian Creanga from Romania.

This issue would not have been possible without the help and support from the associate publisher, John Vassallo, developmental editor, Kristen Helm, and journal manager, Joseph Daniel, along with several other members of the Elsevier staff. My sincere appreciation goes to the Department of Oral Medicine administrative staff, Hazel Dean and Umme Jahani, and my Radiology clinic staff, Carol Walsh, Karen McAdoo Wong, and Roseanne Butts, for accommodating my scheduling conflicts while I was authoring this issue.

I would like to thank my wife, Anitha, and my children, Vamsee and Archana, for putting up with me when I was burning the midnight oil or denying them a promised road trip so that I could catch up with writing my articles. I can say with certainty that this would not have been possible without their patience, understanding, and appreciation of my love to teach and share.

Mel Mupparapu, DMD, MDS
Department of Oral Medicine
University of Pennsylvania School of Dental Medicine
Robert Schattner Center
Suite 214, 240 South 40th Street
Philadelphia, PA 19104, USA

E-mail address:
mmd@dental.upenn.edu

Oral and Maxillofacial Imaging

Mel Mupparapu, DMD, MDS[a],*, Christine Nadeau, DMD, MS[b]

KEYWORDS

- Digital radiography • Cone beam computed tomography
- Multidetector computed tomography • Multislice computed tomography • MRI
- Ultrasound • Bone scan • Single photon emission computed tomography

KEY POINTS

- Digital radiography has led to decreased radiation dose to patients.
- Charge coupled devices/complementary metal oxide semiconductors and photostimulable phosphors systems are currently being used as detectors for digital imaging.
- Although computed tomographic (CT) scanners were used for maxillofacial bone imaging in the 1980s and 1990s, the introduction of cone beam CT (CBCT) in the new millennium revolutionized the use of CT for dental and maxillofacial diagnostics. This has become a modality of choice for all implant-related diagnosis and treatment planning in dentistry.
- MRI is being used for diagnosis of maxillofacial conditions with soft tissue involvement as well as temporomandibular joint–related abnormalities.
- PET, PET/CT, PET/MRI, or PET/CBCT fusion techniques are on the rise for the detection of occult pathoses within jaws as well as diagnosis of osteonecrosis of the jaw.

INTRODUCTION

Imaging is an integral part of the Oral and Maxillofacial diagnostics. Before the beginning of any imaging protocol, the health care provider must ask the question, "Where does the imaging fit in within the diagnostic sequence?" In other words, "Do I need the image?" Once the above question has been properly answered, then the next logical question should be, "What type of images should I get?" The choice of image should be the one that is least invasive and most diagnostic. It is often a compromise between the dose and the optimal resolution, if it is a radiation-based image. Other images are selected based on their diagnostic efficacy.

[a] Department of Oral Medicine, Robert Schattner Center, University of Pennsylvania School of Dental Medicine, 240 South 40th Street, Suite 214, Philadelphia, PA 19104, USA; [b] Faculty of Dental Medicine, Université Laval, 2420, rue de la Terrasse, Québec, Québec G1V 0A6, Canada
* Corresponding author.
E-mail address: mmd@dental.upenn.edu

Dent Clin N Am 60 (2016) 1–37
http://dx.doi.org/10.1016/j.cden.2015.08.001
0011-8532/16/$ – see front matter © 2016 Elsevier Inc. All rights reserved.

Why to Image

Imaging is a universal diagnostic tool. In many cases, images uncover the underlying cause of symptoms and form a basis for scientific investigation. Images support the evidence-based case management. Frequently, images document the presence or absence of disease, leading to further investigations that are histologic, immunologic, molecular, or genetic in nature. Finally, images are used for identification of normal anatomic variations so that unnecessary treatment can be avoided.

When to Image

All radiographs are prescribed after a careful clinical examination. They are prescribed only when the clinician anticipates additional diagnostic details from the image. Radiographs are required when the imaging forms a basis for further intervention and follow-up. Last, images are needed because they are the standard of care and necessary to treat the patient.

Where to Image

Isolation of the correct anatomic area as a "suspect" is important. If the pain is from an occult source, then broad-based imaging is called for. The type of trauma or disease suspicion dictates the type of imaging in most cases. Additional indications in dentistry exist, for instance, before implant bone assessment.

How to Image

The details of imaging are largely left to the radiologist and the technical staff. The decision to go digital is dictated by the availability of the imaging technology at the facility. Clinicians' input in the selection of slice thickness or the viewing angles is extremely important. Examinations with or without contrast or a combination should be identified and requested before the examination. Cine-loop of video recording for magnetic resonance (MR) studies and 3-dimensional (3D) reconstruction for computed tomographic (CT) studies can be requested before the images are acquired.

Although planar radiographs, both film and digital, have become obsolete by the advent of 3D imaging in medicine, planar images continue to be of value, in oral and maxillofacial radiology. Intraoral periapical radiographs and bitewing radiographs continue to be gold standards for assessment of many conditions, especially dental caries and crestal bone loss. 3D imaging has become a necessity for preimplant evaluation of jaws and the diagnosis of pathologic abnormality within the maxillofacial region that was not previously possible with planar radiographs alone.

IMAGING TECHNIQUE AND NORMAL ANATOMY
Intraoral Radiography

Imaging protocols
The paralleling technique is used for geometric accuracy of the images, and a rectangular collimator is used for reducing patient dose as well as increasing the contrast within the image. Intraoral positioning devices are used for achieving the parallelism and stability before any exposure.

Voltage is the potential difference between 2 electrical charges. Within a radiograph tube head, the voltage is measured between the negative cathode and positive anode. Voltage determines the speed of electrons from cathode to anode. When the voltage is increased, the speed of electrons is increased, resulting in the elections striking the target with greater force, resulting in a radiograph beam with a shorter wavelength. Voltage is measured in volts or kilovolts (1 kV = 1000 V). A polychromatic beam is the result of varying kilovoltage in an alternating current (AC) tube. Density and contrast are the 2 most important parameters resulting from radiograph exposure. Density is the overall degree of darkness or blackness of a film or image. If all other factors remain constant, an increase in kilovoltage results in increased density, and a decrease in kilovoltage results in decreased density. Image or film contrast refers to how sharply dark and light areas are differentiated. Radiographic contrast is the combination of subject contrast and film contrast (analog detector). In a digital detector, other factors come into play (like the bit depth), but the kilovoltage peak (kVp) will be the key factor. An adjustment in kilovoltage peak results in a change in the contrast of a dental radiograph. When low kilovoltage settings are used (<70 kVp), a high contrast image will result (**Fig. 1**). An image with high contrast is useful in the detection of caries. When high kilovoltage settings are used (>80 kVp), low contrast results with many shades of gray. An image with low contrast is useful in the detection of periodontal and periapical disease (**Fig. 2**). A compromise between high and low contrasts is highly desirable.[1]

Radiographic exposure parameters are typically between 60 and 70 kV and 5 and 8 mA using direct current (DC) radiographic machines. The AC radiographic machines are no longer recommended for use with the digital sensors.

Table 1 shows the factors that affect the image quality and the resultant variation in image density and contrast. **Table 2** shows the variation in image magnification and sharpness due to variation in geometric factors used to acquire the radiographic image.

In intraoral digital radiography, the resolution of an image is limited by the thickness of the layer, not pixel size. Resolution is measured by line pairs resolved per millimeter (lp/mm) and is also limited by what the human eye can detect. Typically, film resolution is greater than 20 lp/mm; the intraoral photostimulable phosphors (PSP) detector resolution is between 7 and 14 lp/mm, and the charge coupled devices/complementary metal oxide semiconductors (CCD/CMOS) sensor resolution is between 10 and 24 lp/mm. Digital imaging systems are capable of capturing up to 256 different densities,[1] whereas the monitors may or may not even display all of the densities captured in one screen. If the resolution of the monitor is higher than the captured densities, then there will not be an issue displaying those images. However, the human eye can only distinguish 32 or so different densities, which is a limiting factor in the diagnostic process. The ideal sensor (detector) should be able to display a full range of densities in order to have wider latitude. Although the dynamic range of film extends

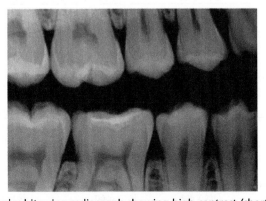

Fig. 1. Right premolar bitewing radiograph showing high contrast (short gray scale).

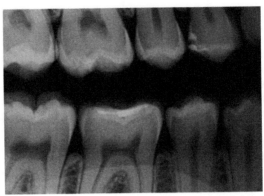

Fig. 2. Right premolar bitewing radiograph demonstrating a low contrast (long gray scale).

to 4 orders of magnitude with hot lighting, the CCD/CMOS sensors extend to 2 orders and PSP sensors extend to 5 orders of magnitude of radiograph exposure. The detector sensitivity is the ability to respond to small amounts of radiation. In intraoral film-based radiography, the sensitivity is directly related to the film speed. The sensitivity of the digital sensors is affected by pixel size and system noise. Although PSP systems allow dose reductions close to 50% compared with F-speed film, the CCD/CMOS sensors have a lesser dose reduction than PSP systems. Modulation transfer factor (MTF) is a measure of the combined sharpness and resolution factors. Generally, the MTF of fast films is superior to the MTF of PSP at high spatial frequencies, which explains the sharpness and higher resolution of E- or F-speed films compared with PSP plates. In terms of contrast, the displayed image provides up to 8 times the amount of information that the human eye can actually resolve.[2]

Table 1
Factors affecting image quality

Factor	Change	Radiographic Density	Radiographic Contrast
kV	Increase >80	Increased (darker)	Low contrast
	Decrease 60–70	Decreased (lighter)	High contrast
mA	Increase	Increased (darker)	No effect
	Decrease	Decreased (lighter)	No effect
Exposure time	Increase	Increased (darker)	No effect
	Decrease	Decreased (lighter)	No effect
Filter thickness	Increase (thick)	Decreased	Decreased
	Decrease (thin)	Increased	Increased
Object density	Increase	Decreased	Varies
	Decrease	Increased	Varies
Ambient light	Increase	No effect	Decreased
	Decrease	No effect	Increased
Glare	Increase	Decreased	No effect
	Decrease	Increased	No effect
Collimator size	Increase	No effect	Decreased
	decrease	No effect	Increased
Target-detector distance	Increase	Decreased	No effect
	Decrease	Increased	No effect

Table 2
List of other geometric factors that affect the image quality (sharpness and magnification)

Geometric Factor	Change	Image Magnification	Image Sharpness
Collimator size	Increase	No effect	Decreased
	Decrease	No effect	Increased
Object-detector distance	Increase	Increased	Decreased
	Decrease	Decreased	Increased
Target-object distance	Increase	Decreased	Increased
	Decrease	Increased	Decreased
Focal spot size	Increase	No effect	Decreased
	Decrease	No effect	Increased

The greatest perceptual sensitivity is about 5 lp/cm (1-mm-wide pixel). It is interesting to note that the sensors can display more than 2.5 times the amount of information that the human eye can actually perceive.

Studies have looked at both natural and simulated carious lesions and tested the resolving power of film and digital intraoral detectors. The conclusion is that the ability to recognize incipient dental caries lesions is not dependent on image receptor (film or digital), the system used, or the manner in which it is displayed. The most important part of lesion diagnosis is knowledge base, training, and to a lesser extent, all other factors, including detector resolution, exposure factors, and display systems.[2]

The kilovoltage peak rule

It is generally recommended that when the kilovoltage peak (for AC machines) is increased by 15, exposure time should be decreased by half when the milliampere is fixed or cannot be altered. When the kilovoltage peak is decreased by 15, exposure time should be doubled. When kilovoltage peak is increased, it results in increased density and hence lower contrast. When the kVp is decreased, it results in lighter density and hence higher contrast, which is recommended for all dental radiographic examinations. When the kilovoltage peak is increased, the milliampere seconds must be decreased in order to maintain the previous radiographic density.[3]

Radiographic images are either stored within a practice management software independently or in a picture archiving and communication system that is connected to a practice management software. This method of storage is especially true when the volume of the radiographic data is high and needs networking for large group practice situations, hospital, or a dental school environment. The stand-along dental practices may simply depend on their native practice management software to accomplish this job.

Imaging findings and pathology

Due to the fact that the anatomic resolution of the digital intraoral periapical radiographs are more than 20 line pairs/mm,[4] the intraoral radiographs are highly recommended for visualization of periapical bone changes or changes related to the tooth. Bitewing radiographs are still the gold standard for the detection of incipient dental caries because most cavitated lesions cannot be observed clinically, which makes the radiograph the only objective source of detection. In a study by Sansare and colleagues,[5] it was noted that the radiographic shallow carious lesions were often cavitated. Occlusal radiographs are recommended for visualization of areas that are not covered by periapical radiographs alone, but due to the fact that size 4 digital CCD or CMOS sensors are not available, the technique has become somewhat obsolete. For localization of pathoses within the jaws, a limited volume cone beam CT (CBCT) is recommended instead.

Diagnostic criteria
The periapical, bitewing, and occlusal radiographs have to be technically accurate without any distortions, digital processing errors, motion artifacts, or any other positioning or exposure errors that make the radiographic image less than ideal to interpret.

Differential diagnosis
The periapical radiographs are frequently used in dental practice for differential diagnosis of apical lesions that result in either demineralization of bone or scleroses of bone. Odontogenic lesions are typically in close association with the offending tooth or teeth. Nonodontogenic lesions could be either in the close vicinity of the teeth or entirely away from the teeth within the jaws. The determination can be made via further investigation or additional imaging modalities. This diagnosis is paramount because the involvement of the tooth in the treatment plan depends on the determination of the odontogenic nature of the lesion.

Pearls, pitfalls, and variations
Intraoral radiographs, although the most frequently used type of radiographs in general dental practices, due to the nature of their 2-dimensionality, cannot be used for the evaluation of bone before implants or to evaluate implants after they are placed, because the third dimension is missing from the radiographs. Intraoral radiographs cannot be used to evaluate bony pathologic abnormality that has spread beyond the apex because the 2-dimensional (2D) radiographs may not show the lesion entirely.

Anatomic variations are numerous and often encountered in radiographic diagnosis. Variation and deviation from normal anatomy are both part of a good differential diagnosis.

Pearls

Intraoral radiographs are the most frequently used radiographs for the diagnosis of odontogenic pathologic abnormality in a dental office.

DC radiograph machines have replaced the AC radiograph machines, especially when digital sensors are used.

Bitewing radiographs are still considered a gold standard for the diagnosis of interproximal incipient caries.

Significant radiation dose reduction can be achieved using digital sensors provided the errors and re-exposures are kept to a minimum.

What the referring dentist needs to know
Because intraoral radiographs are taken in every dental office, unless there is a pathologic finding that is noted beyond the competence of a general dentist, most intraoral radiographs should be interpreted by the general dentist, and the findings need to be recorded in the electronic dental record. The radiographs can be sent for additional interpretation to an oral and maxillofacial radiologist (OMR) when needed, and advanced imaging can be recommended when the clinical situation demands such a need. The advanced radiographic modality is obtained in conjunction with an OMR and is recommended that those images/DICOM volumes be interpreted by such a specialist.[6]

Summary and Conclusions

Intraoral radiographs, both film and digital, are obtained within a dental office. In some states in the United States, they are done exclusively in an imaging center under the guidance of a licensed dentist. In most situations, they are interpreted chair-side by the dentist. The radiographs are obtained via digital sensors, CCD, CMOS, or PSP, using DC radiograph machines, and they are integrated into the practice management software or an electronic dental record.

Extraoral Imaging

Extraoral imaging techniques used in dentistry
Extraoral skull views (plain films and direct digital images)
Tomography (linear and multidirectional) (outdated)
Panoramic imaging, screen/film or digital
CT
CBCT
MRI
PET
PET/CT, PET/CBCT, and PET/MR fusion techniques
Scintigraphy
Sialography and CT sialography
Sialendoscopy

Skull Radiographs

Skull radiography declined with the introduction of CT. The NICE (National Institute for Health and Care Excellence) guidelines do not recommend the use of planar view radiography in the assessment of head injuries. The recommendations from the Royal College of Radiologists (2013) state that plain film/digital skull radiograph images may be used in trauma for triage purposes when CT is unavailable.[7]

Usability of skull views for common anatomic areas
Lateral cephalograms: nasal bones, frontal sinus, and sphenoid sinus
Submentovertex (SMV): zygomatic arch and sphenoid sinus
Waters view: maxillary sinus, frontal sinus, nasal septum, mastoid air cells, zygomatic bone, odontoid process of C2
Posteroanterior (PA) cephalogram: orbit, nasal cavity, and frontal sinus
Reverse Towne: condyles (head and neck)
Lateral oblique body: mandibular body
Lateral oblique ramus: ramus including condyle and coronoid process
Panoramic: mandibular body and ramus, maxilla, upper and lower teeth, glenoid fossa, zygomatic arch, and process

Imaging protocols

The 3 most important planes are depicted in **Fig. 3**. These planes are useful for appropriate positioning of the patient within a cephalostat for skull views.

The canthomeatal (C-M) line is kept perpendicular to the image receptor for acquisition of the PA skull image (**Fig. 4**), whereas for the PA cephalogram, the C-M line forms a 10° angle with the horizontal plane, and the Frankfurt plane is perpendicular to the image receptor. In the lateral skull or lateral cephalogram (**Fig. 5**) acquisition, the detector is kept parallel to the midsagittal plane. The beam is perpendicular to the detector. For the acquisition of Waters view, the C-M line is adjusted so that it is at 37° with the detector and the beam is perpendicular to the detector (**Fig. 6**). For the Reverse Towne view, the C-M line is adjusted so that it is −30° with the detector (**Fig. 7**). The beam is still perpendicular to the detector. For the lateral oblique body, the detector is in contact with the cheek at the molar area, and the radiograph beam is aimed at the premolar-molar area. For the lateral ramus projection, the detector is in contact with the cheek at the ramus area and the radiograph beam is aimed at the ramus area. Although rarely done, for the SMV projection, the C-M line is kept parallel to the detector, and the beam is projected perpendicular to the detector. For detection of maxillary pathoses and skull vault superiorly, an anteroposterior (AP) skull image is preferred (see **Fig. 9**), wherein the C-M line is kept perpendicular to the detector, and the beam is parallel to the C-M plane (see **Figs. 3–7**; **Figs. 8 and 9**).

Imaging findings and pathology

Planar images still have diagnostic value, although they are infrequently obtained in medical centers and hospitals. Demonstration of disseminated systemic skeletal disease like that seen in **Fig. 10** is a great example. The PA radiograph in this figure shows the characteristic punched out lesions of multiple myeloma. The petrous ridge is superimposed over the lower third of the orbital area. The technique is used to assess the orbital borders, the vertex of cranial vault, the inferior border of occiput, and the lateral margins of the cranial vault (**Figs. 11–14**).

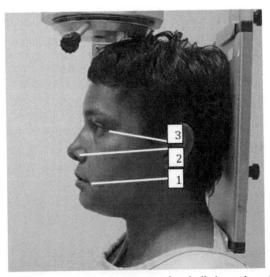

Fig. 3. The 3 important planes used for positioning for skull views: *1.* occlusal plane; *2.* ala-tragus plane; *3.* C-M plane.

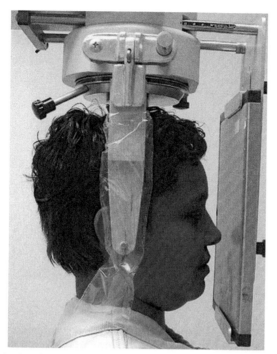

Fig. 4. Head positioning for PA skull within a cephalostat.

Pathologic abnormality detected on skull views

Although infrequently used for the detection of skull pathologic abnormality other than sinus afflictions, skull views are useful and are often the first views to assess the maxillofacial pathoses, used for ruling out trauma and also for selection of the advanced

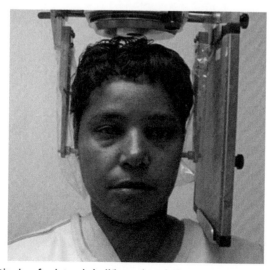

Fig. 5. Head positioning for lateral skull/lateral cephalometric radiograph.

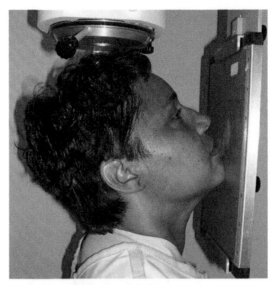

Fig. 6. Head positioning for Waters view of skull.

imaging based on the planar imaging. Lateral oblique views were used with 5 × 7 cassettes to image the mandible and TMJ area of one side. Two lateral oblique views were needed to image both sides of the mandible and TMJ areas. They became outdated after the introduction of panoramic radiography. The skull views are used for overall detection of gross pathoses, to assess symmetry, and to rule out fractures of facial skeleton.

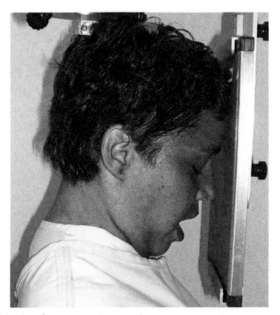

Fig. 7. Head positioning for Reverse Towne view.

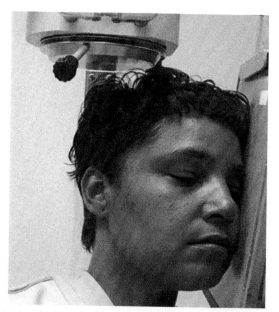

Fig. 8. Head positioning for lateral oblique body of the mandible.

Skull trauma on planar radiographs

Linear skull fractures, the most common form of fractures, involve a break in the bone but no displacement. These fractures are detected on lateral skull views. Depressed skull fractures may be noted on both lateral skull views and SMV views. Depressed skull fractures can be potentially nonaccidental and should be viewed with caution. Diastatic fractures occur along suture lines and are usually noted in newborns and infants in whom fusion of the sutures is not completed yet. In this type of fracture, the

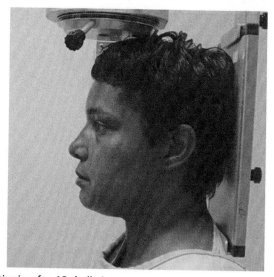

Fig. 9. Head positioning for AP skull view.

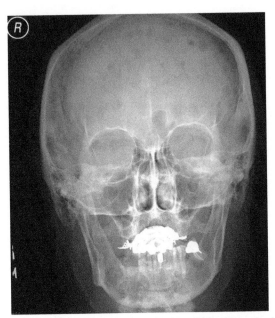

Fig. 10. PA skull radiograph showing a large radiolucency within the body of the right mandible. The diagnosis was plasmacytoma (multiple myeloma). The patient is under care of a physician and an oncologist.

normal suture lines are widened. Basilar skull fractures are the most serious and involve a linear break in the bone at the base of the skull. Most basilar fractures occur at 2 primary locations, the temporal region and the occipital condylar region, which leads to dural tears and cerebrospinal fluid leak. The ping-pong fractures are noted

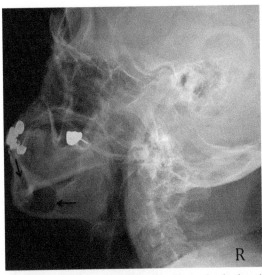

Fig. 11. Right lateral oblique radiograph of the mandibular body showing the large radiolucency within the right body of the mandible consistent with a plasmacytoma. The *arrows* are pointing to plasmacytoma lesion in the mandible.

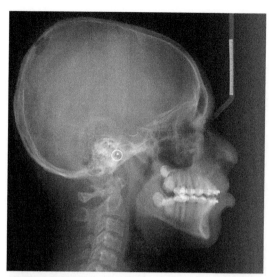

Fig. 12. Lateral cephalometric radiograph. The image includes occipital and frontal bones and vertex of skull, superimposed parietal bones, pituitary fossa, inner table of the frontal bone, and petrous part of the temporal bone. (*From* Mupparapu M, Binder RE, Duarte F. Hereditary cranium bifidum persisting as enlarged parietal foramina (Catlin marks) on cephalometric radiographs. Am J Orthod Dentofacial Orthop 2006;129:836; with permission.)

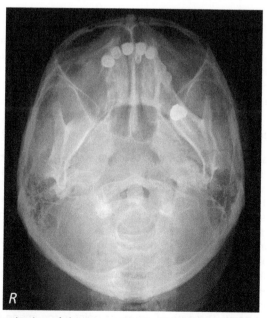

Fig. 13. The SMV projection of the same patient with multiple myeloma noted in **Figs. 10** and **11** demonstrating the skull lesions within frontal bone. The radiograph demonstrates the zygomatic arches bilaterally as well as the coronoid processes, sphenoid sinuses, mastoid air cells, and the odontoid process.

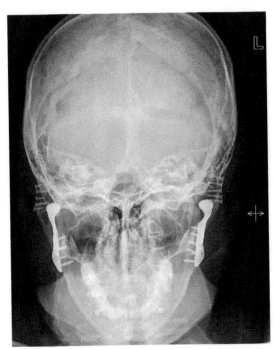

Fig. 14. The AP skull view demonstrates the bilateral total TMJ replacements for cosmetic facial reconstruction. (*Courtesy of* Dr Carl Bouchard, Oral & Maxillofacial Surgery, Faculté de Médecine Dentaire, Université Laval, Québec, Canada.)

in children who fall and injure their skulls against a hard blunt object. It is important to differentiate between normal sutures that are winding, serpiginous lines less than 2 mm in width, have the same width throughout, and do not run a straight line. It is also important to note that about 15% of patients with skull fractures sustain concomitant injury to the cervical spine. Therefore, evaluation of the skull without evaluation of the cervical spine has both clinical and medicolegal implications.

EXTRAORAL RADIOGRAPHY: LINEAR AND COMPLEX MOTION TOMOGRAPHY

Tomography is a specialized radiographic technique whereby the 2 resultant 2D image represents only a slice or a section of the 3D object. The third dimension is the thickness of the slice, which could be as thin as 1 mm. Each tomographic slice shows the tissues within that section sharply defined and in focus. In tomography, the object remains stationary and both the radiograph source and the detector move. Any structures outside the section are blurred and out of focus.

In linear tomography, the radiograph tube moves in one direction along a certain predetermined point of depth (referred to as pivot point or the fulcrum) and the image receptor moves along in the opposite direction. The path of the pivot point along the predetermined depth is known as the object point and is less blurred or unsharp compared with any layer or depth within a patient anterior or posterior, buccal or lingual to the pivot point. The path of the pivot point is the image layer that will be used for diagnosis.

The linear tomography was replaced with complex motion or multidirectional tomography (**Fig. 15**) because linear tomography was not clinically useful in many

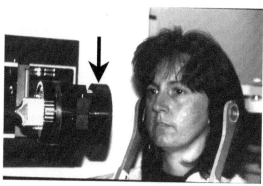

Fig. 15. A patient positioned within a digital complex-motion tomographic machine (Tomax Ultrascan). The arrow points out the CCD of the Tomax Ultrascan.

anatomic areas that are more curved. The complex motion tomography (image), although started as a film-based modality, transformed into a digital modality and was quite popular in the early 1990s before it became outdated. In rotational pantomography, a more complex form of tomography is used for maxillofacial imaging, where the projection of an object point moves along the detector path in the same direction of the radiograph beam (based on a predetermined path or focal trough), thus creating an area of reduced unsharpness compared with the rest of the areas the beam passes through. If the detector moves at the same speed following the moving projection of an object point, this point will always be projected on the same spot on the detector and will not appear unsharp on the resultant image.

Tomographic techniques were used to evaluate bone quantity before implant placement, antral lesions, facial trauma, especially orbital blow out fractures, and TMJ pathologic abnormality (**Fig. 16**). Due to the blurring of structures, the image quality is inferior to that of intraoral radiographs. Eventually, the complex motion tomography was replaced by the CBCT in dentistry.

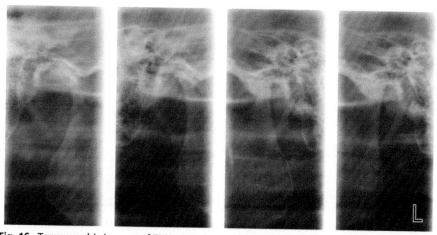

Fig. 16. Tomographic images of TMJ: complex motion tomographic slices of the TMJ in both open and closed positions. Note the significant degenerative changes in both the condyles.

Extraoral Radiography: Panoramic Imaging (Pantomography)

Panoramic imaging (pantomography) is also known as rotational radiography, panoramic radiography, or orthopantomography. The active imaging area is known as the focal trough, which is roughly horseshoe-shaped, matching the shape of the dental arches. A narrow vertical beam (slit beam) is used in rotational pantomography to capture the image layer. Because the objects under investigation are not necessarily perfectly circular and the beam uses one center of rotation (stationary) for the image capture in the maxillofacial region, manufacturers of panoramic radiographic machines developed different movement patterns to capture the average jaw anatomy as accurately as possible. The earliest projection technique that was used for panoramic imaging used one stationary center of rotation at one side of the jaw, projecting the other side of the jaw onto the image receptor (or the detector). Later, as the development of the panoramic radiography technique was refined, continuously moving rotation centers were developed where, the effective projection center, the functional focus is continuously shifted along a defined path. Many manufacturers of panoramic machines used a combination of stationary rotation center and moving rotation centers in their equipment. Early examples of such machines are the Orthopantomograph models OP2 and OP3 made by Siemens and the OrthOralix panoramic machine made by Phillips.

Distortions within panoramic images

It has been shown that the magnification factor in the horizontal dimension in any panoramic machine is a nonlinear function of the object depth, which varies in different regions of the image. Thus, the horizontal dimensions in a panoramic radiograph are very unreliable. In the vertical dimension, the magnification factor varies with the object depth, but the variation is moderate. In panoramic machines that have a constant or nearly constant distance between the ray source and the center of the layer throughout the excursion, the vertical magnification factor at a certain object depth is the same throughout the image. Therefore, it can be summed up from this information that the vertical measurements can be performed in a panoramic radiograph as long as only those distances are measured that, from anatomic factors, are known to be near vertical.[8] **Figs. 17** and **18** are typical examples of panoramic radiography. The images are used for the detection of gross pathologic abnormality within the jaws

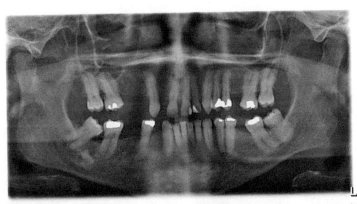

Fig. 17. Panoramic radiograph showing partially edentulous maxilla and mandible. Note the irregular opacity near the root apices of the molars that may not be completely noted on an intraoral radiograph.

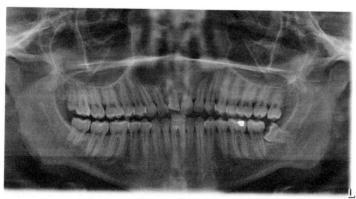

Fig. 18. Partially cropped panoramic radiograph in which 2 fourth molars are noted in the maxilla as well as a large radiolucency in relation to maxillary right central (fractured crown) and lateral incisor apices consistent with an inflammatory cystic lesion extending to the floor of the nasal fossa on the right side.

as well as localization of odontogenic pathologic abnormality and trauma, except incipient dental caries.

Interpretation of panoramic images

The properly exposed digital panoramic radiograph with a properly positioned patient within the machine can be interpreted well on a diagnostic quality computer monitor. The interpretation of film-based panoramic radiograph needs a good-quality light box with properly covered areas for the extraneous light that is not passing through the film. This good-quality light box will increase the diagnostic efficacy of the image because the contrast will be ideal without any extraneous light. The interpretation methodology varies, but a common goal in any interpretative exercise is to be thorough and not miss any area within the image. The ideal diagnostic sequence would be to start with one condyle and end with the other condyle, making sure that the mandible is covered along with the teeth; the maxilla would be interpreted from right to left or left to right with the same thoroughness and the zygomatic processes. Arches as well as bilateral maxillary sinus areas are interpreted along with the midline structures like nasal septum, the conchae, and the nasal fossa, if they are noted without much distortion. Typically, because the positioning of the patient aims at the teeth being centered within the focal trough, the structures either anterior or posterior to the focal trough will be distorted, and these areas should not be interpreted on this image unless accompanied by additional planar or CT images or sections. Suprahyoid and subhyoid regions including the anterior part of the cervical vertebrae are noted in these radiographs, especially between C− and C4 if the patient is properly positioned. This area is interpreted for any notable soft tissue calcifications including but not limited to calcifications of lymph nodes, limbus vertebrae, calcified atherosclerotic plaques within the carotid arteries, and physiologic calcifications like the triticeous cartilages. Also sialoliths, phleboliths, and tonsillar calcifications that are superimposed over the angles of the mandible more superiorly should be further investigated with 3D imaging.

Because structures undergo significant distortions within the panoramic images, the magnification factor supplied by the manufacturer has to be taken into account before performing any measurements. These measurements can never be accurate. Attempts have been made in the past to place root form implants in the mandible and maxilla only using panoramic radiographs without any additional modalities to evaluate the buccolingual width or dimensions. Without this third dimension, the implant placement can be considered very risky because it might lead to the implant endangering the soft tissues around the jaw, entering into the foramina or sinuses inadvertently with devastating results for the patient. A common sequela would be injury to the mandibular (inferior alveolar) nerve, perforation of the maxillary sinus floor, or injury to the incisive or nasopalatine nerve bundles. Injury to the lingual neurovascular bundle in the symphysial region has also been reported during implant placement where a 3D imaging has not been performed before implant placement.[9]

Extraoral Radiography: Multidetector Computed Tomography/Multislice Computed Tomography

The first CT scanner was built and installed at Atkinson-Morley Hospital in England in September of 1971. This first scanner, also known as the EMI device, was a dedicated head and neck scanner developed by Godfrey Hounsfield, who was an engineer with British EMI Corp. The combination of linear translation followed by incremental rotation is called translate-rotate motion, which was the basis for the first-generation scanners. The acquisition time was long, and they were used only for head scanning. In 1974, the second-generation scanners were introduced, which incorporated multiple narrow beams and multiple detectors. The geometry used was still rotate-translate motion. The second-generation scanners were able to attain scan times as low as 20 seconds. The scanners were modified for use of the entire body. In the third-generation CT scanners, the translate motion was removed, and the detector array was linked to the radiograph tube so that both tube and the detectors rotate together around the patient to follow the rotate-rotate geometry. The third-generation scanners reduced the single scan time to as low as 5 seconds.

By 1976, the 1-second scans were achieved with the incorporation of a large stationary ring of detectors, with the radiograph tube alone rotating around the patient. This fourth-generation scanner was developed under contract with the National Institutes of Health. The fourth-generation scanners were limited by the need for large ring diameters (170–180 cm) that were needed to maintain acceptable beam-skin distances. There was a need for at least 1200 detectors to fill the ring, but cost considerations limited the number to 600 initially. The other disadvantage of fourth-generation scanners was its scatter due to design changes from third to fourth generations (**Figs. 19–22**).

Next in the line of CT scanners was the electron beam CT. Ultrafast scan times were achieved by a design using a large bell-shaped radiograph tube. A narrow electron stream from the cathode was electronically steered and swept along an annular target surrounding the patient, producing radiographs at each point impinged by the electron stream. With no moving parts, scan times as short as 10 to 20 ms became a reality.

Further developments in the CT scan technology led to the innovation via the concept of slip-ring design of the CT machine, where a low-voltage ring could pass electrical power to the rotating components in an attempt to reduce interscan delays. Real-time CT fluoroscopy has become a reality with these scans. The developments in CT scanning led to the introduction of multidetector (or multislice) CT in order to maximize the effective use of available radiograph beam. The radiograph beam is widened in the Z-direction (slice thickness), and multiple rows of detectors were used for data acquisition for more than one slice at a time. Using more than one slice at a time would reduce the total number of rotations of the tube head and therefore the scan time. The postprocessing of the volume data from these scanners was almost isotropic, which means that the reformatted images in any plane other than

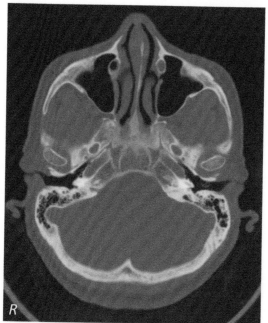

Fig. 19. Axial CT in bone windows at the level of the condyles and skull base.

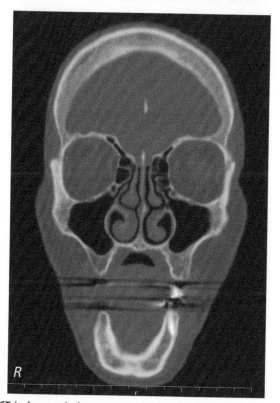

Fig. 20. Coronal CT in bone windows anteriorly showing the nasal, orbital, and maxillary sinus anatomy apart from part of maxilla and mandible.

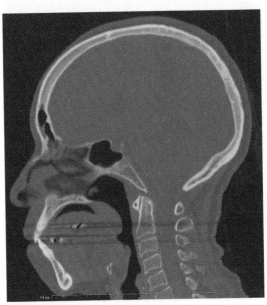

Fig. 21. (Mid) Sagittal CT in bone windows showing the Sella, Clivus, anterior maxilla and mandible, cervical vertebrae, and foramen magnum.

the original plane exhibit spatial resolution (in the Z-direction) that is equal to that of the original images. Submillimeter scanning became a reality after the introduction of the 16-slice scanner in 2002. By 2005, 64-slice scanners were introduced with further lengthening of the detector arrays and z-axis. MDCT is currently used for

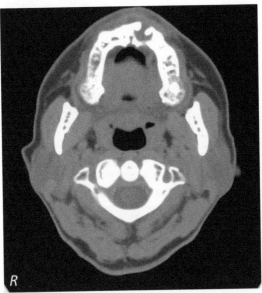

Fig. 22. Axial CT in soft tissue window at the level of the ramus. A radicular cyst is noted in the maxilla in the area of left lateral incisor and canine.

any part of the body anatomy from the head and neck region to the pelvis to the long bones. MDCT has become invaluable for neuroimaging, skeletal imaging, as well as abdominal imaging.[10]

Maxillofacial applications were numerous, including preimplant imaging by using reconstruction software like DentaScan. This Dentascan software is used for the evaluation of jaws and the identification of the proximity of inferior alveolar nerve canal to the impacted teeth and maxillary posterior teeth to the maxillary sinus. It is also intended for use in the presurgical evaluation of dental implants and for diagnosis of diseases of the mandible and maxilla. If the imaging does not have a CBCT machine, then a DentaScan would be appropriate modality, although it imparts higher radiation doses (**Fig. 23**).

The dual-source MDCT scanners were introduced mostly for cardiac imaging; then the next-generation CT scanners, 128-slice and 256-slice scanners, came along. The 256-slice scanner was designed to successfully visualize the coronaries, myocardial contraction, and myocardial enhancement during a single imaging examination without any table motion.

Future of computed tomographic imaging

Fusion imaging technology is the superimposition of images from 2 independent modalities to produce an image that provides greater information. Two structural imaging modalities can be fused (CT-MRI or ultrasound [US]-MRI) or a structural imaging modality can be fused with a functional imaging modality. PET-CT fusion is one of the most clinically relevant forms of fusion. PET-CBCT fusion techniques have been tried as well to see the efficacy of such techniques for early identification of metastatic malignant lesions or medication-related osteonecrosis of the jaw (MRONJ) lesions. Both Image Gently and Image Wisely campaigns advocate the judicious use of radiation in children, to develop separate protocols for pediatric population and education for the users on the risk-benefit ratio, justification, and overall adherence to the selection criteria and protocols. Dentistry is no exception, where the OMRs are the gatekeepers

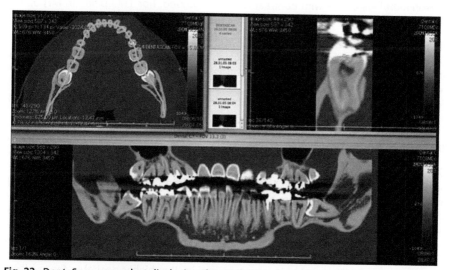

Fig. 23. DentaScan screenshot displaying the axial view, cross-sectional view of a tooth, and the panoramic reconstruction. This was the first software developed with the ability for a panoramic reconstruction using MDCT data before the advent of CBCT.

for such protocols for both advocacy and developing training programs aimed at general dentists.

Indications for prescription of computed tomography (emergent)

- Any sign of basal skull fracture (hemotympanum, cerebrospinal fluid leakage from ear or nose, Battle sign)
- Suspected open or depressed skull fracture
- Focal neurologic deficit
- Posttraumatic seizure
- More than one episode of vomiting
- Amnesia for more than 30 minutes before impact

CT is also indicated for all patients without any loss of consciousness or amnesia following a head trauma, but with additional risk factors, such as:

- Age 65 and over
- Coagulopathy
- Dangerous mechanism of injury, ejections or falls from a height greater than 1 m.

Indications for prescription of maxillofacial computed tomography (nonemergent)

- Suspected benign and malignant lesions of head and neck
- Trauma
- Osteomyelitis and osteonecrosis of the jaw
- Rule out pathologic abnormality before placement of a root form implant

Indications for face computed tomography

CT of the head is recommended for facial trauma (CT without contrast) and sinus disease (CT sinus without contrast). If suspected orbital or intracranial involvement, MR brain and orbits with and without contrast is recommended. For infections, CT maxillofacial with contrast is suggested. With suspected orbit or brain extension, MRI brain and orbits without contrast is the choice of modality. For hearing loss and vertigo, sensorineural loss, MRI with contrast is recommended. For TMJ pain, an MR of the TMJ is suggested if the clinical examination dictates.

Indications for neck computed tomography

For carotid artery or vertebral artery stenosis: CT angiography neck with contrast. MR angiography neck with and without contrast, carotid Doppler US for detection of vessel occlusion.

For neck mass: CT neck with contrast; thyroid nodule: neck US; thyroid cancer: MR neck with and without contrast.[7,11]

EXTRAORAL RADIOGRAPHY: CONE BEAM COMPUTED TOMOGRAPHY NONCONTRAST

CBCT is an advancement in the CT imaging that has now become a potentially low-dose, cross-sectional imaging of choice for visualizing bony structures of the head and neck. The first CBCT system became commercially available for dental and maxillofacial imaging in 2001 with the introduction of New Tom QR DVT 9000 (Quantitative Radiology, Verona, Italy). The CBCT provides high-isotropic spatial resolution acquired only with single-gantry revolution. Efficient use of radiograph beam in CBCT imaging requiring a very low radiograph tube power along with flat panel detector combined with limited anatomic coverage makes this highly desirable for in-office use. CBCT acquisition parameters can be optimized to produce isometric voxels as small as $80 \times 80 \times 80 \ \mu m^3$ at the isocenter.[12,13]

The relatively low patient dose for dedicated dentomaxillofacial scans makes this imaging potentially sought after compared with other high-dose imaging modalities.[13] The effective doses for most CBCT scanners can be categorized between 30 and 80 µSv (broad ranges are between 13 and 498 µSv), depending on the exposure parameters and field-of-view (FOV) size. CBCT is used with increasing frequencies in all branches of dentistry due to its availability, ease of operation, and clinical superiority over the existing 2D modalities like intraoral radiography, panoramic radiography, and skull views (**Fig. 24**). The visualization of the buccolingual or facial-palatal dimension is a major factor in the success of the CBCT imaging. The case shown here illustrates the benefit of CBCT over 2D imaging. A 60-year-old patient underwent root canal treatment of maxillary anterior teeth that did not heal after the endodontic therapy for months and, on suggestion from the endodontist, a CBCT was obtained that showed an extensive cystic lesion that occupied most of the right maxilla (**Figs. 25–28**).

The isotropic voxels combined with the ease of chair-side image reconstructions made this quite popular among dental practitioners. It is suggested that the volumes be read by a trained OMR so as to generate a report for the acquired volumes. Although there are training programs for the general dentist in the interpretation of CBCT volumes, it is a decision that the general dentist or another specialist should take to get the volumes read by an OMR.

The American Dental Association (ADA) in conjunction with the American Academy of Oral and Maxillofacial Radiology (AAOMR) developed certification courses in CBCT to train general dentists who own the CBCT machines and are using them for dental and maxillofacial imaging. The ownership and utilization of CBCT machines have skyrocketed in the past few years. It was estimated that by 2010, more than 3000 CBCT machines and about 30 different models have been sold in the continental United States. No new data are available for 2015 to 2016 regarding the sale of CBCT machines in North America. Although the manufacturers provide some basic training for operation of the CBCT machines, unless the dentists understand responsibilities of owning such equipment and continually educating themselves, the technology is at a risk of being overused. Essentially, there are CBCT machines that are manufactured as small volume machines (use a small FOV and used for dental applications like in periodontics, endodontics, single-implant placements, and identification of pathologic abnormality limited to 1 or 2 teeth) (**Fig. 29**; limited FOV CBCT machine).

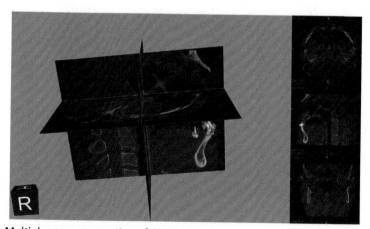

Fig. 24. Multiplanar reconstruction of CBCT data along with 3D display of the data.

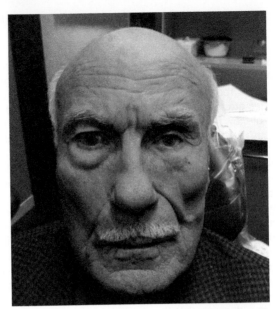

Fig. 25. An endodontic patient who underwent root canal treatment of maxillary right central and lateral incisors. At the time of presentation, he had a diffuse swelling on the right canine fossa area obliterating the nasolabial fold. There was significant discomfort. (*Courtesy of* Dr Elena Kurtz, Endodontist, Philadelphia, PA.)

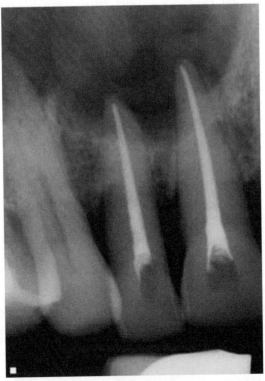

Fig. 26. Maxillary right lateral-canine PA radiograph was obtained that showed the endodontically treated central and lateral incisors and a large radiolucency apical to the root portions. (*Courtesy of* Dr Elena Kurtz, Endodontist, Philadelphia, PA.)

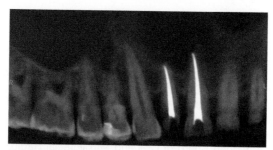

Fig. 27. Limited volume CBCT panoramic reconstruction was sought that showed a large lesion within the right maxilla extending more posteriorly. (*Courtesy of* Dr Elena Kurtz, Endodontist, Philadelphia, PA.)

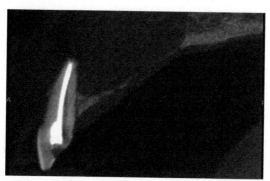

Fig. 28. CBCT sagittal section in the region of the central incisor showing erosion of the palatal bone and possibly even perforation at places. (*Courtesy of* Dr Elena Kurtz, Endodontist, Philadelphia, PA.)

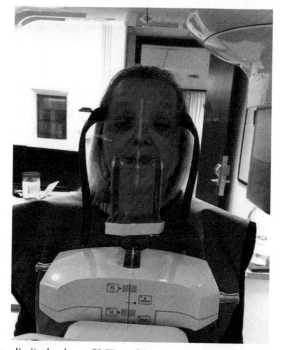

Fig. 29. Patient in a limited volume CBCT machine. Laser beams are used for positioning and selection of volumes. (*Courtesy of* Dr Steven R. Singer, Department of Diagnostic Sciences, Rutgers School of Dental Medicine, Newark, NJ.)

There are other machines that cater to larger FOVs that may acquire medium to large volume data (**Fig. 30**). Currently, there are CBCT machines that are designed to capture many different types of FOVs from small to large. There is an urgent need for appropriate training in the usage and regulation of such machines in the United States. Currently, OMR, either eligible via the commission on dental accreditation or the commission on dental accreditation of Canada (CDAC) certified graduate dental education or certified by the American Board of Oral and Maxillofacial Radiology, are the only ADA-recognized specialists who should interpret and report CBCT, maxillofacial CT, and maxillofacial MR volumes for dental applications. Although general dentists and other dental specialists are using CBCT for clinical applications, reporting of any 3D volumes is within the scope of Oral and Maxillofacial Radiology practice. The AAOMR developed position statements independently and in association with other specialties advocating the judicious use of CBCT and clarifying the role of OMRs in the CBCT interpretative services.[14–16] Any other dental specialist who intends to write their own CBCT reports should consult their liability/malpractice insurance carrier and declare that this is part of their intended dental practice.

EXTRAORAL RADIOGRAPHY: MRI

MRI is an imaging modality that uses static magnetic fields where the hydrogen protons within the patient's body align to the magnetic field created. A radiofrequency (RF) pulse is sent in that is, tuned to a specific range of frequencies at which the hydrogen protons are precessing. Some hydrogen protons result in getting knocked out of the alignment with the static magnetic field and forced into phase with other hydrogen protons. As the energy from the RF pulse weakens, the hydrogen protons will return to alignment with the static magnetic field. The MR signal is captured from the hydrogen protons as they get back into alignment with the magnetic field and fall out of phase with each other. The MR signal is then rearranged and spatially located to produce images.

MRI of the TMJ captures the disk or the meniscus and its relation to the condylar head in both open and closed positions (**Figs. 31** and **32**). The presence of the disk in its normal position is an important observation because any variation from normality would suggest TMJ dysfunction. Because TMJ disk displacement is a common finding even in asymptomatic volunteers, the diagnosis of TMJ dysfunction depends on several other factors, such as joint effusion, ruptured retrodiscal layers, and

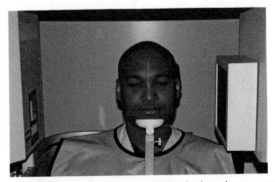

Fig. 30. Patient in a large volume CBCT machine. Note the laser beams used for proper positioning the patient's head in the machine. (*Courtesy of* Dr Steven R. Singer, Department of Diagnostic Sciences, Rutgers School of Dental Medicine, Newark, NJ.)

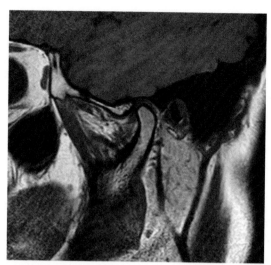

Fig. 31. Left TMJ closed mouth MRI: proton density image in a 46-year-old woman clearly depicting the anatomy of the glenoid fossa and the mandibular condyle. (*Courtesy of* Dr Joanne E. Ethier, Montreal, Canada.)

thickening of the attachment of lateral pterygoid muscles that would suggest early degenerative joint disease (DJD). More advanced DJD would be characterized by osteoarthritic changes within the fossa and the condyle, such as condylar head flattening, osteophytes or decreased joint space, and subchondral sclerosis.

MRI is the standard imaging technique for identifying disk injuries, such as displacement, intrinsic disk lesions, and joint effusion. The joint effusion is generally well depicted with T2-weighted sequences that show the area of effusion as a high-intensity area. When

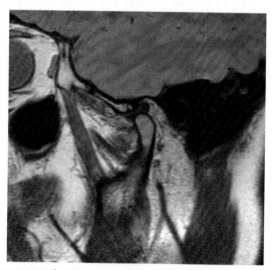

Fig. 32. Left TMJ open mouth MRI: proton density image in a 46-year-old woman showing minimal translation and the position of the disk in relation to the condyle and the articular eminence. (*Courtesy of* Dr Joanne E. Ethier, Montreal, Canada.)

a large amount of fluid accumulates, the effusion gives rise to the effect that simulates the shape of a disk. This process is known as the arthrographic effect.

MRI can also help differentiate between synovial proliferation and joint effusion. Gadolinium-enhanced MRI of TMJ is used to identify proliferating synovium from that of joint effusion, wherein the proliferating synovium enhances well compared with the joint effusion.

MRI Changes in Temporomandibular Joint Dysfunction

The early sign of TMJ dysfunction is the increased thickness of the lateral pterygoid muscle attachments. This increased thickness is followed by disk displacement in closed mouth positions. The disk displacement with a reduction in open-mouth position follows. These changes are followed by joint effusion when the TMJ is sufficiently damaged. The TMJ effusion usually precedes rupture of retrodiscal layers. Next, the disk displacement without reduction in the open mouth is noted. Finally, osteoarthritic changes are evident on the imaging.[17]

The common MR pulse sequences that are used include the following:

- Spin-echo sequences
- T1-weighted images
- T2-weighted images
- Proton density images
- T2-star images
- Diffusion-weighted imaging
- Short tau inversion recovery (STIR)
- Fluid-attenuated inversion recovery
- Fat-suppression techniques (chemical shift selective imaging sequence [CHESS], DIXON (name) sequence, SPIR, and spectral presaturation with inversion recovery [STIR])

EXTRAORAL RADIOGRAPHY: PET SCANNING, PET/COMPUTED TOMOGRAPHY; PET/CONE BEAM COMPUTED TOMOGRAPHY, AND PET/MAGNETIC RESONANCE FUSION TECHNIQUES

PET is an imaging method that uses radiotracer for yielding quantitative images of regional functional anatomy.[18] A short-lived radioactive tracer like the F-18-labeled fluorodeoxyglucose (FDG), a sugar, is injected into the patient. There is a waiting period within which the active molecule becomes concentrated in tissues of interest. The waiting period for FDG is about an hour. Shortly thereafter, the radioisotope undergoes positron emission decay. The emitted positron travels for a short distance within the tissues (a few millimeters) before losing its kinetic energy, decelerates, and interacts with an electron. The interaction annihilates both electron and positron, resulting in a pair of photons that move in opposite directions. These photons are detected when they reach a scintillator in the scanning device, creating a burst of light that is then detected by the photomultiplier tube or silicon avalanche photodiodes; this is how PET images are registered.

An integrated PET-CT scan (PET-CT fusion) combines the images from a PET scan and CT that have been performed at the same time by the same machine. The integrated PET-CT is a diagnostic tool to detect cancer and also helps find the stage of cancer. It is also used to locate the appropriate area for a tissue biopsy. PET scans are read alongside the CT or MR scans via a process called coregistration, giving both anatomic and metabolic information to the investigator. For brain imaging, registration of CT, MR, and PET scans may be accomplished without the need of an integrated PET-CT or PET-MR scanner by using a device known as the N-Scanner, invented by the American physician and computer scientist, Russell Brown.[19]

Sodium fluoride F18 injection ([18]F Naf) is used as a tracer when skeletal imaging is required (**Fig. 33**). The images are used to detect areas of abnormal bone growth associated with tumors that may have metastasized from other organs such as breast or prostate. [18]F Naf is also used recently to detect an area of MRONJ. Recent research conducted in North America validated the use of PET-CBCT fusion to demonstrate a developing MRONJ lesion. Axial CT was coregistered with NaF PET scan.

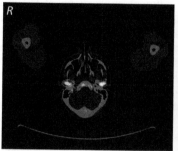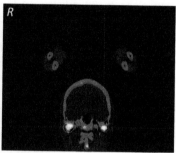

Fig. 33. NaF-PET/CT transaxial (*left*) and coronal projections using the image analysis software, ROVER in a patient with TMJ bilateral rheumatoid arthritis. The ROVER software allows for coregistration of PET and CT scans and helps quantify the radiotracer uptake. (*Courtesy of* Dr Joshua Baker, VA Medical Center, Philadelphia, PA.)

ULTRASOUND

US is the term used to describe the sound of frequencies greater than 20 Hz (MHz). Frequencies of 7.5 to 30 MHz are typical for diagnostic US.[20] Although US has been widely used in medical fields for decades, Baum and colleagues[21] were the first to report the use of diagnostic US in dentistry as a diagnostic aid in visualizing the interior structure of a tooth in 1963. US is based on the evaluation of the reflected echoes from the interface between 2 different tissues having different acoustic properties. Detection of the echoes is made through a transducer, which converts the echoes into an electric signal, producing a real-time black, white, and shades of gray image.[22] An area showing lower echo intensity than surrounding tissue is described as hypoechoic (dark), whereas an area causing a considerable reflection of US is described as hyperechoic (light). Anechoic is an area with no reflection of echoes that can be found, for example, within homogenous liquids.[23,24]

US is a sectional image (or tomography) representing a topographic map of the depth of tissues interfaces, similar to a radar or a sonar picture.[25] The combined utilization of Doppler US with color-flow imaging enables the detection and differentiation of vascular structures (arterial or venous blood flow). For patients with a cardiac pacemaker, metallic prosthesis, or claustrophobia for whom MRI is contraindicated, US can be an interesting alternative diagnostic method.[26]

US is a noninvasive, economical, and painless diagnostic tool for soft tissue investigations of the face and neck, and excellent images can be achieved with high-resolution scan. It is considered the first-choice method of clinical investigation of the salivary glands with indications such as intrinsic and extrinsic swellings to the salivary glands as well as salivary obstruction. Advantages of US include utilization of nonionizing radiation, good soft tissue discrimination (differentiation between solid and cystic mass), excellent sensitivity for superficial mass lesions, identification of radiolucent stones, and possible US-guided fine-needle aspiration biopsy. Drawbacks include no information on fine ductal gland architecture (inability to show the facial nerve relationship to the parotid gland for example) and difficulty in image deeper structures, such as the deep lobes of major salivary glands. Normal salivary glands appear homogenously hyperechoic (light) compared with adjacent muscle, whereas tumors and cysts will be more hypoechoic (dark) than normal parenchyma.

Besides salivary gland investigation, US has been proposed as a complementary diagnostic procedure in dentistry. Marotti and colleagues[27] reviewed the literature and reported close to 60 articles on the different applications of US imaging in dentistry. The different fields explored included dental scanning, caries detection, dental fracture, soft tissue and periapical lesions, maxillofacial fractures, periodontal bony defects, gingival and muscle thickness, temporomandibular disorders, and implant dentistry. Few researchers have also reported the use of US in the examination of bone lesions of endodontic origin.[23,24,28,29] They concluded that US imaging is a useful imaging technique that can give significant diagnostic information in relation to periapical lesions in the anterior region where the buccal bone is thin because thinning or discontinuity in the labial or buccal cortical plate is required for US waves to penetrate and diagnose periapical lesions. Recently, a radiohistopathologic study from Khambete and Kumar[30] assessed the efficacy of US in differential diagnosis of periapical radiolucencies. Although US imaging underestimated the size of the lesions when compared with periapical radiographs, the US diagnosis agreed with the histopathologic diagnosis in all studied cases. They concluded that US can provide accurate information about the nature of intraosseous lesions of the jaws before any surgical procedure (**Fig. 34**).

Table 3 summarizes advantages and disadvantages of US as a potential method of clinical investigation in dentistry. Advantages of US include a real-time imaging that is easy, reproducible, and convenient to use, although the clinician must be trained to take and read the images obtained. It has a lower cost when compared with other advanced imaging modalities. Furthermore, US imaging may prevent unnecessary exposure of the patient to ionizing radiation. Compared with other imaging techniques, such as conventional CT and MRI, US is accepted as one of the most risk-free diagnostic imaging methods. However, because US energy is known to be absorbed and converted into heat between tissues in bony structure, cell-damaging effects cannot be completely ruled out.

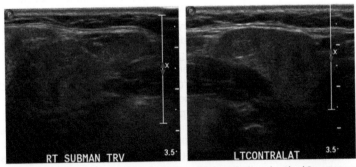

Fig. 34. Transverse US images of right and left submandibular glands. (*Courtesy of* Dr Jaisri R. Thoppay, Virginia Commonwealth University Health System, Richmond, Virginia, USA.)

Table 3	
Ultrasound as a potential method of clinical investigation in dentistry	
Advantages of US	**Disadvantages of US**
• Noninvasive • Nonionizing radiation • Good soft tissue discrimination • Excellent sensitivity for superficial mass lesions • Possible identification of salivary gland, and calculus within ducts • Doppler US and color-flow imaging for blood flow assessment • US-guided fine-needle biopsy of lesions of the neck • Lithotripsy of salivary stones • Good acceptance by patients • Relatively low cost • Can be repeated as required	• Sound waves blocked by bone, limiting the areas for investigation • Technique is operator-dependent • Real-time imaging analysis requires presence of a trained radiologist/clinician during the investigation

RADIOISOTOPE IMAGING (ALSO CALLED BONE SCINTIGRAPHY, RADIONUCLIDE BONE SCAN)

The difference between radioisotope imaging and other imaging techniques, such as radiographs, is the positioning of the radiation source within the body. Diagnostic techniques in radioisotope imaging use radioactive tracers that emit gamma rays from within the body. Several radioisotopes can be used, and the choice of radioisotope is based on their affinity for a particular tissue being investigated (called target tissue). **Box 1** lists the indications, advantages, and disadvantages of radioisotope imaging. **Table 4** summarizes the isotopes used in radioisotope imaging. These short-lived tracer isotopes can be given by injection, inhalation, or orally. Imaging is done using a gamma camera that detects and builds up an image from the points from which radiation is emitted. This image provides a view of the position and concentration of the radioisotope within the body. Malfunction of an organ can be indicated if the isotope is either partially taken up in the organ (called cold spot), or if it is taken up in excess (called hot spot) **(Fig. 35)**. Comparing radioisotope imaging over radiograph techniques, radioisotope imaging has the advantage that both bone and soft tissue can be imaged successfully during one investigation. **Box 1** gives main indications for isotope imaging of the head and neck as well as advantages and disadvantages over conventional radiography modalities.[31]

Technetium (^{99m}Tc) is the most commonly used isotope and has been assessed in different fields of dentistry. Bouquot and colleagues[32] evaluated the association between ^{99m}Tc scintigraphy in patients with idiopathic facial pain (IFP). Their results showed that a positive ^{99m}Tc scan was strongly correlated with the location of pain in IFP and that patients with IFP had significantly more hot spots than controls. Kim and colleagues[33] evaluated the effectiveness of bone scintigraphy in the diagnosis of osteoarthritis of the TMJ. Some investigators have assessed the osteoblastic activity in extraction sockets[34,35] and around dentals implants[36,37] as well as in bisphosphonate-induced osteonecrosis of the jaw.[38,39] ^{99m}Tc salivary gland scintigraphy was also shown to play a substantial role in the diagnosis and differential diagnosis of salivary glands diseases, such as chronic obstructive parotitis, sialolithiasis, and Sjögren syndrome.[40,41]

Box 1
Radioisotope imaging in the head and neck

Indications

Tumor staging (sites and extent of bone metastasis)

Assessment of salivary gland function

Dry mouth particularly common in Sjögren syndrome

Investigation of the thyroid

Investigation of TMJ

Brain scans

Advantages

Investigation of target tissue function

Bilateral comparison and images of all major salivary glands during one bone scan

Computer analysis and enhancement

Can be performed in cases of acute infection

Disadvantages

Relatively high dose of radiation

Time-consuming

Poor image resolution: minimal information on target tissue anatomy

Images are not disease-specific

Adapted from Whaites E, Drage N. Chapter 32. The salivary glands. Essentials of dental radiography and radiology. 5th edition. Edinburgh: Churchill Livingstone Elsevier; 2013.

SIALOGRAPHY (RADIOSIALOGRAPHY)

Radiographic sialography using contrast medium has become an important diagnostic procedure in the evaluation of salivary calculi, fistulae, strictures, sialectasis, and benign tumors affecting parotid and submandibular glands. Both fluoroscopy and tomography were used in the past to image the duct and the gland when the contrast medium had been injected.

The technique of sialography has been described in detail many years ago and essentially remained the same except the developments in the detector technology and the replacement of films with digital sensors. After the identification of the ductal

---

Table 4
Radioisotopes used in nuclear medicine imaging

Radioisotope	Target Tissues	Comment
Technitium (^{99}Tc)	Salivary glands, thyroid, bone, blood, liver, lung, heart	
Gallium (^{67}Ga)	Tumors, inflammation	
Iodine (^{123}I)	Thyroid	
Krypton (^{81}K)	Lung	

Adapted from Whaites E, Drage N. Chapter 32. The salivary glands. Essentials of dental radiography and radiology. 5th edition. Edinburgh: Churchill Livingstone Elsevier; 2013.

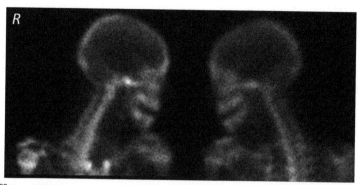

Fig. 35. ^{99m}Tc–MDP scintigraphy in an 18-year-old woman with no significant medical issues, not on any medication, and no known allergies. Notice the increased uptake in the region of the right condyle. (*Courtesy of* Dr Carl Bouchard, Oral & Maxillofacial Surgery, Faculté de MédecineDentaire, Université Laval, Québec, Canada.)

orifice, the orifice is gently dilated before cannulization with a sterile, blunt-tipped, single side-port stainless steel cannula. Care should be exercised not to introduce air bubbles into the contrast medium, which is prefilled in the syringe and extension tubing that is attached to the cannula. The tubing is attached to the skin for stabilization before injecting the contrast material. Although water-soluble contrast material is preferred such as Renograffin, Ethiodol and Renografin-60 were used in the past, which used to give greater density to the ducts and parenchyma. The drawback of Ethiodol is that the contrast medium remains in tissues and cavities for many months and may lead to reactionary granuloma formation. If using fluoroscopy, the medium should be injected gently under direct fluoroscopic control. Multiple sequential fluoroscopic spot images are taken using a small focal spot in varied oblique, lateral, and basal projections during the ductal filling and parenchymal filling phases of the injection. If a stricture, sialectasis, fistula extravasation, or an obstruction is noted, the injection is terminated immediately without any parenchymal filling. If a mass lesion is suspected and the ductal system is normal, the injection is continued until a parenchymal blush is identified.[42]

Standard radiographic views are obtained in the lateral, oblique, and basal projections. With the introduction of CBCT, a large-volume CBCT is performed that images the entire salivary gland (parotid or submandibular) in great detail.

Interpretation of sialograms needs specific training and expertise. Evaluation of intraparenchymal branches can be done with sequential filling before the parenchymal ducts are obscured by the parenchymal blush. The ducts are studied for separation or displacement from each other, obstruction, or invasion by a suspected tumor. Sialograms may reveal a large irregular mass with poorly defined borders, displacement and invasion of the ducts, and pooling of contrast material. If the clinical examination reveals a palpable hard mass, pain, swift growth, and facial nerve palsy, a malignant tumor should be suspected and a histopathologic examination is recommended at that time. Typical commercially available sialography catheter measurements are as noted in **Table 5**.

Digital Subtraction Sialography and Magnetic Resonance Sialography

These 2 techniques have been studied for their efficacy, and it was noted that digital subtraction sialography proved to be superior for imaging extraglanular and intraglandular duct system in one study. The investigators concluded that if digital

Table 5
Typical sialography catheter measurements

Salivary Gland	Tubing Length (cm)	Tip Diameter (inches)	Tip Gage	Side Ports
Submandibular	30	0.012	30	0
Submandibular	30	0.016	27	0
Submandibular	30	0.022	24	0
Parotid	30	0.032	21	1

subtraction sialography could not be performed because of acute inflammation of the gland or if the cannula could not be successfully inserted, noninvasive MR sialography is the next best technique in such situations. A contrast-enhanced MRI is recommended if there is a suspicion of malignancy.[43]

SIALENDOSCOPY

Obstructive sialadenitis, with or without sialolithiasis, represents the major inflammatory disorder of the major salivary glands. Although 60% to 70% of all obstructive disorders are due to stones, stenosis (15%–20%) and sialodochitis (5%–10%) are not uncommon.[44]

Sialendoscopy is a minimally invasive endoscopic procedure developed for the parotid or submandibular ductal system. It is an endoscopic, transoral gland preservation technique. This technique was developed both in Europe by Marchal and his associates[45] and in Israel by Nahlieli and associates.[46]

The removal of submandibular sialoliths smaller than 4 mm and parotid sialoliths smaller than 3 mm is amenable to sialendoscopy with basket or forceps retrieval. Larger stones require the use of other supplemental techniques such as fragmentation.[47]

Diagnostic sialendoscopy and interventional sialendoscopy have become the emerging standard in the diagnosing and locating intraductal obstructions, managing the blockages using basket technique and intracorporeal lithotripsy with a very high success rate.

REFERENCES

1. Horner K, Drage N, Brettle D. 21st century imaging. In: Wilson NH, editor. London: Quintessence Publishing Co, Ltd; 2008. p. 13–78.
2. Cederberg RA, Fredericksen NL, Benson BW, et al. Influence of the digital image display monitor on observer performance. Dentomaxillofac Radiol 1999;28: 203–7.
3. Fosbinder R, Orth D. Essentials of radiologic science. Baltimore: Wolters Kluwer Health/Lippincott Williams & Wilkins; 2011.
4. Udupa H, Mah P, Dove SB, et al. Evaluation of image quality parameters of representative intraoral digital radiographic systems. Oral Surg Oral Med Oral Pathol Oral Radiol 2013;116:774–83.
5. Sansare K, Raghav M, Sontakke S, et al. Clinical cavitation and radiographic lesion depth in proximal surfaces in an Indian population. Acta Odontol Scand 2014;72:1084–8.
6. Carter L, Farman AG, Geist J, et al. American Academy of Oral and Maxillofacial Radiology executive opinion statement on performing and interpreting diagnostic

cone beam computed tomography. Oral Surg Oral Med Oral Pathol Oral Radiol Endod 2008;106:561–2.

7. NICE guidelines (National Institute for Health and Care Excellence, UK). Head injury: Triage, assessment, investigation and early management of head injury in infants, children and adults. Clinical guideline 56, September 2007. Available at: http://www.nice.org.uk/guidance/cg176. Accessed June 10, 2015.
8. Langland OE, Langlais RP, Morris CR. Principles and practice of panoramic radiography. Philadelphia: WB Saunders Company; 1982.
9. Niamtu J 3rd. Near-fatal airway obstruction after routine implant placement. Oral Surg Oral Med Oral Pathol Oral Radiol Endod 2001;92:597–600.
10. Goldman LW. Principles of CT: multislice CT. J Nucl Med Technol 2008;36:57–68.
11. ACR-ASNR guidelines for the performance of CT of the brain. Agency for healthcare research and quality. U.S. Department of health and human services. Available at: http://www.guideline.gov/content.aspx?id=32518. Accessed June 10, 2015.
12. Miracle AC, Mukherji SK. Conebeam CT of the head and neck, part 1: physical principles. AJNR Am J Neuroradiol 2009;30:1088–95.
13. Miracle AC, Mukherji SK. Conebeam CT of the head and neck, part 2: clinical applications. AJNR Am J Neuroradiol 2009;30:1285–92.
14. Available at: http://tech.mit.edu/V130/N56/3ddental.html. Accessed July 5, 2015.
15. American Association of Endodontists, American Academy of Oral and Maxillofacial Radiology. AAE and AAOMR joint position statement. Use of cone-beam computed tomography in endodontics. Pa Dental J (Harrisb) 2011;78:37–9.
16. American Academy of Oral and Maxillofacial Radiology. Clinical recommendations regarding use of cone beam computed tomography in orthodontics. Position statement by the American Academy of Oral and Maxillofacial Radiology. Oral Surg Oral Med Oral Pathol Oral Radiol 2013;116:238–57.
17. Tomas X, Pomes J, Berenguer J, et al. MR imaging of temporomandibular joint dysfunction: a pictoral review. Radiographics 2006;26:765–81.
18. Farwell MD, Pryma DA, Mankoff DA. PET/CT imaging in cancer: current applications and future directions. Cancer 2014;120:3433–45.
19. Brown RA. A computerized tomography-computer graphics approach to stereotactic localization. J Neurosurg 1979;50:715–20.
20. Agni NA, Borle RM. Chapter 6. Diagnosis and diagnostic aids. In: Agni NA, Borle RM, editors. Salivary gland pathologies. 1st edition. New Delhi (India): Jaypee Brothers Medical Publishers ltd; 2013. p. 34–53.
21. Baum G, Greenwood I, Slawski S, et al. Observation of internal structures of teeth by ultrasonography. Science 1963;139(3554):495–6.
22. White FC, Pharoah MJ, editors. Advanced imaging. Oral radiology. Principles and interpretation. 6th edition. St Louis (MO): Mosby Elsevier; 2009. p. 207–24. Chapter 13.
23. Gundappa M, Ng SY, Whaites EJ. Comparison of ultrasound, digital and conventional radiography in differentiating periapical lesions. Dentomaxillofac Radiol 2006;35(5):326–33.
24. Aggarwal V, Logani A, Shah N. The evaluation of computed tomography scans and ultrasounds in the differential diagnosis of periapical lesions. J Endod 2008;34(11):1312–5.
25. Agni NA, Borle RM. Chapter 6. Diagnosis and diagnostic aids. In: Agni NA, Borle RM, editors. Ultrasound-guided procedure and investigations. A manual for the clinician. New york: Taylor & Francis Group; 2006. p. 1–16.
26. Shah N, Bansal N, Logani A. Recent advances in imaging technologies in dentistry. World J Radiol 2014;6(10):794–807.

27. Marotti J, Heger S, Tinschert J, et al. Recent advances of ultrasound imaging in dentistry–a review of the literature. Oral Surg Oral Med Oral Pathol Oral Radiol 2013;115(6):819–32.
28. Cotti E, Campisi G, Ambu R, et al. Ultrasound real-time imaging in the differential diagnosis of periapical lesions. Int Endod J 2003;36(8):556–63.
29. Aggarwal V, Singla M. Use of computed tomography scans and ultrasound in differential diagnosis and evaluation of nonsurgical management of periapical lesions. Oral Surg Oral Med Oral Pathol Oral Radiol Endod 2010;109(6):917–23.
30. Khambete N, Kumar R. Ultrasound in differential diagnosis of periapical radiolucencies: a radiohistopathological study. J Conserv Dent 2015;18(1):39–43.
31. Whaites E, Drage N. Chapter 32. The salivary glands. Essentials of dental radiography and radiology. 5th edition. Churchill Livingstone Elsevier; 2013. p. 447–60.
32. Bouquot JE, Spolnik K, Adams W, et al. Technetium-99mTc MDP imaging of 293 quadrants of idiopathic facial pain: 79% show increased radioisotope uptake. Oral Surg Oral Med Oral Pathol Oral Radiol 2012;114(1):83–92.
33. Kim JH, Kim YK, Kim SG, et al. Effectiveness of bone scans in the diagnosis of osteoarthritis of the temporomandibular joint. Dentomaxillofac Radiol 2012;41(3):224–9.
34. Gurbuzer B, Pikdoken L, Urhan M, et al. Scintigraphic evaluation of early osteoblastic activity in extraction sockets treated with platelet-rich plasma. J Oral Maxillofac Surg 2008;66(12):2454–60.
35. Gurbuzer B, Pikdoken L, Tunali M, et al. Scintigraphic evaluation of osteoblastic activity in extraction sockets treated with platelet-rich fibrin. J Oral Maxillofac Surg 2010;68(5):980–9.
36. Kalayci A, Durmus E, Tastekin G, et al. Evaluation of osteoblastic activity around dental implants using bone scintigraphy. Clin Oral Implants Res 2010;21(2):209–12.
37. Sanchez-Garces MA, Manzanares-Cespedes MC, Berini-Aytes L, et al. Assessment of osteointegrative response around dental implants using technetium 99-methylene diphosphate scintigraphy: a comparison of two implant surfaces in a rabbit model. Int J Oral Maxillofac Implants 2012;27(3):561–5.
38. Dore F, Filippi L, Biasotto M, et al. Bone scintigraphy and SPECT/CT of bisphosphonate-induced osteonecrosis of the jaw. J Nucl Med 2009;50(1):30–5.
39. Fabbricini R, Catalano L, Pace L, et al. Bone scintigraphy and SPECT/CT in bisphosphonate-induced osteonecrosis of the jaw. J Nucl Med 2009;50(8):1385 [author reply: 1385].
40. Taura S, Murata Y, Aung W, et al. Decreased thyroid uptake of tc-99m pertechnetate in patients with advanced-stage Sjögren syndrome: evaluation using salivary gland scintigraphy. Clin Nucl Med 2002;27(4):265–9.
41. Wu CB, Xi H, Zhou Q, et al. The diagnostic value of technetium 99m pertechnetate salivary gland scintigraphy in patients with certain salivary gland diseases. J Oral Maxillofac Surg 2015;73(3):443–50.
42. Kushner DC, Weber AL. Sialography of salivary gland tumors with fluoroscopy and tomography. Am J Roentgenol 1978;130:941–4.
43. Kalinowski M, Haverhagen JT, Rehberg E, et al. Comparative study of MR sialography and digital subtraction sialography for benign salivary gland disorders. AJNR Am J Neuroradiol 2002;23:1485–92.
44. Witt RL, Iro H, Koch M, et al. Minimally invasive options for salivary calculi. Laryngoscope 2012;122:1306–11.
45. Marchal F, Dulguerov P, Lehmann W. Interventional sialendoscopy. N Engl J Med 1999;341:1242–3.

46. Nahlieli O, Neder A, Baruchin AM. Salivary gland endoscopy; a new technique for diagnosis and treatment of sialolithiasis. J Oral Maxillofac Surg 1994;52: 1240–2.
47. Marchal F, Dulguerov P. Sialolithasis management: the state of the art. Arch Otolaryngol Head Neck Surg 2003;129:951–6.

Developmental Disorders Affecting Jaws

Ghada AlZamel, DDS[a],*, Scott Odell, DMD[b], Mel Mupparapu, DMD, MDS[b]

KEYWORDS

- Microdontia • Macrodontia • Syndromes • Hypoplasia • Ectodermal dysplasia
- Hemifacial hypertrophy • Growth disturbances

KEY POINTS

- Teeth are housed in mandible and maxilla and are known to undergo variations in clinical presentation depending on the degree of abnormality during growth and development. It is essential to identify these variations in normal anatomy so that appropriate treatment is initiated to address the anomaly.
- This article focuses on the diagnostic radiographic interpretation and strategies to include pertinent differential diagnosis.
- The developmental anomalies can range from mere increase or decrease in the number of teeth to that of atrophy or hypertrophy of the entire jaws. These changes might be accompanied by several systemic abnormalities that constitute a "syndrome." Dentists may encounter such patients in their dental practice and should be prepared to diagnose and manage such cases.
- Also discussed is the importance of advanced imaging and its appropriateness in the diagnosis and interpretation.

DEVELOPMENTAL DEFECTS OF TEETH SIZE
Macrodontia

In macrodontia the teeth are larger than normal.[1,2] Generalized macrodontia, which is a rare condition, is characterized by the appearance of enlarged teeth throughout the dentition.[1,2] This may be absolute, as seen in pituitary gigantism, or it may be relative because of relatively small maxilla and mandible, which could result in crowding of teeth and possibly an abnormal eruption pattern caused by insufficient arch space.[1,2]

[a] King Abdulaziz Medical City-Dental Center, Departmet of Dental Care Services, Division of Oral Medicine, PO Box-5101, Riyadh 11422, Kingdom of Saudi Arabia; [b] Department of Oral Medicine, University of Pennsylvania School of Dental Medicine, 240 S 40th Street, Philadelphia, PA 19104, USA
* Corresponding author.
E-mail address: Ghada.alzamel@gmail.com

Dent Clin N Am 60 (2016) 39–90
http://dx.doi.org/10.1016/j.cden.2015.08.002
0011-8532/16/$ – see front matter © 2016 Elsevier Inc. All rights reserved.

dental.theclinics.com

Localized macrodontia is characterized by an abnormally large tooth or group of teeth (**Fig. 1**).[1,2] This relatively uncommon condition usually is seen with mandibular third molars.[1,2] In the rare condition known as hemifacial hypertrophy, teeth on the affected side are abnormally large compared with the unaffected side.[1,2]

Radiographic findings
Radiographs reveal the increased size of unerupted and erupted macrodont teeth. The shape of the tooth is usually normal but in some cases may exhibit a mildly distorted morphology that may resemble gemination or fusion.[1]

Treatment
Microdontic teeth require no treatment other than cosmetic intervention. Orthodontic treatment may be necessary in case of malocclusion.[1]

Microdontia
Affected teeth are smaller than normal.[1,2] As in macrodontia, it may involve all teeth or be limited to a single tooth or group of teeth.[1,2] In Generalized microdontia all teeth in the dentition appear smaller than normal and can be absolute as seen in patients with pituitary dwarfism, or relative, where teeth appear smaller in relation to large maxilla and mandible.[1,2]

In localized microdontia, a single tooth is affected and appears smaller than normal.[1,2] The shape of these microdont is often altered with the reduced size.[1,2] This phenomenon is most commonly seen with maxillary lateral incisors where the

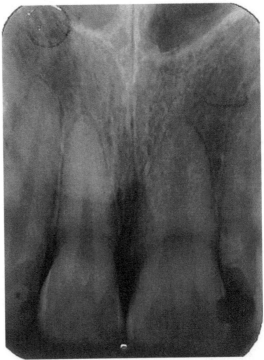

Fig. 1. Maxillary central periapical radiograph showing macrodontia affecting left central incisor.

tooth crown appears cone or peg shaped (peg lateral).[1,2] The second most commonly seen microdont is the maxillary third molar, followed by supernumerary teeth.[1,2]

Treatment

Restorative or prosthetic treatment may be considered to create a more normal-appearing tooth, especially when considering esthetic concerns in the anterior dentition.[1]

DEVELOPMENTAL DEFECTS OF TEETH NUMBER
Hypodontia/Anodontia

The congenital absence of teeth may be referred to as hypodontia when one or several teeth are missing or anodontia when there's a complete absence of one or both denti-tion.[3,4] Although it's rare for a primary tooth to be congenitally absent it is likely that in such cases the permanent successional tooth also fails to form.[3,4] Third molars, per-manent maxillary lateral incisors, and mandibular second premolars are the teeth most frequently involved and a hereditary trait can sometimes be shown with missing maxil-lary lateral incisors.[3,4]

The prevalence of any type of hypodontia in the general population is 4.6%, and there is no significant difference between males and females. The prevalence of maxil-lary lateral incisor absence is 2.1% and is significantly lower in males than in females. The prevalence of absence of the second premolars is 1.9% for the general popula-tion, with no significant difference between males and females. The prevalence of hypodontia in primary dentition is between 0.1% and 2.4%.[3]

Complete anodontia is rare but is often associated with a syndrome known as he-reditary ectodermal dysplasia, which usually is transmitted as an X-linked recessive disorder and results in the absence of at least two ectodermally derived structures, such as sweat glands, hair, skin, nails, and teeth.[1,2] When the teeth are involved, the condition may present with multiple missing and/or malformed teeth that often have a conical or canine shape or a notable decrease in tooth size (**Fig. 2**).[1,2]

Treatment

Dental implants have been used to replace missing teeth with good success. Tradi-tionally, dental prosthetics have provided patients with improved esthetics and masti-catory function.[3]

Supernumerary Teeth

Extra, or supernumerary, teeth in the dentition most probably result from continued proliferation of the permanent or primary dental lamina to form a third tooth germ.[5,6]

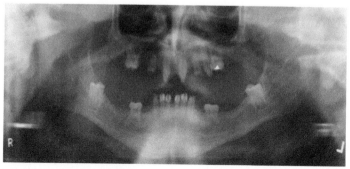

Fig. 2. Panoramic radiograph demonstrating anodontia in a clinically suspected case of ectodermal dysplasia.

The reported prevalence of supernumerary teeth ranges from 0.2% to 0.8% in the deciduous dentition, and from 0.5% to 5.3% in the permanent dentition with geographic variations.[5,7] Supernumerary teeth are more prevalent among men than women in a proportion of 2:1.[6–8] The cause of supernumerary teeth is multifactorial, a combination of environmental and genetic factors.[7]

Supernumerary teeth are estimated to occur 8.2 times more frequently in the maxilla than the mandible.[6] The anterior midline of the maxilla is the most common site, in which case the supernumerary tooth is known as a mesiodens.[5] The maxillary molar area (fourth molar or paramolar) is the second most common site.[5]

Complications associated with supernumerary teeth include impaction, delayed eruption, ectopic eruption, overcrowding, spacing anomalies, and the formation of follicular cysts.[6,7] Some cases of supernumerary teeth are asymptomatic and detected incidentally in the course of radiographic examination.[7]

Both clinical and radiographic examinations are essential for detecting supernumerary teeth, although recently computerized tomography (CT) has been used as a complimentary diagnostic test.[7]

Radiographic features

The radiographic features of supernumerary teeth are variable. They may appear entirely normal in size and shape, but they may also be smaller in size compared with the adjacent normal dentition or have a conical shape.[5] In extreme cases, the supernumerary teeth may appear grossly deformed. Most are isolated events, although some may be familial and others may be syndrome associated (Gardner syndrome and cleidocranial dysplasia [CCD]).[6,7] In addition to periapical radiography, occlusal radiographs may aid in determining the location and number of unerupted supernumerary teeth. Care should be taken to review panoramic radiographs for supernumerary teeth.[7] Cone-beam CT is used to precisely determine the location of each supernumerary tooth (**Fig. 3**).[7]

Treatment

The usual treatment is to extract the supernumerary tooth, although repositioning it in the dental arch may be an alternative option.[6,7] Extraction must be performed with care, avoiding any damage to blood vessels and nerves or to anatomic structures, such as the maxillary sinus, pterygomaxillary space, or the orbit and possible fracture of the maxillary tuberosity.[6,7] Another therapeutic option is to keep the supernumerary tooth under observation as long as it does not provoke any complication and does not interfere with function or aesthetics.[6,7]

DEVELOPMENTAL DEFECTS OF TEETH SHAPE
Fusion

Fusion is the joining of two developing tooth germs, resulting in a single large tooth structure.[9,10] The fusion process may involve the entire length of the teeth, or it may involve the roots only, in which case cementum and dentin are shared.[9,10] Root canals may also be separate or shared.[9,10] The cause of this condition is unknown, although trauma and genetics have been suggested.[9]

Fusion results in a reduced number of teeth in the arch. Although more common between deciduous teeth, fusion may also occur in the permanent dentition and it is more common in anterior teeth of both dentitions.[9] Fusion may be differentiated from gemination when the number of teeth is reduced by one, except in the unusual case in which a normal tooth and a supernumerary tooth have fused.[11]

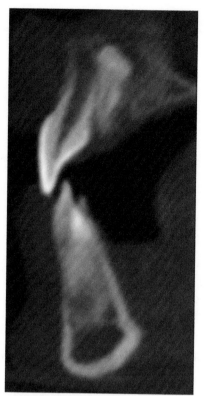

Fig. 3. Sagittal section of anterior maxilla showing the palatal location of mesiodens on this limited volume cone-beam computerized tomography (CBCT).

Radiographic features

Radiographs disclose the unusual shape or size of the fused teeth (**Fig. 4**).[1] The true nature and extent of the union are frequently more evident on the radiograph than can be determined by clinical examination.[1] Fused teeth may also show an unusual configuration of the pulp chamber or root canal.[1]

Treatment

The management of a case of fusion depends on which teeth are involved, the degree of fusion, and the morphologic result. If the affected teeth are deciduous, they may be retained as they are.[9] If the clinician contemplates extraction, it is important first to determine whether the permanent teeth are present.[9] In the case of fused permanent teeth, the fused crowns may be reshaped with a restoration that mimics two independent crowns.[9] Endodontic therapy may be necessary and perhaps may be difficult or impossible if the root canals are of unusual shape.[9] In some cases it is most prudent to leave the teeth as they are.[9]

Gemination

Gemination is the fusion of two teeth from a single enamel organ.[9,10] The typical result is partial cleavage, with the appearance of two crowns that share the same root canal.[9,10] Although trauma has been suggested as a possible cause, the cause of gemination is unknown, but some evidence suggests that it is familial.[9] These teeth may be

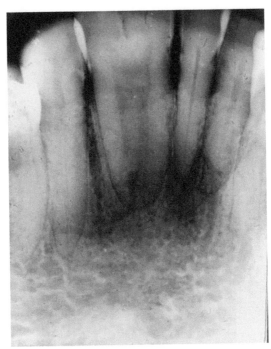

Fig. 4. Mandibular central incisor periapical radiograph (PA) showing the fusion of central and lateral incisor on the right side.

cosmetically unacceptable and may cause crowding.[9] Although gemination may occur in the deciduous and permanent dentitions, it more frequently affects the primary teeth, usually in the incisor region.[9]

Radiographic findings
Radiographs reveal the altered shape of the hard tissue and pulp chamber of the geminated tooth (**Fig. 5**).[1] Radiopaque enamel outlines the clefts in the crowns and invaginations and thus accentuates them.[1] The pulp chamber is usually single and enlarged and may be partially divided.[1] In the rare case of premolar gemination, the tooth image suggests a molar with an enlarged crown and two roots.[1]

Treatment
A geminated tooth in the anterior region may compromise arch esthetics and arch length.[1] Areas of hypoplasia and invagination lines or areas of coronal separation represent caries-susceptible sites that may in time result in pulpal inflammation.[1] Affected teeth can cause malocclusion and lead to periodontal disease. Consequently, the affected tooth may be removed (especially if it is deciduous), the crowns may be restored or reshaped, or the tooth may be left untreated and periodically examined to preclude the development of complications.[9] Before treatment is initiated on a primary tooth, the status of the permanent tooth and configuration of its root canals should be determined radiographically.[1]

Concrescence
Concrescence occurs when the roots of two or more primary or permanent teeth are fused by cementum (**Fig. 6**).[12,13] Although its cause is unknown, many authorities

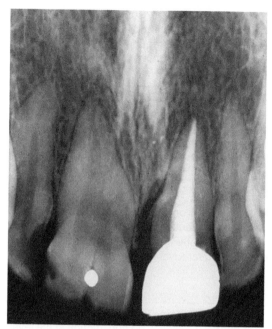

Fig. 5. Maxillary central incisor PA showing the gemination of right central incisor. Note the prominent notching in the middle.

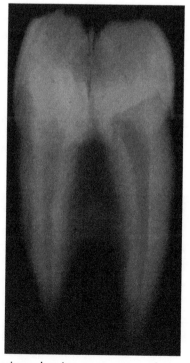

Fig. 6. Radiograph of a specimen showing concrescence of two mandibular anterior teeth.

suspect that space restriction during development, local trauma, excessive occlusal force, or local infection after development play an important role.[12]

Maxillary molars are the teeth most frequently involved, especially a third molar and a supernumerary tooth.[13] Involved teeth may fail to erupt or may erupt incompletely. The sexes are equally affected.

Radiographic features

A radiographic examination may not always distinguish between concrescence and teeth that are in close contact or that are simply superimposed.[12] When the condition is suspected on a radiograph and extraction of one of the teeth is being considered, additional projections at different angles may be obtained to better delineate the condition.[12]

Treatment

Concrescence affects treatment only when the decision is made to remove one or both of the involved teeth because this condition complicates the extraction.[1,13] The clinician should warn the patient that an effort to remove one might result in the unintended and simultaneous removal of the other.[1]

Taurodontism

A taurodont tooth (bull-like tooth) is one where the pulp chamber has a greater apico-occlusal height than in normal teeth, with no constriction at the level of the cementoenamel junction (**Fig. 7**).[14,15] The result is that the chamber extends apically, well beyond the neck of the tooth.[14,15] The anomaly affects multirooted teeth and is thought to be caused by the failure of Hertwig sheath to invaginate at the proper horizontal level.[14,16]

Taurodontism may be seen as an isolated incident; in families; and in association with syndromes, such as Down syndrome and Klinefelter syndrome.[14,16] Although taurodontism is generally an uncommon finding, it has been reported to have a relatively high prevalence in Eskimos, and incidence has been reported to be 11% in a Middle Eastern population.[14,15]

Radiographic features

The distinctive morphology of taurodont teeth is quite apparent on radiographs. The features are the elongated pulp chamber, the apically positioned furcation, and the shortened roots and root canals. The dimensions of the crown are normal.[14,16]

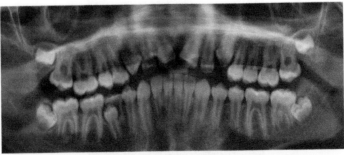

Fig. 7. Cropped panoramic radiograph demonstrating taurodontism in mandibular premolars.

Treatment

Taurodontism is of little clinical significance unless the tooth becomes nonvital, in which case it becomes a challenging endodontic problem[14,16] For the prosthetic treatment of a taurodont tooth, it has been recommended that post placement be avoided for tooth reconstruction. Because less surface area of the tooth is embedded in the alveolus, a taurodont tooth may not have much stability when used as an abutment for either prosthetic or orthodontic purposes. The lack of a cervical constriction would deprive the tooth of the buttressing effect against excessive loading of the crown.[16] From a periodontal standpoint, taurodont teeth may, in specific cases, offer favorable prognosis. Where periodontal pocketing or gingival recession occurs, the chances of furcation involvement are considerably less than those in normal teeth because taurodont teeth have to demonstrate significant periodontal destruction before furcation involvement occurs.[16]

Dens Invaginatus

Dens invaginatus is a developmental anomaly affecting permanent and, less commonly, primary dentition.[17] It is characterized by the inversion or infolding of the enamel and dentin toward the pulp chamber, usually appearing as an opening on the surface of the crown (**Fig. 8**).[17,18]

This defect ranges in severity from superficial, in which only the crown is affected, to deep, in which the crown and the root are involved.[18] The permanent maxillary lateral incisors are most commonly involved, although any anterior tooth may be affected.[18] Bilateral involvement is commonly seen.[17,18] The cause of this developmental condition is unknown.[17]

Radiographic features

The infolding of the enamel lining is more radiopaque than the surrounding tooth structure and can easily be identified as an inverted teardrop-shaped radiolucency with a radiopaque border.[19] Less frequently the radicular invaginations appear as poorly defined, slightly radiolucent structures running longitudinally within the root (**Fig. 9**).[19]

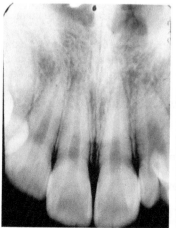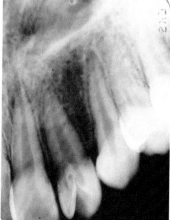

Fig. 8. Maxillary left lateral incisor in this central incisor PA view and left lateral-canine PA view showing both dens evaginatus and dens invaginatus.

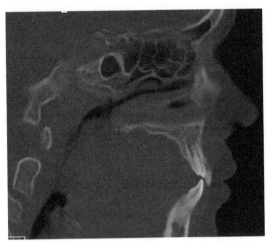

Fig. 9. Sagittal CBCT view showing dens invaginatus of maxillary left lateral incisor (both coronal and radicular types within the same tooth).

Treatment

Because the defect cannot be kept free of plaque and bacteria, dens invaginatus predisposes the tooth to early decay and subsequent pulpitis.[17,19] Prophylactic filling of the pit is recommended to avoid this complication.[19] Failure of early identification and hence treatment may result in premature tooth loss or the requirement for root canal therapy.[19]

Dens Evaginatus

Dens evaginatus is a relatively common developmental condition affecting predominantly premolar teeth (Leung premolars).[11] It has been reported almost exclusively in Asians, Inuits, and Native Americans (see **Fig. 8**).[20]

Mupparapu and colleagues[18] noted that this condition was previously referred to as talon cusp in the anterior teeth. The talon cusp is an entity that is somewhat different than the dens evaginatus because the talon-like evagination in talon cusp is perpendicular to the lingual surface and usually in the midline. Dens evaginatus appears like an overgrowth of a cusp. Hence these two entities must be differentiated from one another.

The defect, which is often bilateral, is an anomalous tubercle, or cusp, located at the center of the occlusal surface.[20,21] Because of occlusal abrasion, the tubercle wears quickly, causing early exposure of an accessory pulp horn that extends into the tubercle.[20] This may result in periapical pathology in young, caries-free teeth, often before completion of root development and apical closure, making root canal fillings more difficult.[20]

Radiographic features

The radiographic image shows an extension of dentin tubercle on the occlusal surface unless the tubercle is already worn down.[11] The dentin core is usually covered with opaque enamel.[11] A fine pulp horn may extend into the tubercle, but this may not be visible radiographically.[11]

Treatment

Judicious grinding of the opposing tooth or the accessory tubercle to stimulate secondary dentin formation may prevent the periapical sequelae associated with this defect. Sealants, pulp capping, and partial pulpotomy have been suggested as measures to allow complete root development.[11,20,21]

Enamel Pearls

Droplets of ectopic enamel may occasionally be found on the roots of teeth.[22] They occur most commonly in the bifurcation or trifurcation of teeth but may also appear on single-rooted premolar teeth.[22] Maxillary molars are more commonly affected than mandibular molars.[23] These deposits are occasionally supported by dentin and rarely may have a pulp horn extending into them.[22,23]

This developmental disturbance of enamel formation may be detected on radiographic examination.[22] It generally is of little significance except when located in an area of periodontal disease.[22] In such cases, it may contribute to the extension of a periodontal pocket, because a periodontal ligament attachment would not be expected and hygiene would be more difficult.[22]

Dilaceration

Dilaceration is an extraordinary curving or angulation of tooth roots.[24,25] The cause of this condition has been related to trauma during root development.[24,25] Movement of the crown or of the crown and part of the root from the remaining developing root may result in sharp angulation after the tooth completes development (**Fig. 10**).[24,25] Extraction may be difficult and if root canal fillings are required in these teeth, the procedure is challenging.[24]

Radiographic features

Radiographs provide the best means of detecting a radicular dilaceration.[24] If the roots dilacerate mesially or distally, the condition is clearly apparent on a periapical radiograph.[24] However, when the roots are dilacerated buccally (labially) or lingually, the apical end of the root may have the appearance of a circular or oval radiopaque area with a central radiolucency (the apical foramen and root canal), giving the appearance of a bull's eye.[24] The periodontal ligament (PDL) space around this dilacerated portion may be seen as a radiolucent halo encircling the radiopaque area.[25]

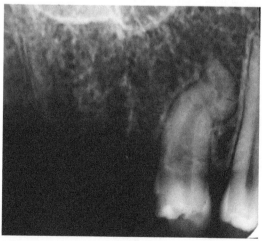

Fig. 10. Maxillary right premolar PA showing the dilaceration of the second premolar.

Differential diagnosis

Occasionally dilacerated roots may be difficult to differentiate from fused roots, sclerosing osteitis, or a dense bone island. These can usually be discerned by radiographs made at different angles.[25]

DEFECT OF ENAMEL
Amelogenesis Imperfecta

Amelogenesis imperfecta (AI) is a group of hereditary conditions affecting enamel formation.[26] According to the Witkop's classification, there are four main forms of AI: (1) hypoplastic, (2) hypocalcified, (3) hypomatured, and (4) AI with tarudontism. Differences among the various types are related to the phase of enamel formation when the disturbance occurred.[26]

Hypoplastic AI is characterized by defects in the secretary process of ameloblasts resulting in thin or pitted enamel, which may be normal or altered in structure or composition.[26] Hypocalcified AI results from an inability of crystallites to nucleate properly, causing abnormal crystallite growth and decreased mineral enamel content.[26] Abnormal processing of the matrix proteins during maturation causes hypomatured AI, resulting from either abnormal cleavage of enamel matrix proteins or abnormal proteinase activity.[26]

Because the hypoplastic types are caused by reduction in the amount of matrix protein secreted, the clinical presentation is usually thin enamel, surface pitting, or vertical grooving.[27] In contrast, the hypomineralized and hypomaturation types are characterized by the presence of normal amounts of enamel matrix that is deficiently mineralized.[27] Hypomineralized AI shows soft enamel, whereas hypomaturation AI usually presents as opaque and discolored enamel that fractures easily (**Figs. 11 and 12**).[27]

AI can be inherited as autosomal-dominant, autosomal-recessive, or X-linked forms.[26] All types of AI affect the deciduous and permanent dentitions and most of the enamel on all of the teeth is involved.[26]

Clinical presentation

The clinical appearance of AI varies considerably among different AI types.[26,28] Enamel in hypoplastic AI more frequently appears pitted, thin, and tinged with a yellow-brown color, and has a hard texture.[26,28] Radiographically, the enamel contrasts normally from dentine.[28] Enamel is soft opaque, and mottled white, yellow, or brown in hypomature AI.[26,28] Radiographically, it is similar radiodensity as dentine.[28] In hypocalcified AI, enamel is generally abraded and easily detachable from the

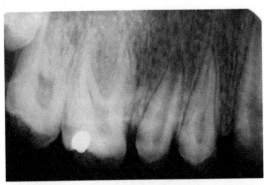

Fig. 11. Maxillary right premolar PA showing enamel defects in a case of amelogenesis imperfecta (hypocalcified type).

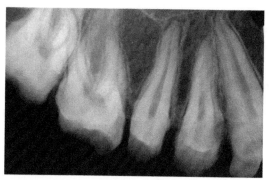

Fig. 12. Maxillary right premolar PA showing radiographic features of amelogenesis imperfecta (hypoplastic type).

underlying dentine.[26,28] Radiographically, enamel is less radiopaque than dentine.[28] In the hypomature-hypoplastic AI with taurodontism, clinical features show mixed hypomaturation and hypoplasia appearance with taurodont teeth.[28]

In addition, clinical features of AI include delay in dental eruption, microdontia, root resorption, short roots, enlarged pulp chamber, pulp stones, dens in dente, tooth agenesis, crowding of teeth, gingival enlargement, gingivitis, and periodontitis.[28] Additionally there are other reported skeletal abnormalities, such as overbite, overjet, and crossbites (discussed later).[28] The primary clinical problems present in AI patients, regardless of subtype, are unsatisfactory esthetics, dental sensitivity, and loss of occlusal vertical dimension caused by the rapid wear of dentition.[26,27]

Treatment

Teeth affected by AI are otherwise sound and are not more caries prone than normal teeth except for their exposed dentin. Cosmetic dentistry in the anterior dentition and occlusal coverage in the posterior dentition are indicated.[1]

Materials that can bond to both dentine and enamel, such as resin modified glass-ionomer cements and polyacid modified composite resins, are likely to be successful for restoration of teeth with enamel defects.[27,29] Although composite resins have good aesthetics, direct adhesion of the composite resins to teeth with minimal or poorly mineralized enamel is usually difficult to achieve.[27,29]

In contrast to plastic restorations, stainless steel crowns are highly durable for restoring and protecting primary and permanent molars affected by enamel hypoplasia.[27,29] Complete coverage of the teeth with stainless steel crowns reduces tooth sensitivity, prevents cusp fractures, and helps maintain space and crown height. The crowns are best inserted using a conservative technique with minimal removal of tooth structure.[27,29]

DEFECT OF DENTIN
Dentinogenesis Imperfecta I, II, III

Three types of dentinogenesis imperfecta are recognized: type 1, which is associated with osteogenesis imperfecta; type II, where only the teeth are affected; and type III, which only occurs in a rare racial isolate in the United States. Type II is the commonest type.[1,2,27]

Dentinogenesis type I

Dentinogenesis type I is associated with osteogenesis imperfecta and although the two conditions are closely related they are genetically distinct.[1,2,27] In many patients with osteogenesis imperfecta the appearances of the teeth in the primary dentition are indistinguishable from those seen in dentinogenesis type II.[1,2,27] However, the involvement of the permanent dentition in type I (associated with osteogenesis imperfecta) is variable and tooth discoloration and attrition do not occur to the same extent.[1,2,27]

Dentinogenesis imperfecta type II

Dentinogenesis imperfecta type II is an autosomal-dominant disorder with variable expressivity and is the most common dental genetic disease, involving approximately 1 in 6000 to 1 in 8000 of the population.[1,2,27] Both the deciduous and permanent dentitions are affected.[1,2,27] On eruption the teeth have a normal contour but an opalescent amber-like appearance.[1,2,27] Subsequently, they may have an almost normal color, following which they become translucent, and finally gray or brownish with bluish reflections from the enamel.[1,2,27] Although in most cases the enamel is structurally normal, it is rapidly lost and the teeth then show marked attrition.[1,2,27] Radiologic examination shows short, blunt roots with partial or even total obliteration of the pulp chambers and root canals by dentine (**Fig. 13**).[1,2,27]

Dentinogenesis imperfecta type III

A similar appearance is seen in dentinogenesis type III, which occurs in a particular racial isolate group in southern Maryland (the Brandywine isolate).[1,2,27] In type III, only dental defects occur.[1,2,27] This type is similar to type II, but has some clinical and radiographic variations.[1,2,27] Features of type III that are not seen in types I and II include multiple pulp exposures, periapical radiolucencies, and a variable radiographic appearance.[1,2,27]

Radiographic findings

Radiographically, types I and II exhibit identical changes.[1,2,27] Opacification of dental pulps occurs as the result of continued deposition of abnormal dentin.[1,2,27] The short roots and the bell-shaped crowns are also obvious on radiographic examination.[1,2,27] In type III, the dentin appears thin and the pulp chambers and root canals extremely large, giving the appearance of thin dentin shells, hence the previous designation of "shell teeth."[1,2,27]

Treatment

Treatment is aimed at protecting teeth from caries and wear.[1,2,27] Most patients seek cosmetic dental improvement. Although the dentin is defective and the enamel is also secondarily abnormal, full crowns and veneer restorations are possible and very serviceable.[1,2,27] Because the dentin is structurally somewhat brittle, excessive

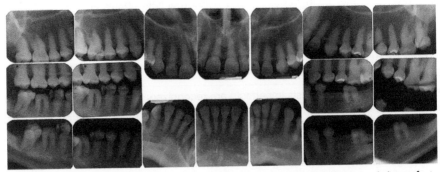

Fig. 13. Intraoral full mouth radiographic series demonstrating dentinogenesis imperfecta.

occlusal forces on a single tooth or teeth used as abutments for fixed partial dentures are not recommended because of risk for fracture.[1,2,27]

Dentine Dysplasia

Dentin dysplasia I, II

Dentine dysplasia type I is a rare condition that shows normal-appearing crowns and short roots in primary and permanent dentitions and causes mobility and early tooth loss.[1,2,27] The pulps are reduced in size, and may have crescent shapes that run parallel to the cementoenamel junction, and associated with periapical radiolucencies.[1,2,27] The genetic changes are unknown.[27]

In dentine dysplasia type II, the crowns of the primary dentition are opalescent because of large dentinal tubules (thistle tube dentin) and abnormal globules of dentin. The permanent teeth appear clinically normal although they often show enlarged pulp chambers (thistle-shaped pulps) with pulp stones.[1,2,27] Occasionally, other abnormalities, such as dental discolorations, bulbous crowns, and pulp obliterations, may be encountered.[1,2,27]

Radiographic findings

Radiographically, in dentin dysplasia type I, roots appear extremely short and pulps are almost completely obliterated.[1,2,27] Residual fragments of pulp tissue appear typically as horizontal lucencies.[1,2,27] Periapical lucencies are typically seen; they represent chronic abscesses, granulomas, or cysts.[1,2,27] In dentin dysplasia type II, deciduous teeth are similar in radiographic appearance to those in type I, but permanent teeth exhibit enlarged pulp chambers that have been described as thistle tube in appearance.[1,2,27]

Treatment

Teeth with reasonable root lengths may be treated with full crown coverage.[1,2,27] Those with short roots often require removal and replacement with dental implant-retained fixed crowns or removable tissue-borne prostheses.[1,2,27]

Regional Odontodysplasia (Ghost Teeth)

This is an uncommon developmental disorder of unknown cause associated with abnormalities of enamel, dentine, pulp, and the dental follicle.[30,31] Both deciduous and permanent dentitions are affected and the number of teeth and number of quadrants involved varies.[30,32] The defect occurs most frequently in the anterior part of the maxilla and is usually unilateral.[30,32] The teeth appear to be discolored, hypoplastic, and hypocalcified.[30,31] The thin enamel is soft on probing and teeth are typically discolored, yellow or yellowish brown.[30,31] Affected teeth are more susceptible to caries and are extremely friable, fracturing at the slightest trauma. Tooth eruption is delayed or does not occur.[30,32] The most frequent clinical symptoms after eruption of teeth with regional odontodysplasia are gingival swelling, periapical infection, and abscess formation in the absence of caries. There is a range of severity with this condition.[30,31]

The cause of this rare dental abnormality is unknown, although numerous causative factors have been suggested, including trauma, nutritional deficiency, infection, metabolic abnormality, systemic disease, local vascular compromise, and genetic influences.[30–32]

Radiographic findings

Radiographically, the affected teeth show a "ghostlike" appearance caused by reduced thickness and radiodensity of enamel and dentin.[31,32] A demarcation between hypomineralized dentin and hypomineralized enamel is not visible.[31,32] The teeth tend to be shorter, have short roots with wide open apices, and abnormally wide pulp chambers and canals.[30–32]

Treatment

The treatment plan has to be based on degree of involvement and functional and esthetic needs of a patient.[30] Older reports have uniformly advised extraction and replacement.[30] However, the newer cases in literature especially with milder forms of disease have tried various treatment modalities.[30] Conservative treatments have tried to retain the involved teeth for a long time without extraction.[30] Auto transplantation has been suggested as a good partial treatment option during period of mixed dentition in some cases.[30] Implants have been suggested as the definite treatment option when the patient reaches adulthood.[30]

DEFECTS OF CEMENTUM
Hypercementosis

Hypercementosis may be idiopathic or the result of local or general disorders.[1,2] It may affect one or several teeth and may be associated with root ankylosis, when cementum is directly continuous with the alveolar bone, or with concrescence.[1,2]

Causes of Hypercementosis

Periapical inflammation
Resorption of cementum as a result of an inflammatory process may stimulate the apposition of cementum. This produces a generalized thickening of the cementum or a localized knob-like enlargement.[1,2]

Mechanical stimulation
Excessive forces applied to a tooth may produce resorption, but mechanical stimulation below a certain threshold may stimulate apposition of cementum.[1,2]

Functionless and unerupted teeth
Such teeth may show areas of cementum resorption, but excessive apposition of cementum may also occur. In unerupted teeth the cementum may even extend over the surface of the enamel if the reduced enamel epithelium is lost.[1,2]

Paget's disease of bone
Hypercementosis is often seen in teeth of patients with Paget disease, the thickened cementum showing a mosaic appearance analogous to that seen in the bone.[1,2] The cementum forms irregular masses and ankylosis is common.[1,2]

DEVELOPMENTAL DISORDERS OF THE JAWS
Exostosis and Tori

Tori and exostosis are nodular, nonpathologic, localized protuberances of cortical bone, the precise designation of which depends on anatomic location.[33,34] Torus palatinus and torus mandibularis are the two most common intraoral osseous outgrowths; the less common form of tori is torus maxillaris.[33,34]

Torus Palatinus

The torus palatinus is located along the longitudinal ridge of the hard palate and can be flat, nodular, spindle-shaped, and lobular.[34] The flat type is the most common torus (49%) and is described as smooth and symmetrically distributed on either side of the median raphe.[34] The nodular variety, being the least common (6.5%), has multiple prominences each protruding from its own base.[34] The spindle-shaped type appears as a ridge divided by the longitudinal medial groove and can be either confined to a limited area or may extend to the posterior end of the hard palate. The lobular form is usually the largest and is characterized by a broad base with multiple vertical and horizontal furrows.[34] The size varies greatly among patients, because some individuals have a torus that is barely discernible, whereas others have a very large exostosis that may warrant removal, especially if the patient is planning for denture construction.[34]

The literature varies with regards to the prevalence of the torus palatinus, especially among different populations. However, it is found in about 20% of the US population and more frequently among American Indians and Eskimos.[34] Females are affected about 1.7 times as often as males in similar populations.[34] The torus palatinus seems to be most prevalent between the third and fourth decade of life, although it can occur at any age.[34]

Etiology

The most common understanding is that the gene for torus palatinus is autosomal-dominant. The trait is also described as having variable expressivity and a penetrance of 85%.[34,35] Environmental factors are also recognized as contributing to the incidence of the torus palatinus. Many studies show that torus formation is influenced by stress on the palatine bone caused by masticatory hyperfunction.[34,35]

Dental considerations

The torus palatinus is usually benign, and there is rarely a reason for removal.[34] It can, however, cause irritation when the patient moves the tongue or masticates.[34] The fragility of the thin mucosal layer covering the torus palatinus can lead to abrasion or laceration, exposing the bone.[34] Dentures can sometimes irritate the torus and cause ulceration of the mucosa. This condition may warrant removal of the torus if the dentures cannot be constructed to avoid such an interaction.[34] The torus may be useful in some cases, because of its ability to be harvested for grafting of periodontal or alveolar ridge defects.[34] Sometimes the torus may contain an air space, which with subsequent excision could cause wound breakdown and form an oronasal fistula.[34] This is a serious condition and can be difficult to correct.[34]

Torus Mandibularis

Torus mandibularis is a bony protuberance located on the lingual aspect of the mandible, commonly in the canine and premolar areas.[33,34] Most studies show that the torus mandibularis is less common than the torus palatinus with a general prevalence of about 6% with a bilateral presentation in about 80% of cases.[34] It can appear as a single elevation or as a group of fused tubercles varying in size (**Fig. 14**).[34] Some studies simply classify the size of the torus as "palpable, visible, or large."[34]

Most sources document the prevalence of the torus mandibularis between 6% and 40%.[34] Some literature claims there is no gender predilection, but some have found it slightly more common in men.[34]

Etiology

Most literature cites genetics as having at least some effect on its occurrence, but it is difficult to link this torus to a simple autosomal-dominant pattern of inheritance.[34,35] In comparison with the torus palatinus, the mandibularis seems to have a higher functional component because of stress placed on the jaw during mastication.[34,35] Studies have shown that clenching and grinding the teeth leads to a higher prevalence of torus mandibularis.[34,35] Studies also show a correlation between the

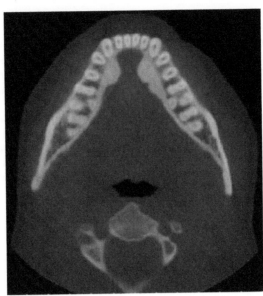

Fig. 14. Axial CBCT of mandible at the midroot level of teeth demonstrating mandibular tori bilaterally.

torus mandibularis and the number of teeth in patients, suggesting that the mandibular torus is protected from resorption throughout life by the functional capacity of the teeth.[34,35]

Dental considerations

Because of its benign nature, most patients do not recognize its existence and diagnosis is found on incidental observations during dental visits.[34] The torus mandiularis can lead to disturbances in speech and mastication if exceptionally large.[34] Ulcerations of the mucosa are not uncommon, and the pocket formed under the torus can lead to food retention.[34] The most frequent reason for removal is the delivery of a dental prosthesis in edentulous patients.[34] In some cases the torus mandibularis has been used as a bone graft for periodontal or alveolar ridge defects.[34] High incidences of large exostoses could be a factor in the delayed healing of gingivectomy wounds.[34]

Buccal and Palatal Exostosis (Torus Maxillaris)

Buccal and palatal exostosis is multiple bony nodules that occur less frequently than tori.[33,34] Buccal exostosis occur along the buccal aspect of the maxilla or mandible, usually in the premolar and molar areas. Palatal exostoses are found on the palatal aspect of the maxilla, and the most common location is the tuberosity area.[33] It is seen in 2.5% to 17% of the population and the prevalence of maxillary tori increases with age.[34]

Etiology

As with tori, many theories describe the cause of exostoses.[34,35] It has been suggested that the bony out-growth represents a reaction to increased or abnormal occlusal stress to the teeth in the involved areas.[34,35]

Dental considerations

Similar to the other oral tori, maxillary exostoses are relatively benign and usually do not warrant removal.[34] A maxillary torus can cause difficulty in mastication and can lead to irritation or ulceration of the surrounding mucosa when consuming hard food.[34] Reasons for removal could be difficulty in speech or interference with the delivery of prosthesis, such as a complete full mouth denture.[34] In periodontal surgery, a maxillary torus can interfere significantly with the repositioning of a mucoperiosteal flap.[34]

Hemifacial Hyperplasia

Facial hemihyperplasia, formerly known as hemihypertrophy, is a rare congenital anomaly that causes asymmetry resulting from the exaggerated growth of all tissues or part of the tissues on the affected side.[36,37] True facial hemihyperplasia is defined as overgrowth of all tissues of one side of the face (skin, bone, nerves, vessels, and adipose tissue), whereas in partial facial hemihyperplasia, overgrowth of one or more, but not all, facial structures is observed.[36,37] Asymmetry is noted at birth and becomes more evident over the years. This disproportional growth continues until complete cessation of the patient's growth, resulting in permanent asymmetry.[36,37] The prevalence rate of hemifacial hyperplasia is 1 in 86,000 live births.[38] It affects men more commonly than women with the right side of the face more commonly affected than left side, as observed in the present case.[38] White persons are more commonly affected than black persons.[38] Hemifacial hyperplasia may be associated with other conditions, such as acromegaly and pituitary gigantism, or with hypertrophy of other parts of the body.[38]

Etiology

The cause of hemifacial hyperplasia is unknown, but various causes have been put forward to explain it including vascular or lymphatic malformations, endocrine disorders, neurocutaneous lesions, neural abnormalities, central nervous system lesions leading to altered neurotropic action, abnormal intrauterine environment, somatic mutations, mechanical influences, and congenital syphilis.[37,38]

Dental considerations

Involvement of orofacial structures is related to asymmetric morphogenesis of teeth, bone, and soft tissues. Tooth size enlargement is random with the frequency of involvement more in canines followed by premolars and first molars and least occurring in incisors, second molars, and third molars.[39] Usually enlargement does not exceed 50% of the normal size.[39] Root size and shape may be proportionally enlarged.[39] Skeletal findings may be in the form of an asymmetric growth of the frontal bone, maxilla, palate, mandible, or condyles.[39] Abnormal occlusal relationships, such as midline deviation, unequal occlusal plane level, open bite, and widely spaced teeth on the involved side, have been reported.[39] The tongue, which is commonly involved, may show a bizarre picture of enlargement of fungiform papillae with unilateral enlargement and contralateral displacement.[39] Other soft tissues, such as lips, buccal mucosa, uvula, and tonsils, are also affected.[39]

Treatment

The treatment of hemifacial hyperplasia continues to be limited. The main aim is to follow the patient for a prolonged period until the growth has stopped.[37,39] During this time, any functional corrections can be performed.[37,39] Esthetic correction according to the patient need is done only after the physiologic growth has ceased.[37,39] Procedures include reconstructive procedures, such as osteotomies or orthognathic surgical procedure, and soft tissue debulking by excision of excess masticatory and subcutaneous tissues, with preservation of neuromuscular functions.[39]

Hemifacial Atrophy (Parry-Romberg Syndrome)

Parry-Romberg syndrome (PRS) is an infrequent, acquired disorder characterized by progressive hemiatrophy of the skin and soft tissue of the face and, in some cases, results in atrophy of muscles, cartilage, and the underlying bony structures.[40,41] Early facial changes usually begin during the first decade and spread slowly and progressively to involve soft tissue, muscle, cartilage, and underlying bone.[36,40] It is typically restricted to one-half of the face but occasionally involves the arm, trunk, and leg (**Fig. 15**).[36,40]

This syndrome seems to have higher incidence among women and to affect most often the left side of the face.[40,41] It is believed to be sporadic, although some rare familial cases have been reported.[40,41]

Etiology

The pathogenesis of PRS is not well understood and seems to be heterogeneous; trauma, infection, cranial vascular malformation, immune-mediated processes, disturbance of fat metabolism, and sympathetic dysfunction has been proposed.[40,41] Trauma has been hypothesized to be at the origin of PRS in 24% to 34% of patients, whether accidental traumas; operative traumas, such as thyroidectomy or dental avulsion; or obstetric traumas, such as forceps or vacuum maneuvers.[40] Occasional PRS cases are familial and point to a genetic predisposition.[40] Some authors have suggested the mode of inheritance to be autosomal-dominant with incomplete penetrance.[40]

Clinical manifestations

PRS is associated with several developmental and congenital deformities, such as neurologic, ophthalmologic, cardiac, endocrine, autoimmune, craniomaxillofacial, and orthodontic abnormalities.[41] PRS is clinically characterized by mostly unilateral facial atrophy of the skin, soft tissues, muscles, and underlying bony structures that

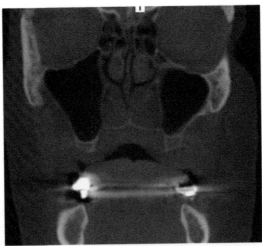

Fig. 15. Coronal CBCT of a patient with hemifacial atrophy (*left side*). Note the smaller maxilla and smaller maxillary sinus on the left.

may be preceded by cutaneous induration.[36,40–42] Skin discoloration (eg, hyperpigmentation or depigmentation) and cicatricial alopecia may also be observed in the affected areas.[36,40–42] There is progressive shrinking and deformation of one side of the face, resulting in unilateral facial atrophy, ipsilateral enophthalmos, and deviation of the mouth and nose toward the affected side.[36,40–42] Neurologic manifestations, such as trigeminal neuralgia, epilepsy, facial paresthesia, and migraine, may be associated with this condition.[41]

Several oral manifestations could be associated with PRS.[41] The oral mucosa and tongue can be affected, also jaws, salivary glands, and teeth.[41] There is deviation of the mouth and nose toward the affected side.[40,41] Atrophy of superior lip led to exposure of anterior teeth.[36,40,41] Unilateral atrophy of muscle of the tongue is seen with PRS.[36,40,41] Deficiencies of the soft and hard palates in all dimensions, shortness and deficiency of the mandibular body and ramus, delayed tooth eruption, root atrophy, and retarded tooth formation may also be observed.[41] However, the affected teeth are normal and vital clinically.[41] Frequently, there is unilateral posterior crossbite as a result of jaw hypoplasia and delayed teeth eruption.[41] Communication disorders and dysphonia have also been reported.[40]

Treatment

The disease is self-limiting and has no definite cure.[41] The patients affected should have multidisciplinary attendance, involving such experts as dermatologists, dentists, and psychologists.[41] The treatment is usually based on reposition of adipose tissue that was lost because of atrophy.[41] Autogenously fat grafts, cartilage grafts, silicone injections and prostheses, bovine collagen, inorganic implants, and recently cell fat mixed with platelet gel are some alternatives to esthetic correction of the atrophy.[41]

Correction of malocclusion is restored by orthodontic movement of teeth.[41] Cone-beam CT, along with the mirror image of the unaffected side superimposed on the affected side, were found to be very helpful in making clear linear, angular, and volumetric measurements and assess the degree of asymmetry, giving the orthodontist insight to the therapeutic possibilities.[41] Prosthetic intervention or additional surgery for the jaws can be used also as a mean to recover the dental occlusion.[41]

Condylar Hyperplasia

Condylar hyperplasia (CH) is characterized by a slowly progressive unilateral enlargement of the condyle, the condylar neck, the ramus, and body of the mandible, leading to facial asymmetry and deviation of the chin to the unaffected side (**Figs. 16** and **17**).[42–44] CH usually occurs after puberty and is completed by 18 to 25 years.[43,44] There is no reported sex or race predilection.[44,45]

Etiology

The cause of CH is controversial and not well-understood. Suggested theories include neoplasia, hormonal influences, hypervascularity, excessive proliferation in repair, or a response to infection or to abnormal loading.[43–45] Other factors that have been advanced as possible etiologic factors are hereditary and intrauterine influences. A possible genetic role in CH is also frequently suggested.[44]

Diagnosis consideration

The diagnosis and treatment of mandibular asymmetry is quite difficult because of the morphologic complexity of the deformity.[43] Careful history, clinical, and radiographic examination usually reveal the true nature of the condition.[43]

CT has contributed to establishing the pathology and condylar morphology (comparing both condyles), making it possible to recognize and classify the different

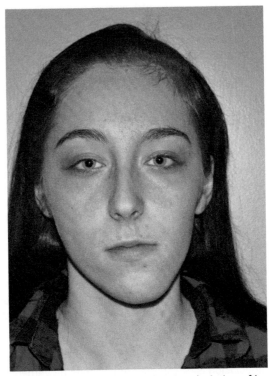

Fig. 16. Patient with right condylar hyperplasia showing deviation of jaw to the left. (*Courtesy of* Dr Carl Bouchard, Université Laval, Quebec, Canada.)

degrees of the disease.[46] Before CT, serial radiographic images were taken in follow-up, which enabled the size and shape of the condyle to be compared at 6-month intervals to determine whether the CH was growing or if this growth had stopped.[46] Nevertheless, it is the nuclear medicine studies that are most associated with the diagnosis of CH; the use of technetium 99 m diphosphonate bone scans may assist in the differential diagnosis by assessing the degree of bone turnover in the affected

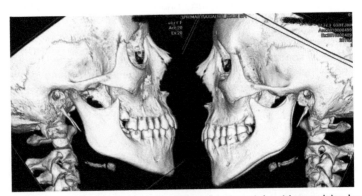

Fig. 17. CBCT three-dimensional reconstructions showing right side condylar hyperplasia and normal left side. (*Courtesy of* Dr Carl Bouchard, Université Laval, Quebec, Canada.)

areas.[45,46] Active CH exhibits increased uptake of radionuclide on the hyperplastic side.[45,46]

Clinical features

Prominent features of CH include an enlarged mandibular condyle, elongated condylar neck and ramus of the mandible of the mandible on the affected side, causing fullness of the face on that side and flattening of the face on the contralateral side and giving a prognathic appearance.[42–45] The prominence of the chin is shifted to the unaffected side.[43–45] There is a compensatory eruption of the maxillary teeth and downward growth of the maxillary alveolar bone to maintain occlusion.[42] There is also compensatory eruption of the mandibular teeth, resulting in increased alveolar height and a bowing effect on the inferior border of the mandible.[42]

Treatment considerations

Because the treatment is influenced by the patients' growth, it is important to determine whether growth is still occurring.[43] If growth has ceased, the mandibular asymmetry is treated by orthognathic surgery and if growth is still occurring a partial condylectomy should be performed.[43] Sufficient cartilage and bone has to be removed to eradicate the condylar growth site and permit rotation of the mandible into normal occlusion.[43] The decision of whether condylectomy is required involves consideration of evidence of active change in the hyperplastic condyle or radiographic and clinical suggestions of pathologic conditions, such as chondroma, osteoma, or other neoplasm that may warrant tissue diagnosis.[43]

Condylar Hypoplasia or Aplasia

Hypoplasia or aplasia of the mandibular condyle indicates underdevelopment or nondevelopment associated mainly with various craniofacial abnormalities.[45] These may be either congenital or acquired. Congenital condylar hypoplasia is characterized by unilateral or bilateral underdevelopment of the mandibular condyle, and usually occurs as part of some systemic condition originating in the first and second branchial arches, such as mandibulofacial dysostosis.[45] Acquired (secondary) condylar hypoplasia may be caused by local factors (trauma, infection of the mandibular bone or middle ear, irradiation) or by systemic factors (toxic agents, rheumatoid arthritis, mucopolysaccharoidosis).[45]

Bilateral aplasia and hypoplasia of the mandibular condyle lead to the underdevelopment of the mandible, resulting in a lack of symmetric growth of the mandible, micrognathia characterized by bird face, and a markedly short mandible. As a result of severe micrognathia the teeth may be markedly crowded and anterior open bite may develop.[42,45] In unilateral condylar hypoplasia, the continued growth of the contralateral side causes deviation toward the affected side and results in a crossbite relationship of the teeth.[42,45] On the affected side, the ramus and body of the mandible remain underdeveloped.[42,45]

Coronoid Process Hyperplasia

Coronoid hyperplasia is enlargement of one or both coronoid processes causing impingement of the enlarged coronoid processes on the zygomatic bones.[42,47,48] The primary complaint and clinical feature is opening restriction.[42,47]

The pathogenesis of coronoid hyperplasia is unclear.[47] Trauma is thought to be a factor in some cases of coronoid process hyperplasia. Restricted opening usually happens after trauma and results in hyperplasia of the coronoid processes.[47] Increased activity of the temporal muscles is considered as a pathogenic factor. In some pathologic conditions, such as where the patient underwent condyle process resection, the continuous distraction of the temporal muscle to the coronoid process without the balance from the condyle process can cause hyperplasia.[47]

It has been reported that the osteoma responsible for constriction may be considered to be a localization of neurogenic paraosteoarthropathies.[47] Endocrine abnormality may result in coronoid process hyperplasia. There has been a reported case occurring in two members of one family, indicating that heredity may play a role in coronoid process hyperplasia.[47]

Chronic temporomandibular joint disk displacement has been proposed as an etiologic factor of coronoid process enlargement.[47] Consequently, the clinician easily neglects coronoid process hyperplasia when temporomandibular disease exists in the same patient.[47]

Diagnostic consideration
Panoramic radiography can reflect the morphologic change of the coronoid process.[47] CT provides detailed imaging of coronoid hyperplasia in axial and coronal planes; it also shows the precise site of impingement between the coronoid process and the zygomatic arch and the relationship between coronoid process and surrounding tissues giving the exact information for interpretation and treatment guidance.[47,49] Three-dimensional CT reconstructions have the definite advantage of showing the angle at which the enlarged coronoid process impinges.[47,49]

Preoperative MRI, although superior to CT because of its multiplanar capabilities and superior tissue contrast, is not necessary for surgical planning. It is of advantage in the postoperative follow-up in young patients because it avoids high-dose CT.[49]

Treatment and follow-up
Hyperplasia of the coronoid process is usually treated by intraoral coronoidectomy.[47,49] A coronal incision is considered when the coronoid process hyperplasia is accompanied by temporomandibular disorder; the intraoral incision is not used, because serious opening restriction usually exists in this situation.[47]

The prognosis depends on postoperative mouth opening training and exercises. It is important to give appropriate physiotherapy after operation.[47] Postoperative follow-up of patients with complete functional recovery requires only a panoramic radiograph with the mouth open.[49] Follow-up of patients with incomplete or absent recovery of function requires panoramic radiography and MRI.[49] The former demonstrates incomplete bony resections and/or the inability of the mandibular condyles to translate.[49] However, MRI can detect complications at the site of surgery, such as hematomas, fibrosis, and atrophy of the muscles of mastication; furthermore, it allows the assessment of the anatomic continuity between the tendon of the temporalis muscle and the ramus of the mandible.[49]

GENETIC CONDITIONS AFFECTING THE JAWS
Cleidocranial Dysplasia

CCD is an autosomal-dominant malformation syndrome[1] primarily affecting bones that undergo intermembranous ossification (ie, generally the calvarian and clavicular bones).[50] It has variable expressivity and almost complete penetrance.[1]

Clinical features
The adverse general health effects of CCD are usually not very severe or debilitating and there is no associated impairment in cognitive or intellectual functioning in affected persons.[50] Clinical features of CCD are summarized in **Table 1**.

Table 1 Clinical features in cleidocranial dysplasia	
Organ/System	**Clinical Features**
Skull	Brachycephalic skull Maxillary hypoplasia Frontal and parietal bossing Underdeveloped paranasal sinuses Delayed closure of cranial sutures Broad and depressed bridge of the nose Hypertelorism
Clavicles	Aplasia or hypoplasia Excessive mobility of shoulder griddle
Thoracic cage	Small and bell-shaped thoracic cage Short ribs
Pelvis	Delayed closure of wide symphysis pubis
Skeleton	Shorter stature Short terminal phalanges Spinal malalignment
Dental	Hyperdontia "major feature" Prolonged retention of primary teeth Delayed eruption of permanent dentition Dentigerous cyst Taurodontia

Data from Refs.[1,50,51]

Radiographic features

Skull The characteristic skull findings are brachycephaly, delayed or failed closure of the fontanels, open skull sutures, and multiple wormian bones (small, irregular bones in the sutures of the skull that are formed by secondary centers of ossification in the suture lines).[1,51] In the most severe cases, very little formation of the parietal and frontal bones may occur.[1,51]

Clavicles and skeleton Typically the clavicles are underdeveloped to varying degrees and, in approximately 10% of cases, they are completely absent.[1] Other bones also may be affected, including the long bones, vertebral column, pelvis, and bones of the hands and feet.[1]

Jaws In CCD the maxilla and paranasal sinuses characteristically are underdeveloped, resulting in maxillary micrognathia. The mandible is usually normal size. A patent (open) mandibular symphysis has been reported in 3% of adults and 64% of children.[1] The alveolar bone overlying unerupted teeth is being denser than usual, with a coarse trabecular pattern in the mandible.[1]

Teeth The unerupted teeth develop most commonly in the anterior maxilla and premolar regions of the jaws. Many resemble premolars and these unerupted teeth may develop dentigerous cysts.[1] Three-dimensional CT imaging is used to visualize the size and thickness of bony defects of the skull and plan for harvesting of bone graft material from other parts of the skull for surgical treatment to address esthetic concerns.[1]

Treatment and management considerations

The aim of dental management in CCD is to achieve an optimal functional and cosmetic result by early adulthood.[51] A multidisciplinary approach is necessary. **Box 1** summarizes some strategies used in dental treatment.

Box 1
Dental strategies in the management of patients with cleidocranial dysplasia

- Removal of primary and supernumerary teeth for spontaneous eruption of permanent teeth
- Removal of bone overlying permanent teeth to expose the crown when half of the root is formed to aid in their eruption
- Dental rehabilitation with dental implants
- Autotransplantation in older patients has been reported as a successful strategy

Data from Refs.[1,50,51]

The commitment of the patient to the treatment plan is also crucial.[51] Ideally patients should be identified early, before the age of 5 years, to take advantage of combined orthodontic-surgical treatment.[1] Because of the long duration of some dental procedures, speech therapy is sometimes required.[51]

Surgical procedures are usually uneventful in CCD but atlantoaxial subluxation with consequent damage to the spinal cord has been documented.[51]

Crouzon Syndrome

Crouzon syndrome is characterized by premature craniosynostosis, usually affecting the coronal suture in combination with craniosynostosis of the sagittal and/or lambdoid sutures, and midface malformations notably ocular proptosis.[52] Craniosynostosis may be present at birth but usually develops during the first year of life.[52,53] It has a prevalence of 1 in 25,500 live births.[53,54] It is inherited in an autosomal-dominant manner and caused by mutations in *FGFR2*.[52]

Clinical features

Individuals with Crouzon syndrome exhibit several characteristic physical abnormalities, including maxillary hypoplasia, craniosynostosis, mid-face complex underdevelopment, ocular proptosis, and shallow orbits.[53] Nearly all cases of Crouzon syndrome have craniosynostosis of the coronal suture and this is usually in combination with craniosynostosis of the sagittal and lambdoid sutures.[52,54] Craniosynostosis leads to the development of a wide variety of cranial malformations that depend on the order and rate of suture closure. These malformations are explained in **Table 2**. Tracheal abnormalities may occur in patients with Crouzon syndrome. The malformation may present as isolated fusion of the tracheal rings or the whole trachea may present as a solid

---

Table 2
Types of craniosynostosis based on the order and rate of suture closure

Malformation	Shape/Description	Associated Sutures
Brachycephaly	Broad and short in the anteroposterior direction	Coronal or lambdoid sutures
Scaphocephaly	Narrow and elongated from anterior to posterior	Sagittal suture
Trigonocephaly	Triangular shape with pointed forehead	Metopic suture
Cloverleaf	Trilobed	Pansynostosis

Data from Refs.[50–53]

cartilaginous tube. The abnormality may extend into the bronchi.[52] Clinical characteristics of Crouzon syndrome and percentage of prevalence are shown in **Table 3**.

Dental features

Crouzon syndrome has many specific intraoral physical characteristics. Lateral palatal swellings, short upper lip, cleft lip, cleft palates, and bifid uvulas.[53] Crouzon patients have a hypoplastic maxilla and the palate is narrow and high vaulted (**Fig. 18**). These physical abnormalities of the palate and maxilla contribute to dental crowding, malocclusion, a significant openbite and prognathic mandible.[52,53] The most common malocclusions are unilateral and bilateral posterior crossbites, and class III incisor and molar relationships.[52] Ectopic eruption of permanent first molar has been observed in nearly half of the cases of Crouzon syndrome.[52,53] Delayed eruption of the primary and permanent teeth has been observed.[53] The anterior open bite increases the likelihood of chronic mouth breathing, angular cheilitis, drooling, and chapped lower lips.[53] Chronic mouth breathing also can increase the patient's potential for respiratory infections, persistent periodontitis, and a dry or chapped tongue.[53]

Radiographic features

Skull The earliest radiographic signs of cranial suture synostosis are sclerosis and overlapping edges.[1] Premature fusion of the cranial base leads to diminished facial growth. In some cases, prominent cranial markings are noted.[1] These markings may be seen as multiple radiolucencies appearing as depressions of the inner surface of the cranial vault, which results in a beaten metal appearance.[1]

Jaws The lack of growth in an anteroposterior direction at the cranial base results in maxillary hypoplasia, creating a class III malocclusion in some patients.[1] The mandible is typically smaller than normal but appears prognathic in relation to the severely hypoplastic maxilla (**Fig. 19**).[1]

Table 3
Clinical characteristics of Crouzon syndrome and percentage of prevalence

System/Organ	Clinical Characteristics	Percentage(%)
Eyes	Ocular proptosis[4]	100
	Extropia	77
Oral/dental	Lateral palatal swelling 3–4	50
	Cleft lip	2
	Cleft palate	3
	Bifid uvula	9
	Unilateral or bilateral crossbite	67
	Anterior openbite	32
	Ectopic eruption of maxillary first molar	47
Ears	Conductive hearing loss 3	50
	Atresia of external auditory meatus 3	13
Vascular	Stenosis of jugular foramen and associated obstruction of jugular vein 3	60
Skeletal	Fusion of cervical vertebrae (C2-C3/C5-C6) 3	22
Neurologic	Hydrocephalus (headaches and seizures) 2	9–26
	Chiari malformation 3	
Mental	Varying degrees of intellectual disabilities 4	3

Data from Refs.[50–52]

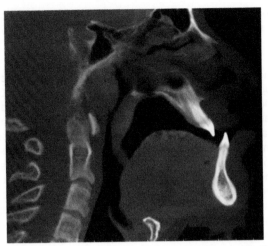

Fig. 18. Sagittal CBCT showing high palatal vault in a patient with Crouzon syndrome. (*Courtesy of* Dr Mansur Ahmad, University of Minnesota School of Dentistry, Minneapolis, MN.)

Treatment and management considerations

The craniofacial features of Crouzon syndrome worsen over time because of the abnormal craniofacial growth. Early diagnosis permits surgical and orthodontic treatment from infancy through adolescence.[53] Patients with Crouzon syndrome should have an orthodontic evaluation at 3 or 4 years of age; at that time, corrective treatment should be considered.[53] Underdeveloped midface complex usually is corrected when the patient is 4 to 6 years of age by advancing it to a predetermined point using standard surgical techniques (**Figs. 20 and 21**).[53]

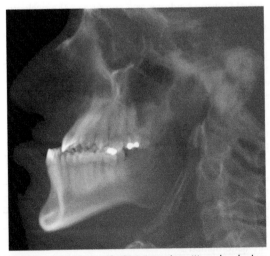

Fig. 19. CBCT sagittal view (20-mm cut) showing class III malocclusion with retrognathic maxilla and prognathic mandible in a patient with Crouzon syndrome. (*Courtesy of* Dr Mansur Ahmad, University of Minnesota School of Dentistry, Minneapolis, MN.)

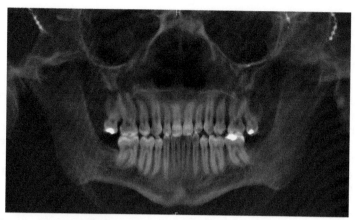

Fig. 20. Panoramic reconstruction of CBCT showing surgical intervention in the region of orbital rim and temporal bone. (*Courtesy of* Dr Mansur Ahmad, University of Minnesota School of Dentistry, Minneapolis, MN.)

The objectives of these treatments are to allow normal brain growth and development by preventing increased intracranial pressure, protect the eyes by providing adequate bony support, and improve facial esthetics and occlusal function.[1,53]

Treacher Collins Syndrome

Treacher Collins syndrome (TCS) or mandibulofacial dysostosis is a rare autosomal-dominant disorder of craniofacial development.[1,54,55] It is generally characterized by bilaterally symmetric abnormalities of structures within the first and second branchial arches occur during histodifferentiation morphogenesis between approximately the 20th day and the 12th week of intrauterine life.[56,57] It affects approximately 1 in 50,000 live births.[58] It is an autosomal-dominant condition with variable expressivity;

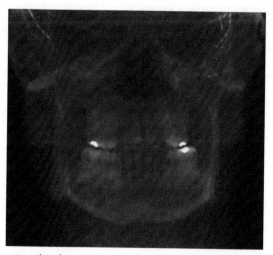

Fig. 21. CBCT reconstruction in anteroposterior dimension showing surgical intervention. (*Courtesy of* Dr Mansur Ahmad, University of Minnesota School of Dentistry, Minneapolis, MN.)

males and females are equally affected.[56] In cases of full expression of the syndrome, the diagnosis is easily made based on clinical characteristics alone.[57] TCS patients have normal intelligence. As a result of distorted physical appearance, patients often experience significant psychosocial challenges and social stigma.[54]

Clinical and radiographic features

Individuals with TCS have a wide range of anomalies, depending on the severity of the condition.[1] Severe cases of TCS may result in perinatal death because of a compromised airway. Some individuals may be so mildly affected that it can be difficult to establish an unequivocal clinical diagnosis.[58] **Tables 4** and **5** summarize the clinical and radiographic features of this condition and treatment recommendations. **Table 6** explains the uses of different radiographic modalities in the diagnosis and management of TCS (**Figs. 22** and **23**).

Management considerations

An extensive range of surgical interventions is used to secure respiratory function, ensure proper feeding, improve hearing, and reconstruct profound periorbital and craniofacial defects.[55] Nasal reconstruction uses nasal hump reduction, and

Table 4
Clinical features of Treacher Collins syndrome and treatment recommendations for each

	Clinical Features	Treatment
Skull	Underdevelopment/absence of zygomatic bones Narrow face Downward inclination of palpebral fissure	—
Eye/Vision	Lower eyelid colobomas with absence of the eyelash medially Strabismus Vision loss Amblyopia	Complaints concerning the eyelids were most frequently managed by lateral canthopexy Lower eyelid reconstruction
Ear/Hearing	Hypoplasia or atresia of external ears, auditory canal, and ossicles of middle ear may result in partial or complete deafness	Treatment of external ear defects may involve plastic and reconstructive surgery or maxillofacial prosthetics Hearing aids or cochlear implants may be used to treat the hearing loss
Jaw/Dental	Mandibular hypoplasia and steep angle of mandible Angle class II with anterior open bite malocclusion Hypoplastic maxilla with high arched palate Cleft palate in 30% of cases Temporomandibular joint ankylosis as a result of the combined effect of maxillary and mandibular hypoplasia Tooth agenesis predominantly affecting mandibular second premolar Enamel opacities	Conservative treatment including orthodontics, tooth extraction, and implants Coordinated orthodontics and orthognathic surgery Including bilateral distraction osteogenesis of the mandible Le Fort I with bilateral sagittal split osteotomy Palatoplasty is used for the management of cleft palate during the first year of life

Data from Refs.[1,54–58]

Table 5	
Radiographic features of Treacher Collins syndrome	
Skull	Hypoplastic or missing zygomatic bones
	Hypoplastic lateral aspect of the orbit
	Underdeveloped or absent maxillary sinuses
Ears	Malformation of the auditory ossicles with fusion between rudiments of the malleus and incus
	Partial absence of the stapes and oval window
	Complete absence of the middle ear and epitympanic space
Jaw	Hypoplastic maxilla and mandible
	Steep mandibular angle and accentuation of the antegonial notch
	Short ramus
	Absent or smaller than usual mastoid air cells and articular eminence
	Posteriorly and inferiorly positioned condyles

Data from Refs.[1,54–58]

rhinoplasty, septoplasty, and nasal tip reconstruction.[1,55] Refer to **Table 4** for treatment options.

Hemifacial Microsomia

Hemifacial microsomia (HFM) is the second most common developmental craniofacial anomaly after cleft lip and palate.[1] Patients with HFM typically display reduced growth and development of half of the face as a result of abnormal development of the first and second branchial arches.[1] During Week 4 of gestation, the neural crest cells from the neural tube migrate into the pharyngeal arches. Each arch consists of three different layers: (1) the endoderm, (2) the ectoderm, and (3) the mesoderm. Disturbances of this migration lead to deformities of the face, ear, and maxilla.[54] This malformation sequence is usually unilateral but occasionally may involve both sides (craniofacial microsomia).[1] It affects approximately 1 in 3500 to 5600 live births.[1,54]

Table 6	
Different imaging modalities uses in diagnosis, management, and follow-up of patients with craniofacial syndromes: Treacher Collins syndrome	
Imaging Modality	**Uses**
Computer tomography	Used in diagnosis and planning of surgical intervention
	Axial and coronal images should be obtained to accurately delineate the bony labyrinth, middle ear, and facial nerves
	Help identify contraindications to surgical procedure, such as gross anomalies of the inner ear
	Measure the amount of bone generated in patients during distraction osteogenesis of the mandible or maxilla
Plain film (occipital view)	Identifying aplasia or hypoplasia of the zygomatic arch
Occipitomental view (Water view) and orthopantogram films	Identifying mandibular hypoplasia
Cephalometric radiographs	Determine the extent of mandibular retrognathia

Data from Dixon J, Trainor P, Dixon MJ. Treacher Collins syndrome. Orthod Craniofac Res 2007;10(2):88–95.

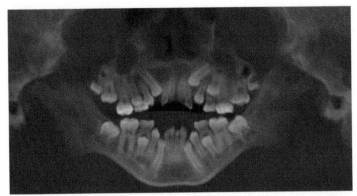

Fig. 22. CBCT panoramic reconstruction showing features of Treacher Collins syndrome: steep mandibular angle, shallow articular eminence, and posteriorly and inferiorly positioned condyles. (*Courtesy of* Dr Mansur Ahmad, University of Minnesota School of Dentistry, Minneapolis, MN.)

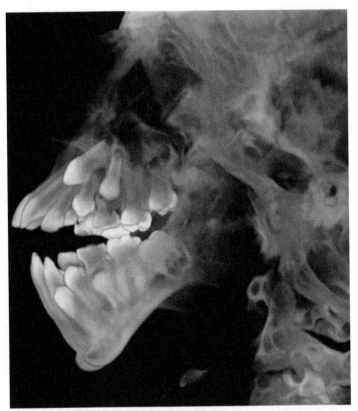

Fig. 23. CBCT maximum intensity projection showing features of Treacher Collins syndrome: hypoplastic maxilla and mandible, steep mandibular angle. (*Courtesy of* Dr Mansur Ahmad, University of Minnesota School of Dentistry, Minneapolis, MN.)

Most cases occur spontaneously, but familial cases demonstrating autosomal-dominant inheritance have been reported. There is a male predominance of 3:2 and a right side predominance of 3:2.[1]

Clinical and radiographic features

HFM is marked by phenotypic variability, ranging from simple preauricular skin tags to severe facial asymmetry with microtia or anotia.[54] HFM is usually apparent at birth.[54] Patients with this condition have a striking appearance caused by progressive failure of the affected side to grow.[54] Clinical and radiographic features for patients with HFM are summarized in **Table 7**. The different radiographic modalities used in the diagnosis and treatment planning of patients with HFM are explained in **Table 8**.

Management

Treatment of craniofacial microsomia depends on the severity of the disease. In milder cases, in which only skin tags are present, removal at an appropriate age is warranted.[54] It is important to be wary of the facial nerve when removing skin tags because the cartilage remnants can be closely associated.[54] The ear abnormalities may be repaired by plastic surgery or corrected with maxillofacial prosthetics, and the hearing loss may be partly corrected by hearing aids. In bilateral cases with profound hearing loss, cochlear implants may be used to correct severe hearing loss.[1] The mandibular abnormalities may be corrected by conventional orthognathic surgery or distraction osteogenesis to lengthen the ramus on the affected side. Orthodontic intervention may correct or prevent malocclusion.[1,59]

Ectodermal Dysplasia

Ectodermal dysplasia (ED) represents a large, complex group of inherited disorders comprising more than 192 different conditions, which are defined by primary defects in the development of two or more tissues derived from embryonic ectoderm.[60] Included are the hair, sebaceous glands, eccrine and apocrine glands, nails, teeth, lenses and conjunctiva of the eyes, anterior pituitary gland, nipples, and the ears.[61]

Table 7	
Clinical and radiographic features for patients with hemifacial microsomia	
Appearance	Reduced dimension of the involved side of the face/skull Curved midsaggital plane of the face toward affected side Defects of the second branchial arch involving the facial nerve and facial muscles of the affected side
Ear/Hearing	Aplasia or hypoplasia of external ear Missing ear canal Underdevelopment of the osseous component of auditory system Diminished or absent external auditory meatus Hearing loss caused by previously mentioned characteristics
Jaw/Dental	Malocclusion on the affected side Occlusal plane is canted up to the affected side Cleft palate and velopharyngeal insufficiency Dental crowding in the affected side Unilateral crossbite Delayed tooth development in the affected side Enamel hypoplasia in primary incisors

Data from White SC, Pharoah MJ. Oral radiology: principles and interpretation. 7th edition. St Louis (MO): Mosby/Elsevier, 2014; and Buchanan EP, Xue AS, Hollier LH Jr. Craniofacial syndromes. Plast Reconstr Surg 2014;134(1):128e–53e.

Table 8
Different radiographic modalities used in the assessment of patients with HFM

Modality	Findings
Panoramic radiograph	Overview of the osseous structures of the mandible and maxillofacial complex
	Reduction in the size of the bones on the affected side
	Reduced or lack of any development of the condyle, coronoid process, or ramus
	The dentition on the affected side may show a reduction in the number or size of the teeth
Occlusal radiographs	Depict the osseous integrity of the palatal vault
Lateral cephalometric radiographs	The relationship of the mandible and maxilla to the cranial base
Frontal skull radiograph (posteroanterior view)	Depict the degree of osseous asymmetry of the face
Computed tomography	Shows a reduction in the size of the muscles of mastication and muscles of facial expression
	Hypoplasia or atresia of the auditory canal and ossicles of the middle ear
	Abnormal course of the facial nerve

Data from White SC, Pharoah MJ. Oral radiology: principles and interpretation. 7th edition. St Louis (MO): Mosby/Elsevier, 2014; and Buchanan EP, Xue AS, Hollier LH Jr. Craniofacial syndromes. Plast Reconstr Surg 2014;134(1):128e–53e.

It is usually transmitted as an X-linked recessive trait where the gene is carried by the female and manifested in males.[62] All racial groups have been afflicted by this condition.[61] However, it is most often observed in white persons.[60] The incidence of this disease is 1 in 100,000, with a mortality rate of 30% in infancy or early childhood because of intermittent hyperpyrexia.[60]

Clinical features
Table 9 summarizes clinical features in patients with ED (**Fig. 24**).

Treatment
ED patients often need a multidisciplinary approach to treatment planning and dental treatment to regain esthetics and functioning.[60] The optimal dental treatment should be commenced as soon as possible to improve the sagittal and vertical skeletal relationship during craniofacial growth and development and to provide improvements in esthetics, emotional well-being, stomatognathic efficiency, and temporomandibular joint function.[60] **Box 2** summarizes dental treatment modalities in patient with ED.

Ehlers-Danlos Syndromes

Ehlers-Danlos syndromes (EDS) comprise a clinically and genetically heterogeneous group of heritable disorders of connective tissue, of which the principal clinical features are caused by varying degrees of tissue fragility of the skin, ligaments, blood vessels, and internal organs.[63] The first genetic defect was identified as a deficiency of lysyl hydroxylase, a collagen-modifying enzyme.[63] An EDS diagnosis encompasses any of six types of connective tissue disorders, each of which is heritable and involves a unique defect in collagen metabolism.[64] The prevalence of EDS is between 1 in 5000 and 1 in 10,000, but the epidemiology of the specific types is largely unknown.[64] EDS

Table 9
Clinical features in patients with ectodermal dysplasia

Systemic	Hypohidrosis (fever of unknown origin)
	Increased susceptibility to allergic disorders (eg, asthma and eczema)
Skin	Partial or complete absence of sweat and sebaceous glands
	Smooth, soft, dry, and thin skin
	Fine linear wrinkles and increased pigmentation around the eyes and mouth
	Hyperkeratosis of the palms of the hands and soles of the feet
Hair and nails	Hair over the scalp is often blond, fine, stiff, and short
	Normal beard but spare axillary and pubic hair
	Missing eyebrows and eyelashes
	Nails appear normal or spoon-shaped
Skull	Frontal bossing
	Depressed mid-face
	Malar hypoplasia
	Prominent supraorbital ridges
	Saddle nose
	Large low-set ears
	Prominent chin
Eyes/Vision	Impaired lacrimal gland functions
	Glaucoma
Jaw development	Lack of alveolar ridge development
	Reduced vertical dimension
	High palatal arch with possibility of cleft palate
Oral/Dental	Protuberant lips
	Hypodontia or anodontia of primary or permanent teeth
	Loss of function and esthetics
	Anomalies of tooth shape, size, and structure

Data from Refs.[60–62]

is observed throughout the world, affecting both sexes without racial predisposition.[64] Early diagnosis by means of biochemical and molecular testing is now feasible for most EDS variants, and may prove important for adequate follow-up and genetic counseling.[63] Classifications of EDS are summarized in **Table 10**.

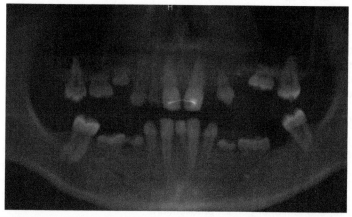

Fig. 24. CBCT panoramic reconstruction in a patient with ectodermal dysplasia showing hypodontia. (*Courtesy of* Dr Mansur Ahmad, University of Minnesota School of Dentistry, Minneapolis, MN.)

> **Box 2**
> **Dental treatment options for patients with ectodermal dysplasia**
>
> - Most frequent prosthetic treatment is removable prosthodontics
> - Overdentures can be fabricated when teeth are present to add the advantage of alveolar bone preservation
> - Dental implants are the ideal treatment option for the adult patient depending on the amount of alveolar bone available
> - Implant-supported oral rehabilitation in pediatric patients has been reported of benefit
>
> *Data from Refs.*[60–62]

Clinical and radiographic features

Features include skin hyperextensibility, delayed wound healing with atrophic scarring, joint hypermobility, easy bruising, and generalized fragility of the soft connective tissues.[63] Skin hyperextensibility is characteristic for all EDS subtypes, except the vascular type where the skin appears thin and transparent, showing the venous pattern over the chest, abdomen, and extremities.[63] General characteristics of all subtypes of EDS are listed in **Box 3**. Features specific for the vascular subtype of EDS are listed in **Box 4**. Oral and dental manifestations are listed in **Table 11**.

Management

Preventive and management guidelines in all subtypes of EDS are listed in **Box 5**. The dental considerations for the management of patients with EDS are listed in **Table 12**.

Papillon-Lefèvre Syndrome

Definition

Papillon-Lefèvre syndrome is an autosomal-recessive disorder caused by mutations on the cathepsin C gene characterized by a diffuse palmoplanter hyperkeratosis and rapidly progressive and devastating periodontitis, affecting the primary and permanent dentition.[68,69] The onset of disease usually coincides with the eruption of primary teeth.[69] Boys and girls are equally affected, with no racial predominance.[69] Clinical and radiographic features of Papillon-Lefevre syndrome are summarized in **Table 13**.

Treatment considerations

Careful attention to oral hygiene and periodontal care are essential; however, disease is progressive even with conventional approaches to periodontal disease.[68] It has been recommended that compromised primary teeth should be extracted 6 months before eruption of the permanent dentition.[68]

Down Syndrome

Down syndrome is an easily recognized congenital, autosomal anomaly characterized by generalized growth and mental deficiencies affecting 1 in 600 to 1 in 1000 live births.[70,71] Approximately 95% of Down syndrome cases have the extra chromosome 21, making the chromosome count 47 instead of the normal 46.[70,71] Maternal age plays an important role in the frequency of Down syndrome. There seems to be no racial, social, economic, or gender predilection.[70]

Clinical characteristics

The physical characteristic features of Down syndrome include[71]

Table 10
Classification of Ehler-Danlos syndrome

Villefranche Type	Corresponding Berlin Types	Collagen Defects	Characteristics
Classical	I (gravis) II (mitis)	Type V	Marked skin hyperextensibility Widened atrophic scars Joint hypermobility Molluscoid pseudotumors (calcified hematomas) Periodontitis
Hypermobility	III (hypermobile)	Unknown	Joint hypermobility "dominant feature" The hyperextensibility and/or smooth velvety skin Bruising tendencies Periodontitis
Vascular	IV (arterial-ecchymotic)	Type III	Thin and translucent skin with visible veins The facial characteristics: large eyes, thin nose, lobeless ears, short stature, thin scalp hair Decrease in subcutaneous tissue of face and extremities Easy bruising manifested by spontaneous ecchymosis Arterial/intestinal/uterine fragility or ruptures are common
	V	Unknown	It has been described in a single family "rare" Women are only carriers X-linked
Kyphoscoliosis	VI (ocular-scoliotic)	Lysyl hydroxylase	Generalized joint laxity, severe muscle hypotonia, and scoliosis at birth Tissue fragility, atrophic scars, easy bruising Micro cornea Radiologically considerable osteopenia
Arthrochalasia	VIIa (arthrochalasis multiplex congenita) VIIb (arthrochalasis multiplex congenita)	Type I	Congenital hip dislocation Generalized joint hypermobility with recurrent subluxations Skin hyperextensibility with easy bruising Tissue fragility including atrophic scars Muscle hypotonia; kyphoscoliosis Radiologically mild osteopenia
Dermatosparaxis	VIIc (human dermatosparaxis)	Procollagen N-peptidase	Severe skin fragility and substantial bruising Normal wound healing and scars formation Skin texture is soft and doughy Redundant facial skin Large hernias (umbilical, inguinal) The oral findings are alterations in teeth and severe periodontitis

(continued on next page)

Table 10 (continued)			
Villefranche Type	Corresponding Berlin Types	Collagen Defects	Characteristics
Periodontitis type	VIII	Unknown	Similar to the classical type except that it also presents as periodontal friability
			The periodontal problems appear at puberty and usually lead to loss of the teeth before age 30
			Rare
			Generalized early onset periodontitis (dominant)
			Large patches of scar tissue on the shins, similar to diabetic ulcers or varicose veins
			Hyperelasticity of the skin and hypermobility of the joints are moderate
			Facial characteristics include hypertelorism, widening of the root of the nose, a narrow curved nose, narrow face, and scarring on the forehead and chin

Data from Refs.[64–67]

- Below-average weight and length at birth
- Reduced muscle tone resulting in hypotonia in infancy, which improves spontaneously with age
- Generalized growth defect resulting in a short, broad stature
- Brachycephalic skull resulting in a flattened face and occiput
- Legs and arms that are short in relation to the rest of the body
- Broad hands with short fingers and a little finger that curls inward
- Underdevelopment of the middle third of face slanting eyes and prominent epicanthic folds
- Delayed speech development
- Low-pitched voice
- Learning disability

Box 3
General characteristics of all subtypes of EDS
• Joint hypermobility and related problems, such as congenital clubfoot, joint effusion, and premature osteoarthritis
• Unilateral or bilateral hip dislocation at birth
• Primary muscle hypotonia and delayed motor development
• Chronic musculoskeletal pain in some adults
• Easy bruising, spontaneous ecchymoses, and prolonged bleeding tendency
• Structural cardiac malformations, such as mitral valve prolapse and tricuspid valve prolapse "uncommon"
Data from Refs.[64–67]

Box 4
Additional features of patients with vascular EDS

- Skin appears thin and transparent showing the venous pattern over the chest, abdomen, and extremities
- Increased risk of life-threatening complications and a decreased life expectancy
- At risk of arterial rupture, which may occur spontaneously or may be preceded by aneurysm, arteriovenous fistulae, or dissection
- Spontaneous rupture of the bowel, intestine, or gravid uterus
- Patients with vascular EDS who are pregnant should be followed in a high-risk obstetric program

Data from Refs.[64–67]

Medical conditions affecting patients with Down syndrome are summarized in **Table 14**. Oral manifestations and common dental anomalies in patients with Down syndrome are summarized in **Boxes 6** and **7**.

Considerations for dental treatment include the following[71,74]:

- Careful medical history and updated laboratory testing should be taken to assess any hematologic or immunologic alteration before any invasive dental procedure.
- The need for antibiotic prophylaxis based on the procedure and the cardiac condition of the patient.

Table 11
Clinical and radiographic oral manifestations of Ehlers-Danlos syndrome

Mucosa and periodontal tissues	Fragile mucosa that tears easily with ulcerations
	Sutures do not hold
	Fibrinoid deposits
	Absence of inferior labial and lingual frena
	Early onset generalized periodontitis that causes primary and permanent teeth mobility and premature loss
	Increased bleeding tendency
Teeth	Enamel hypoplasia
	Deep fissures and long cusps of premolars and molars
	Microdontia
	Dentin structural irregularities
	Short, malformed, dilacerated roots
	Pulpal calcifications and pulp stones
	Congenitally missing teeth
	Multiple supernumerary teeth
Tongue	Gorlin sign (tip of tongue touching tip of nose)
Palate	High vaulted palate
Temporomandibular joint	Laxity
	Pain
	Trismus
	Clicking or crepitus
	Locking

Data from De Coster PJ, Martens LC, De Paepe A. Oral health in prevalent types of Ehlers-Danlos syndromes. J Oral Pathol Med 2005;34(5):298–307; and Létourneau Y, Pérusse R, Buithieu H. Oral manifestations of Ehlers-Danlos syndrome. J Can Dent Assoc 2001;67(6):330–4.

Box 5
Preventive and management guidelines in all subtypes of EDS

- Protective pads and bandages are useful in preventing skin lacerations, bruises, and hematomas
- Dermal wounds should be closed without tension, preferably in two layers
- Deep stitches should be applied generously
- Cutaneous stitches should be left in place twice as long as usual
- Patients with pronounced bruising are advised to avoid contact sports and heavy exercise
- Supplementation of ascorbic acid can decrease bruising tendency
- A physiotherapeutic program is important in hypotonia and delayed motor development
- Anti-inflammatory drugs that interfere with platelets function and acetylsalicylic acid should be avoided in patients with pronounced bruising
- Antibiotic prophylaxis for bacterial endocarditis should be considered in patients with mitral valve prolapse and regurgitation
- Surgical interventions are generally discouraged and conservative therapy is recommended
- If surgery is unavoidable, manipulation of vascular and other tissues should be done with extreme care
- Emotional support and behavioral and psychological therapy can be useful

Data from Refs.[64–67]

Table 12
Dental considerations for the management of patients with Ehlers-Danlos syndrome

Procedure	Precaution/Consideration
General	Consider resting temporomandibular joint frequently during lengthy therapy Inferior alveolar nerve blocks should be given with great care to avoid causing hematoma
Surgery	Dental and maxillofacial surgery should be avoided if possible Test blood coagulation values before proceeding with surgery Check for mitral valve prolapse and consider prophylaxis antibiotic if indicated Prepare for risk of hemorrhage with perioperative hemorrhage control, such as desmopressin Careful flap manipulation Suture with less tension and large section of tissue Consider placing prefabricated acrylic plate over surgical site
Orthodontics	Increased risk for mucosal ulceration related to bracket position Increased risk for rapid migration and teeth mobility Consider longer period of retention
Endodontics	Check for pulp stones, pulpal calcifications, and abnormal root morphologies

Data from Abel MD, Carrasco LR. Ehlers-Danlos syndrome: classifications, oral manifestations, and dental considerations. Oral Surg Oral Med Oral Pathol Oral Radiol Endod 2006;102(5):582–90; and Létourneau Y, Pérusse R, Buithieu H. Oral manifestations of Ehlers-Danlos syndrome. J Can Dent Assoc 2001;67(6):330–4.

Table 13	
Clinical and radiographic features of Papillon-Lefevre syndrome	
System/Organ	**Clinical and Radiographic Features**
Skull	Calcified falx and choroid plexus in some cases
Skin	Palmoplantar erythema and hyperkeratosis
	Abscess formation caused by superimposed infections on defective skin
Jaw development	Retrognathic and hypoplastic maxilla
	Class III skeletal relationship
	Decreased lower facial height
Oral/Dental	Lucencies surrounding the roots of maxillar and mandibular teeth
	Alveolar bone resorption
	Hypermobility and exfoliation of teeth
	No signs of root resorption
	Tooth loss follows sequence of eruption
	Normal-appearing oral mucosa
	Pain during chewing
	Fetid mouth odor
	Retroclination of mandibular incisor to compensate for maxillary retrognathia
	Lip retrusion caused by jaw relationship

Data from Jose J, Bartlett K, Salgado C, et al. Papillon-Lefèvre syndrome: review of imaging findings and current literature. Foot Ankle Spec 2015;8(2):139–42.

- Careful manipulation of the neck to avoid atlantoaxial instability and spinal injury during intubation or surgical procedures.
- Careful management of the airway to avoid aspiration or obstruction.
- Careful examination of the oral tissue to detect any changes associated with leukemia.
- Encourage maintaining good oral hygiene with frequent dental visits at least every 6 months.
- Consider the use of chlohexidine mouthwash for the control of periodontal disease.
- Detection of erosions of the teeth can be attributed to gastric reflux or vomiting. Referral to a gastroenterologist and education of the family and caregivers minimizes dental destruction and dentinal hypersensitivity.
- Daily oral hygiene is an important strategy for prevention of pneumonia. Dental treatment should be delayed for patients with acute pneumonia.
- Bronchodilating inhalers should be readily available during the treatment of patients with bronchitis or asthma.
- For many patients, it is possible to carry out simple restorative treatment and preventive measures using behavioral management techniques, such as tell-show-do, positive reinforcement, modeling, distraction, and verbal and nonverbal communication.
- Keep appointments short and focus on a specific treatment for each consultation.
- The dentist's primary concern in using an antianxiety agent in individuals with hypothyroidism should be excessive central nervous system depression.
- In younger patients the use of space maintainers or referral to orthodontic and speech therapy is recommended if necessary.
- Replacement of missing teeth (anteriors) improves the speech quality.

Table 14
Medical conditions affecting patients with Down syndrome and effect on dental treatment

System	Characters	Effect on Dental Treatment
Cardiac	Congenital heart defects: atrioventricular septal defects, atrial septal defect, patent ductus arteriosus, ventricular septal defect, tetralogy of Fallot	Increased risk of infective endocarditis Antibiotic prophylaxis
Immune Hematologic	Impaired immunity Increased susceptibility to infections (skin, gastrointestinal, and respiratory systems) High risk of hepatitis B infection (risk factors: institutionalization and predisposition) Leukemia (acute lymphoblastic type)	Periodontitis Infection control Oral manifestations of leukemia
Skeletal	Atlantoaxial instability Short neck Rib anomalies	Careful manipulation of neck during surgery and intubation
Nervous	Delayed motor function Dementia/Alzheimer disease Epilepsy	Oral hygiene maintenance Avoid epilepsy triggers
Mental and behavior	Wide range of mental deficiency Delayed expressive language Natural spontaneity, genuine warmth, gentleness, patience, and tolerance Anxiety and stubbornness (in few patients)	Most can be easily treated in general setting Some require behavioral management, conscious sedation, or general anesthesia for dental treatment
Vision	Refractive errors: myopia, hyperopia, astigmatism, and cataracts	—
Auditory	Accumulation of fluid in the middle ear causes mild to moderate hearing loss Middle ear infections	Delayed speech
Endocrine	Hypothyroidism Diabetes mellitus	Increased susceptibility to periodontitis and oral infections
Gastroesophageal	Gastroesophageal reflux Vomiting	Teeth erosions
Respiratory	Abnormal airway anatomy: upper airway narrowing, congenital malformations of larynx, trachea, and bronchi	Risk of aspiration or obstruction

Data from Refs.[70–72]

- Patients should be evaluated for orthodontic and surgical correction of malocclusion.
- Prosthodontic appliances or implants may be considered depending on the individual patient.
- Hypocalcified teeth should be observed for early onset of decay.

> **Box 6**
> **Oral manifestations in patients with Down syndrome**
>
> Palate is reduced in length, height, and depth because of midface deficiency
>
> Hypotonia of oral musculature results in significant facial features including pulled down angle of the mouth and everted lower lip
>
> Mouth is open because of the underdevelopment of midface, relatively large tongue, and muscle hypotonia
>
> Mouth breathing, drooling, and angular cheilitis
>
> Chronic periodontitis caused by mouth breathing
>
> Bifid uvula
>
> Cleft lip and palate
>
> Enlarged tonsils and adenoid
>
> Thin oral mucosal lining because of the reduction of salivary flow that may result in xerostomia
>
> Scalloped or crenated tongue caused by the abnormal pressure of the tongue on the teeth
>
> Fissured tongue on the dorsal surface of the anterior two-thirds of the tongue, and can occur in combination with geographic tongue
>
> *Data from* Refs.[70,71,73]

- In cases of bruxism, active treatment is rarely commenced in preschool age child. For active treatment a "mouth guard" type appliance may be used. The nature of the appliance depends on individual needs.

Gorlin Syndrome (Nevoid Basal Cell Carcinoma Syndrome)

Gorlin syndrome, also called nevoid basal cell carcinoma syndrome or basal cell nevus syndrome, was first reported by Gorlin and Goltz in 1960.[75] It is an

> **Box 7**
> **Dental anomalies noted in Down syndrome**
>
> Microdontia in primary and secondary dentitions (35%–55%) that results in spacing
>
> Hypoplasia and hypocalcifications
>
> Congenitally missing teeth; the only teeth not missing are first molars
>
> Taurodontism with the mandibular second molar is the most frequently involved tooth in the dentition
>
> Low prevalence of dental caries
>
> Delayed eruption in timing and sequence of primary and permanent teeth
>
> Gingivitis and generalized periodontitis
>
> Malocclusion in primary and permanent dentitions
>
> Jaw relationship abnormalities include incisal class III relationships, anterior open bite, anterior and posterior crossbite
>
> Bruxism
>
> *Data from* Desai SS. Down syndrome: a review of the literature. Oral Surg Oral Med Oral Pathol Oral Radiol Endod 1997;84(3):279–85; and Shukla D, Bablani D, Chowdhry A, et al. Dentofacial and cranial changes in Down syndrome. Osong Public Health Res Perspect 2014;5(6):339–44.

autosomal-dominant neurocutaneous disease with a high level of penetrance and variable expressivity characterized by developmental defects including bifid ribs and palmar pits, and a predisposition to various tumors including basal cell carcinoma, medulloblastoma, ovarioma, cardiac fibroma, and keratocystic odontogenic tumor.[75,76] The gene responsible for Gorlin syndrome is the human homologue of the Drosophila patched gene, PTCH1.[75] Gorlin syndrome has been reported from all over the world with the estimated prevalence varies from 1 in 57,000 to 1 in 256,000, with a male-to-female ratio of 1:1.[75] Intellectual deficit is present in up to 5% of cases.[75] Diagnostic criteria of Gorlin syndrome are summarized in **Table 15**.

Clinical features of Gorlin syndrome

Developmental defects commonly seen in Gorlin syndrome include rib anomalies, falx calcifications, palmar and plantar pits, and tumorigenesis. These features are explained in **Tables 15–17**.[75–77]

Oral manifestation of Gorlin syndrome is keratocystic dontogenic tumor KCOT (formerly termed odontogenic keratocyst), which are benign cystic lesions, slowly progressive, locally destructive with high recurrence rate. KCOTs in nevoid basal cell carcinoma syndrome have a high potential for recurrence (60%) as compared with nonsyndromic KCOT (28%). Radiographic features and dental management are summarized in **Table 16**.[75–77]

Gardner Syndrome

Gardner syndrome, a variant of familial adenomatous polyposis, is a rare autosomal-dominant condition with complete penetrance and variable expressivity characterized by gastrointestinal polyps, multiple osteomas, and skin and soft tissue tumors including a characteristic retinal lesion.[78–80] Approximately 10% of familial adenomatous polyposis individuals are affected by Gardner syndrome. Gardner syndrome and familial adenomatous polyposis are caused by mutations in Adenomatous Polyposis

Table 15 Diagnostic criteria of Gorlin syndrome (nevoid basal cell carcinoma syndrome)	
Diagnosis of Gorlin Syndrome is Made in the Presence of Two Major or One Major and Two Minor Criteria	
Major criteria	Multiple (>2) basal cell carcinoma, or one in a patient younger than 20 y Odontogenic keratocysts of the jaws proved by histopathology Three or more palmar or plantar pits Bilamellar calcification of the falx cerebri Bifid, fused, or markedly splayed ribs First-degree relative with nevoid basal cell carcinoma syndrome
Minor criteria	Macrocephaly determined after adjustment for height Congenital malformations: cleft lip or palate, frontal bossing, "coarse face," moderate or severe hypertelorism Other skeletal abnormalities: Sprengel deformity, marked pectus deformity, marked syndactyly of the digits Radiologic abnormalities: bridging of the sella turcica, vertebral anomalies, such as hemivertebrae, fusion or elongation of the vertebral bodies, modelling defects of the hands and feet, or flame-shaped lucencies of the hands or feet Ovarian fibroma Medulloblastoma

Data from Refs.[75–77]

Table 16
Clinical features of Gorlin syndrome (nevoid basal cell carcinoma syndrome)

Clinical Characteristic	Clinical and Radiographic Features
Rib anomalies	Reported in 30%–60% of patients Bifid (40%), splayed, or fused
Falx calcification	Reported in 65% of patients Not detected in early childhood Aging gradually accelerates the calcium deposition on the falx cerebri and cerebelli
Palmar and plantar pits	Most characteristic findings of Gorlin syndrome Small multiple pits 2–3 mm in diameter and 1–3 mm in depth seen on the palms (77%) and soles (50%) The color of the base: red in white persons and black in Africans Prevalence: between 30% and 65% by the age of 10 y, 80% by the age of 15 y, and 85% of patients older than the age of 20 y
Macrocephaly	From the neonatal period Often associated with nonspecific cerebral ventricular dilatation proved on brain computed tomography or MRI Surgical ventricle–peritoneal shunt operation is subsequently performed

Data from Refs.[75–77]

Coli gene at 5q21.[78,80] Gardner syndrome affects 1 in 8300 individuals and 1 in 7500 births in the United States.[80]

Clinical presentation

The characteristic features of the syndrome are multiple adenomatous polyposis of the large intestine, multiple osteomas, dental abnormalities, and fibrous dysplasia of the skull.[79] These are summarized in **Table 18**.[78–80]

Osteomas

Presence of osteomas is required to make the diagnosis of Gardner syndrome. Osteomas are usually asymptomatic and are typically localized in the mandible, but can also appear in the skull and long bones.[79] Osteomas precede the clinical and radiographic evidence of colonic polyposis of Gardner syndrome; therefore, they may be sensitive markers for the disease.[80]

Skin tumors

The most common cutaneous finding in patients with Gardner syndrome is epidermoid cysts, which tend to be numerous and are present in the multiple forms in 50% to 65% of the patients.[80] Several factors differentiate cutaneous cysts associated with Gardner syndrome from ordinary cysts.[80] These lesions occur at an earlier age than ordinary cysts, which occur around puberty.[80] They also appear in less common locations, such as the face, the scalp, and the extremities.[80] Similar to epidermal inclusion cysts, the cysts in Gardner syndrome are usually asymptomatic; however, they may become purulent and/or inflamed, and they may rupture.[80] Other skin signs include presence of fibromas, lipomas, leiomyomas, neurofibromas, or pigmented skin lesions.[79,80]

Oral and dental manifestation

Dental anomalies are present in 30% to 75% of patients with Gardner syndrome, and may include impacted or unerupted teeth, hypodontia, abnormal tooth morphology,

Table 17
Tumorigenesis features in nevoid basal cell carcinoma syndrome

Tumor	Age of Onset (Mean)	Characteristics
Cardiac fibroma	0–1 mo	Stable and non–life threatening but occasionally causes fatal arrhythmia
Medulloblastoma	2–3 y	Relatively low prevalence (1%–4%) Desmoplastic subtype, which is relatively benign
Basal cell carcinoma	3–53 y (21.4 y)	Most characteristic tumor in Gorlin syndrome Rate increases with age (51.4% for patients >20 y and 71.7% for patients >40 y) Clinically they may vary from flesh-colored papules to ulcerating plaques[2] The most common locations are the face, the back, and the chest; the waist and extremities are rarely involved[2] Correlated with exposure to UV radiation[2,3] Importance of early diagnosis
Keratocystic dontogenic tumor (formerly termed odontogenic keratocyst)	6–12 y (15.5 y)	Benign cystic lesions Slowly progressive, locally destructive, with high recurrence rate KCOTs in nevoid basal cell carcinoma syndrome have a high potential for recurrence (60%) as compared with nonsyndromic KCOT (28%) Early treatment is crucial for adequate jaw function Most common site is mandibular molar ramus region Radiographic features include radiolucent lesions, unilocular/multilocular, with smooth/scalloped borders, associated with impacted/displaced teeth and tendency to grow along the internal aspect of the jaws causing minimal expansion On CT examination, KCOTs appear as minimally expansile benign lesions, with scalloped borders and high attenuation of contents, which do not enhance with contrast; the high attenuation is because of dense proteinacious material like keratin within the lesion On MRI, the contents of the lesion appear as low to intermediate signal intensity on T1 and high signal intensity on T2 images KCOTs are treated by marsupialization/enucleation/osseous resection en block with adjunctive therapies, such as aggressive curettage, cryotherapy, or application of Carnoy solution Regular follow-up every year for the first 5 y and thereafter every 2 y has been recommended
Ovarian fibroma	16–45 y (30.6 y)	Rarely noticed Often bilateral (75%), overlapping medially and calcified in the nodular subtype

Data from Refs.[75–77]

Table 18 Clinical and radiographic presentation of Gardner syndrome	
System/Organ	**Clinical and Radiographic Presentation**
Gastrointestinal	Multiple adenomatous polyposis of the large intestine Usually appear by the early to mid-teenage years By age 35, almost all with this disease have polyps
Cutaneous/skin	Epidermoid cysts: numerous and are present in multiple forms (in 50%–65% of the patients) Desmoid tumors Fibromas Lipomas Neurofibromas Atypical skin pigmentation
Dental	Impacted or unerupted teeth Hypodontia Abnormal tooth morphology Supernumerary teeth Hypercementosis Compound odontomas Dentigerous cysts Central or lobulated osteomas In the mandible

Data from Refs.[78–80]

supernumerary teeth, hypercementosis, compound odontomas, dentigerous cysts, fused molar roots, long and tapered molar roots, and multiple caries.[78] Osteomas occur in 68% to 82% and are generally located in the paranasal sinuses and mandible. They can also affect the skull and long bones. In the mandible, central or lobulated osteomas can be observed; central osteomas are characteristically near the roots of the teeth, and lobulated types arise from the cortex and most commonly at the mandibular angle.[78] Because the clinical and radiologic features in the maxillofacial region, dental practitioners and radiologists should be familiar with the manifestations of this syndrome (**Figs. 25** and **26**).[80]

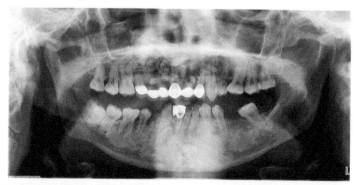

Fig. 25. CBCT panoramic reconstruction in a patient with Gardner syndrome: multiple impacted teeth and odontomas. (*Courtesy of* Dr Steven R. Singer, Rutgers School of Dental Medicine, Newark, NJ.)

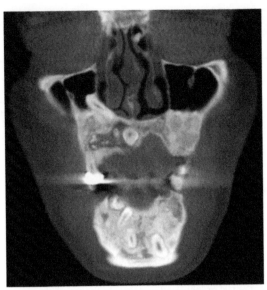

Fig. 26. Coronal CBCT view showing multiple impacted teeth in a patient with Gardner syndrome. (*Courtesy of* Dr Steven R. Singer, Rutgers School of Dental Medicine, Newark, NJ.)

Dental considerations

Often general dentists or orthodontists are the first health care professionals to suspect the diagnosis and refer to the oral and maxillofacial surgeon.[78] Dental professionals can play a significant role in early diagnosis, treatment of mandibular or other facial osteomas, and management of impacted or unerupted teeth and cysts of the jaws or face.[80]

REFERENCES

1. White SC, Pharoah MJ. Oral radiology: principles and interpretation. 7th edition. St Louis (MO): Mosby/Elsevier; 2014.
2. Ongole R, Praveen BN. Textbook of oral medicine, oral diagnosis and oral radiology. 2nd edition. New Delhi: Elsevier; 2013.
3. Rakhshan V. Congenitally missing teeth (hypodontia): a review of the literature concerning the etiology, prevalence, risk factors, patterns and treatment. Dent Res J (Isfahan) 2015;12(1):1–13.
4. Rakhshan V. Meta-analysis and systematic review of factors biasing the observed prevalence of congenitally missing teeth in permanent dentition excluding third molars. Prog Orthod 2013;1(14):33.
5. Wang XP, Fan J. Molecular genetics of supernumerary tooth formation. Genesis 2011;49(4):261–77.
6. Amarlal D, Muthu MS. Supernumerary teeth: review of literature and decision support system. Indian J Dent Res 2013;24(1):117–22.
7. Ata-Ali F, Ata-Ali J, Peñarrocha-Oltra D, et al. Prevalence, etiology, diagnosis, treatment and complications of supernumerary teeth. J Clin Exp Dent 2014; 6(4):e414–8.
8. Anthonappa RP, King NM, Rabie AB. Prevalence of supernumerary teeth based on panoramic radiographs revisited. Pediatr Dent 2013;35(3):257–61.
9. Tuna EB, Yildirim M, Seymen F, et al. Fused teeth: a review of the treatment options. J Dent Child (Chic) 2009;76(2):109–16.

10. Shah P, Chander JM, Noar J, et al. Management of "double teeth" in children and adolescents. Int J Paediatr Dent 2012;22(6):419–26.
11. de Siqueira VC, Braga TL, Martins MA, et al. Dental fusion and dens evaginatus in the permanent dentition: literature review and clinical case report with conservative treatment. J Dent Child (Chic) 2004;71(1):69–72.
12. Romito LM. Concrescence: report of a rare case. Oral Surg Oral Med Oral Pathol Oral Radiol Endod 2004;97(3):325–7.
13. Neves FS, Rovaris K, Oliveira ML, et al. Concrescence: assessment of case by periapical radiography, cone beam computed tomography and micro-computed tomography. N Y State Dent J 2014;80(3):21–3.
14. Jafarzadeh H, Azarpazhooh A, Mayhall JT. Taurodontism: a review of the condition and endodontic treatment challenges. Int Endod J 2008;41(5):375–88.
15. Bharti R, Chandra A, Tikku AP, et al. "Taurodontism" an endodontic challenge: a case report. J Oral Sci 2009;51(3):471–4.
16. Dineshshankar J, Sivakumar M, Balasubramanium AM, et al. Taurodontism. J Pharm Bioallied Sci 2014;6(Suppl 1):S13–5.
17. Alani A, Bishop K. Dens invaginatus. Part 1: classification, prevalence and aetiology. Int Endod J 2008;41(12):1123–36.
18. Mupparapu M, Singer SR. A review of dens invaginatus (dens in dente) in permanent and primary teeth: report of a case in a microdontic maxillary lateral incisor. Quintessence Int 2006;37(2):125–9.
19. Bishop K, Alani A. Dens invaginatus. Part 2: clinical, radiographic features and management options. Int Endod J 2008;41(12):1137–54.
20. Levitan ME, Himel VT. Dens evaginatus: literature review, pathophysiology, and comprehensive treatment regimen. J Endod 2006;32(1):1–9.
21. Rao YG, Guo LY, Tao HT. Multiple dens evaginatus of premolars and molars in Chinese dentition: a case report and literature review. Int J Oral Sci 2010;2(3):177–80.
22. Romeo U, Palaia G, Botti R, et al. Enamel pearls as a predisposing factor to localized periodontitis. Quintessence Int 2011;42(1):69–71.
23. Moskow BS, Canut PM. Studies on root enamel (2). Enamel pearls. A review of their morphology, localization, nomenclature, occurrence, classification, histogenesis and incidence. J Clin Periodontol 1990;17(5):275–81.
24. Nabavizadeh M, Sedigh Shamsi M, Moazami F, et al. Prevalence of root dilaceration in adult patients referred to Shiraz Dental School (2005-2010). J Dent (Shiraz) 2013;14(4):160–4.
25. Jafarzadeh H, Abbott PV. Dilaceration: review of an endodontic challenge. J Endod 2007;33(9):1025–30.
26. Markovic D, Petrovic B, Peric T. Case series: clinical findings and oral rehabilitation of patients with amelogenesis imperfecta. Eur Arch Paediatr Dent 2010;11(4):201–8.
27. Seow WK. Developmental defects of enamel and dentine: challenges for basic science research and clinical management. Aust Dent J 2014;59(Suppl 1):143–54.
28. Gadhia K, McDonald S, Arkutu N, et al. Amelogenesis imperfecta: an introduction. Br Dent J 2012;212(8):377–9.
29. Ng FK, Messer LB. Dental management of amelogenesis imperfecta patients: a primer on genotype-phenotype correlations. Pediatr Dent 2009;31(1):20–30.
30. Gauri Srindhi G, Raghavendra SS. Regional odontodysplasia: report of a rare case and review of literature. J Int Dent Med Res 2011;4(3):145–9.
31. Matsuyama J, Tanaka R, Iizawa F, et al. Clinical and radiographic findings and usefulness of computed tomographic assessment in two children with regional odontodysplasia. Case Rep Dent 2014;2014:764393.

32. Magalhães AC, Pessan JP, Cunha RF, et al. Regional odontodysplasia: case report. J Appl Oral Sci 2007;15(6):465–9.
33. Jainkittivong A, Langlais RP. Buccal and palatal exostoses: prevalence and concurrence with tori. Oral Surg Oral Med Oral Pathol Oral Radiol Endod 2000; 90(1):48–53.
34. Loukas M, Hulsberg P, Tubbs RS, et al. The tori of the mouth and ear: a review. Clin Anat 2013;26(8):953–60.
35. Sonnier KE, Horning GM, Cohen ME. Palatal tubercles, palatal tori, and mandibular tori: prevalence and anatomical features in a U.S. population. J Periodontol 1999;70(3):329–36.
36. Cohen MM Jr. Perspectives on craniofacial asymmetry. IV. Hemi-asymmetries. Int J Oral Maxillofac Surg 1995;24(2):134–41.
37. Jagtap RR, Deshpande GS. Gingival enlargement in partial hemifacial hyperplasia. J Indian Soc Periodontol 2014;18(6):772–5.
38. Bhuta BA, Yadav A, Desai RS, et al. Clinical and imaging findings of true hemifacial hyperplasia. Case Rep Dent 2013;2013:152528.
39. Deshingkar SA, Barpande SR, Bhavthankar JD. Congenital hemifacial hyperplasia. Contemp Clin Dent 2011;2(3):261–4.
40. El-Kehdy J, Abbas O, Rubeiz N. A review of Parry-Romberg syndrome. J Am Acad Dermatol 2012;67(4):769–84.
41. Al-Aizari NA, Azzeghaiby SN, Al-Shamiri HM, et al. Oral manifestations of Parry-Romberg syndrome: a review of literature. Avicenna J Med 2015;5(2):25–8.
42. Sarnat BG. Some selected dental and jaw aberrations. Ann Plast Surg 2006; 57(4):453–61.
43. Shankar U, Chandra S, Raju BH, et al. Condylar hyperplasia. J Contemp Dent Pract 2012;13(6):914–7.
44. Angiero F, Farronato G, Benedicenti S, et al. Mandibular condylar hyperplasia: clinical, histopathological, and treatment considerations. Cranio 2009;27(1):24–32.
45. Kaneyama K, Segami N, Hatta T. Congenital deformities and developmental abnormalities of the mandibular condyle in the temporomandibular joint. Congenit Anom (Kyoto) 2008;48(3):118–25.
46. Olate S, Netto HD, Rodriguez-Chessa J, et al. Mandible condylar hyperplasia: a review of diagnosis and treatment protocol. Int J Clin Exp Med 2013;6(9):727–37.
47. Zhong SC, Xu ZJ, Zhang ZG, et al. Bilateral coronoid hyperplasia (Jacob disease on right and elongation on left): report of a case and literature review. Oral Surg Oral Med Oral Pathol Oral Radiol Endod 2009;107(3):e64–7.
48. Totsuka Y, Fukuda H. Bilateral coronoid hyperplasia. Report of two cases and review of the literature. J Craniomaxillofac Surg 1991;19(4):172–7.
49. Pregarz M, Fugazzola C, Consolo U, et al. Computed tomography and magnetic resonance imaging in the management of coronoid process hyperplasia: review of five cases. Dentomaxillofac Radiol 1998;27(4):215–20.
50. Golan I, Baumert U, Hrala BP, et al. Dentomaxillofacial variability of cleidocranial dysplasia: clinicoradiological presentation and systematic review. Dentomaxillofac Radiol 2003;32(6):347–54.
51. Roberts T, Stephen L, Beighton P. Cleidocranial dysplasia: a review of the dental, historical, and practical implications with an overview of the South African experience. Oral Surg Oral Med Oral Pathol Oral Radiol 2013;115(1):46–55.
52. Rice DP. Craniofacial sutures. Development, disease and treatment. Preface Front Oral Biol 2008;12:xi.
53. Horbelt CV. Physical and oral characteristics of Crouzon syndrome, Apert syndrome, and Pierre Robin sequence. Gen Dent 2008;56(2):132–4.

54. Buchanan EP, Xue AS, Hollier LH Jr. Craniofacial syndromes. Plast Reconstr Surg 2014;134(1):128e–53e.
55. Kadakia S, Helman SN, Badhey AK, et al. Treacher collins syndrome: the genetics of a craniofacial disease. Int J Pediatr Otorhinolaryngol 2014;78(6): 893–8.
56. Posnick JC, Ruiz RL. Treacher Collins syndrome: current evaluation, treatment, and future directions. Cleft Palate Craniofac J 2000;37(5):434.
57. Magalhães MH, da Silveira CB, Moreira CR, et al. Clinical and imaging correlations of Treacher Collins syndrome: report of two cases. Oral Surg Oral Med Oral Pathol Oral Radiol Endod 2007;103(6):836–42.
58. Dixon J, Trainor P, Dixon MJ. Treacher collins syndrome. Orthod Craniofac Res 2007;10(2):88–95.
59. Monahan R, Seder K, Patel P, et al. Hemifacial microsomia. Etiology, diagnosis and treatment. J Am Dent Assoc 2001;132(10):1402–8.
60. Aydinbelge M, Gumus HO, Sekerci AE, et al. Implants in children with hypohidrotic ectodermal dysplasia: an alternative approach to esthetic management: case report and review of the literature. Pediatr Dent 2013;35(5):441–6.
61. Itthagarun A, King NM. Ectodermal dysplasia: a review and case report. Quintessence Int 1997;28(9):595–602.
62. Deshmukh S, Prashanth S. Ectodermal dysplasia: a genetic review. Int J Clin Pediatr Dent 2012;5(3):197–202.
63. Callewaert B, Malfait F, Loeys B, et al. Syndromes and Marfan syndrome. Best Pract Res Clin Rheumatol 2008;22:165–89.
64. Abel MD, Carrasco LR. Ehlers-Danlos syndrome: classifications, oral manifestations, and dental considerations. Oral Surg Oral Med Oral Pathol Oral Radiol Endod 2006;102(5):582–90.
65. Kaurani P, Marwah N, Kaurani M, et al. Ehlers danlos syndrome - a case report. J Clin Diagn Res 2014;8(3):256–8.
66. De Coster PJ, Martens LC, De Paepe A. Oral health in prevalent types of Ehlers-Danlos syndromes. J Oral Pathol Med 2005;34(5):298–307.
67. Létourneau Y, Pérusse R. Buithieu H.Oral manifestations of Ehlers-Danlos syndrome. J Can Dent Assoc 2001;67(6):330–4.
68. Fantasia JE. Syndromes with unusual dental findings or gingival components. Atlas Oral Maxillofac Surg Clin North Am 2014;22(2):211–9.
69. Dhanrajani PJ. Papillon-Lefevre syndrome: clinical presentation and a brief review. Oral Surg Oral Med Oral Pathol Oral Radiol Endod 2009;108(1):e1–7.
70. Desai SS. Down syndrome: a review of the literature. Oral Surg Oral Med Oral Pathol Oral Radiol Endod 1997;84(3):279–85.
71. Fiske J, Shafik HH. Down's syndrome and oral care. Dent Update 2001;28(3): 148–56.
72. Jose J, Bartlett K, Salgado C, et al. Papillon-Lefèvre syndrome: review of imaging findings and current literature. Foot Ankle Spec 2015;8(2):139–42.
73. Shukla D, Bablani D, Chowdhry A, et al. Dentofacial and cranial changes in down syndrome. Osong Public Health Res Perspect 2014;5(6):339–44.
74. Abanto J, Ciamponi AL, Francischini E, et al. Medical problems and oral care of patients with Down syndrome: a literature review. Spec Care Dentist 2011;31(6): 197–203.
75. Fujii K, Miyashita T. Gorlin syndrome (nevoid basal cell carcinoma syndrome): update and literature review. Pediatr Int 2014;56(5):667–74.
76. Lo Muzio L. Nevoid basal cell carcinoma syndrome (Gorlin syndrome). Orphanet J Rare Dis 2008;25(3):32.

77. Gupta SR, Jaetli V, Mohanty S, et al. Nevoid basal cell carcinoma syndrome in Indian patients: a clinical and radiological study of 6 cases and review of literature. Oral Surg Oral Med Oral Pathol Oral Radiol 2012;113(1):99–110.

78. Klein OD, Oberoi S, Huysseune A, et al. Developmental disorders of the dentition: an update. Am J Med Genet C Semin Med Genet 2013;163C(4):318–32.

79. Subasioglu A, Savas S, Kucukyilmaz E, et al. Genetic background of supernumerary teeth. Eur J Dent 2015;9(1):153–8.

80. Madani M, Madani F. Gardner's syndrome presenting with dental complaints. Arch Iran Med 2007;10(4):535–9.

Radiologic Assessment of the Periodontal Patient

Jonathan Korostoff, DMD, PhD*, Ali Aratsu, DMD, MS, Brian Kasten, DMD, Mel Mupparapu, DMD, MDS

KEYWORDS

- Periodontics • Radiology • Periapical • Bitewing
- Cone beam computed tomography

KEY POINTS

- A typical periodontal examination involves evaluation of soft and hard tissue parameters to gauge gingival inflammatory changes and quantify the extent of attachment loss.
- Conventional dental radiographs can be used to assess the presence of calculus and factors contributing to plaque accumulation, crestal bone heights, infrabony defects, furcation bone loss, and root anatomy.
- All of these factors must be taken into consideration to accurately establish a diagnosis, prognosis, and periodontal treatment plan.
- The advent of high-resolution cone beam computed tomography offers three-dimensional images that might overcome the limitations of two-dimensional images.

INTRODUCTION

A complete and thorough periodontal evaluation consists of both clinical and radiographic examinations. Owing to the nature of the periodontal diseases, an accurate assessment of the supporting bone and level of attachment are critical to make a proper diagnosis of periodontal health or disease. Clinical attachment level can and must be assessed through periodontal probing. However, bone levels and morphology can only be truly evaluated through radiographic examination. Although a radiographic series can only impart the current status of the patient's periodontal morphology, radiographs can serve as a reference point for both past and future radiographs to understand the progression of the disease. In this review, we discuss the use of conventional radiographic techniques as well as cone beam computed tomography (CBCT) for evaluating, diagnosing, and planning treatment for patients

Departments of Periodontics and Oral Medicine, University of Pennsylvania School of Dental Medicine, 240 South 40th Street, Philadelphia, PA 19104, USA
* Corresponding author. University of Pennsylvania School of Dental Medicine, Room NW3 Evans Building, 240 South 40th Street, Philadelphia, PA 19104-6030.
E-mail address: jkorosto@pobox.upenn.edu

Dent Clin N Am 60 (2016) 91–104
http://dx.doi.org/10.1016/j.cden.2015.08.003
0011-8532/16/$ – see front matter © 2016 Elsevier Inc. All rights reserved.

presenting for periodontal therapy. We focus first on conventional radiographic approaches as a group; CBCT imaging is discussed as a distinct entity in a separate section.

CONVENTIONAL RADIOGRAPHY IN PERIODONTICS

Although conventional radiographs are two-dimensional images of three-dimensional structures, they are an indispensable resource and an accurate assessment of a patient periodontal status cannot be made without them.

Film and Sensor Characteristics

Unlike the radiographs taken for caries detection, which require high-contrast images, the radiographs taken for periodontal evaluation and diagnosis require a long scale of contrast. Images with a longer scale of contrast show more shades of gray and allow the evaluator to see changes in bone quality and quantity more easily.[1] Digital sensors with high kilovoltage provide longer shades of gray (long-scale contrast). The recommended beam energy for periodontal evaluation is greater than 65 kVp.[1] With the use of digital radiography, the contrast can be changed after image acquisition via gamma enhancement, and can be optimized before interpretation for the needs of the clinician.

In periodontal radiographic interpretation, image geometry is of key importance. Images should be taken with the extension cone paralleling instruments that use a paralleling technique to reflect the true horizontal bone levels most accurately. The bisecting angle technique more likely leads to "foreshortening" or "elongation" of the teeth. Distortion and inaccurate assessment of the true horizontal bone height is a common problem when a bisecting angle technique is used.

Conventional Radiographic Options and Selection Criteria

Radiographs are a key compliment to the clinical examination of the patient, but should never be exposed without an appropriate and thorough clinical examination first to determine the type and number of images that are necessary for a particular patient. The periodontal examination requires both bitewing and periapical radiographs of all remaining teeth. If the patient has a full dentition, this requires either 18 or 20 images, depending on film or sensor sizes used. Some clinicians use a panoramic radiograph to gain a general scope of the patient's maxillofacial structures. Although intraoral images are typically the preferred method for bone level and morphology assessment, owing to the improved image quality, the panoramic image has been reported in the literature to be adequate. If a high-quality panoramic image is to be used, it should be supplemented with either horizontal or vertical bitewings of remaining posterior teeth for a more detailed investigation of interproximal bone.

The bitewing images can be taken in either a vertical or horizontal fashion. The bitewings taken for interproximal caries detection are typically of the horizontal nature because they include more tooth surfaces in each image (**Figs. 1** and **2**). These images are appropriate for patients with early or mild periodontal disease, in which the interproximal bone is visible in its entirety. When attachment loss has reached a moderate to severe level, as well as when vertical bony defects are suspected, the vertical bitewing is best used to visualize the interproximal bone. Selection of the appropriate type of bitewing can only be done through clinical examination, which is why the clinical examination should precede all radiographs.

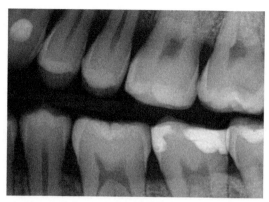

Fig. 1. A left premolar horizontal bitewing radiograph showing the contact points from distal of the canines to the distal of first molars. The alveolar crest can be evaluated effectively using the bitewings.

Interpretation and diagnosis

Interpretation of a dental radiograph should always be done by a trained dental professional. As discussed, radiographs are inherently tied to all aspects of dentistry. In the field of periodontology, periapical, bitewing, and panoramic radiographs all provide different types of information for diagnostic purposes. In this section, we limit our discussion to conventional radiographic techniques. A complete set of periapical and bitewing radiographs are usually the initial radiographs used for developing a periodontal diagnosis (**Fig. 3**). Periapical pathologies or any variation from normal bone tooth, or sinus appearance should be evaluated either via an intraoral or a panoramic radiograph (**Fig. 4**). The patient should be informed of any variation from normal, and an appropriate referral should be given to the patient for further consultation and treatment of nonperiodontal pathology.

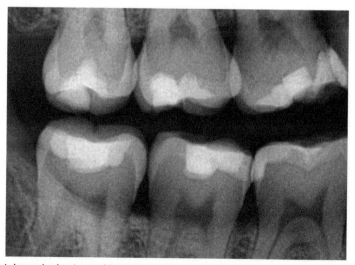

Fig. 2. A right molar horizontal bitewing radiograph showing the contact points of the first and second molars and the distal of the third molars.

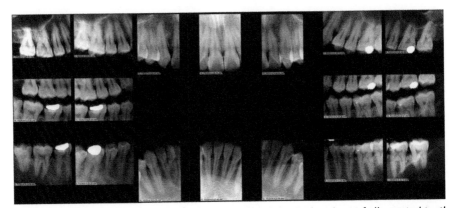

Fig. 3. Full mouth radiographic series demonstrating the apical regions of all erupted teeth and contact points of the posterior teeth.

Once nonperiodontal sources of pathology have been ruled out, the actual periodontal examination can begin. The radiographic evaluation of changes in alveolar bone usually begins with the interdental septum of bone. The most useful intraoral radiograph for this is the vertical bitewing, because it shows significantly more bone than a horizontal bitewing. A bitewing also offers the most perpendicular visualization of the dentition and adjacent supporting structures. This view decreases elongation of both the tooth and bone defects. Depending on the angulation of a periapical radiograph, furcation involvement or vertical bone defects may be completely hidden. These findings should still be confirmed clinically in either case. When examining the interdental septum, an imaginary line can be drawn from the cementoenamel junction of one tooth to that of the adjacent tooth. If this line is parallel to the crest of bone between the two teeth, then any bone loss would be considered horizontal in nature. If the lines are not parallel, then the bone loss is considered vertical in nature. Typically,

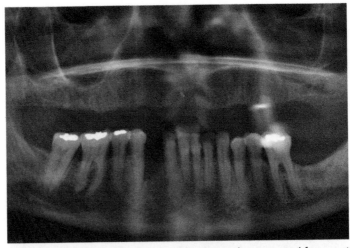

Fig. 4. A panoramic radiograph of a 69-year-old woman who presented for a routine dental examination. Note the area between the right mandibular lateral incisor and the first premolar with an infrabony defect and significant sclerosis.

the distance between the cementoenamel junction and alveolar crest is 2 mm and anything greater than this is indicative of crestal bone loss.[2]

After evaluation of the interdental septum is the examination of the lamina dura. The crest of bone normally presents a thin, radiopaque border that follows the outline of the root surface in a radiograph. This is known as the lamina dura, adjacent to the periodontal ligament (PDL). The ligament occupies the dark space seen between the lamina dura and the cementum of the root. A widened PDL space can be seen in a patient with a form of occlusal traumatism. Toward the apex of a tooth, a widened PDL space can also be seen when a periapical infection is present. A complete loss of the PDL space can sometimes signify an ankylosed tooth, which is an important consideration in an extraction or orthodontic case.

Because bitewings are two-dimensional radiographs, it is difficult to obtain an accurate depiction of the facial/buccal and lingual/palatal bone around a tooth. Frequently, a light pattern of bone superimposed on the tooth may reflect a circular or craterlike defect around a tooth. These craterlike defects must be confirmed by CBCT,[3] clinically, or as a last resort, surgically. Bitewing radiographs do provide reasonably good images of a furcation defect in the form of a radiolucent area between the roots of multirooted teeth. Such a finding suggests that bone no longer occupies 100% of a furcation between the roots of a tooth. Although a clinician cannot state accurately how significant the bone loss is in a furcation based on a bitewing, there are clues that can help with a diagnosis. If the furcation entrance looks slightly less radiopaque than the crest of bone on either side of a tooth, then there is likely a mild furcation involvement. A radiographic "black triangle" usually indicates a more significant involvement of the furcation. However, it should be stressed that a radiolucency in the furcation area does not always correlate with furcal bone loss, such that clinical evaluation of the involved tooth is necessary to confirm such bone loss. There are a number of different classification systems available for diagnosing the extent of furcation bone loss that are based on clinical criteria, but none that use radiographic findings.[4]

Because maxillary molars usually have roots organized in a tripod configuration, it becomes more difficult to assess furcation involvement in these areas, using a vertical bitewing. For example, furcal bone loss between the mesiobuccal and palatal roots may be superimposed by adequate bone on the buccal portion of the tooth. A cone beam computed tomography is more helpful in this regard.

The next factor to consider is that of root morphology and anatomy. Periapical radiographs give a good understanding of a tooth's root morphology. This information is helpful when analyzing a tooth for extraction purposes. A tooth with a dilacerated root may require a different approach to extraction relative to that of a tooth with a straight root. Moreover, the distance between the roots of adjacent teeth should be evaluated. Closely approximated roots generally have less interdental bone between them. Therefore, a small amount of bone loss may seem significant in these situations owing to lack of access for adequate oral hygiene.[4] Furthermore, in such instances it may very difficult to achieve ideal surgical outcomes when attempting to reduce infrabony defects or provide additional clinical crown length for restorative purposes.

As with furcal bone loss, the root morphology becomes slightly more difficult to assess on maxillary molars owing to the typical presence of three roots. The tripod configuration of the roots, interseptal bone, and occasional pneumatized maxillary sinus can make analysis of this area challenging. Careful consideration should be taken when evaluating images of this area. A clinical examination and radiographic examination may differ significantly (**Figs. 5** and **6**), but they should both be used to most accurately determine the diagnosis, prognosis, and appropriate treatment plan for a given

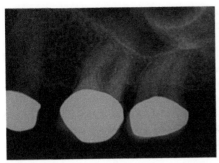
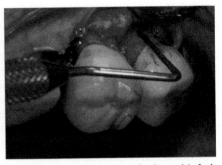

Fig. 5. Maxillary left molar periapical radiograph failing to demonstrate the buccal infrabony defect that was noted during surgical exposure of the site.

tooth.[5] When evaluating vertical bitewings, another important consideration is the presence of calculus. Calculus deposits typically present as radiopaque irregularities or spikes adjacent to or apical to the cementoenamel junction. Radiographically, the root surface is usually a smooth surface that is, contiguous with the crown of the tooth. However, calculus generally creates a radiographic disturbance in the smooth root form and appears as a radiopaque irregularity. When seen on a radiograph, a clinician can be certain that there is a significant amount of calculus present on that surface of the tooth. Crestal bone loss may or may not be present in areas where calculus is radiographically present (**Fig. 7**).

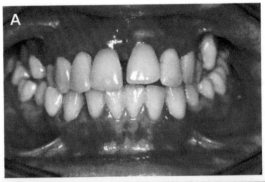

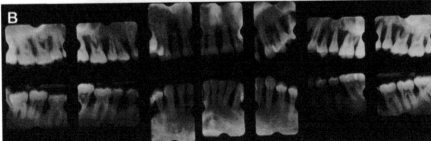

Fig. 6. (*A*) Intraoral photograph of a patient's teeth in occlusion showing only signs of marginal gingival inflammation and a malpositioned maxillary left central incisor. (*B*) Full mouth series of the same patient as in (*A*) showing the extensive generalized alveolar bone loss. The patient was 17 years old at the time of initial presentation and was subsequently diagnosed with generalized aggressive periodontitis.

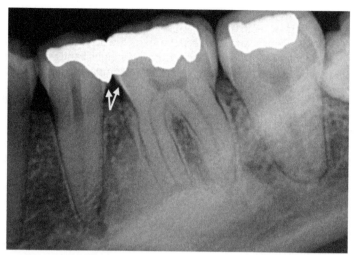

Fig. 7. A mandibular left molar periapical radiograph showing subgingival calculus (*arrows*) below the contact point between the second premolar and first molar.

Local tooth-related factors such as open margins or overhanging margins are also important to diagnose. These restorative features can sometimes trap plaque, and harbor periodontopathic bacteria. Again, bone loss may or may not be present in these cases, but these features should be addressed when treating the patient, owing to their ability to contribute to periodontal disease.[4]

CONE BEAM COMPUTED TOMOGRAPHY IN PERIODONTICS

A typical periodontal examination involves evaluation of a number of soft and hard tissue parameters that enable the clinician to gauge gingival inflammatory changes and quantify the extent of attachment loss. Conventional dental radiographs (periapical, bitewing, and panoramic) are vital components of this process. However, the two-dimensional nature of these images often limits their utility in certain aspects of a periodontal assessment, including the measurement of crestal bone heights, mapping of infrabony defect morphology, and appraisal of furcation involvement. This is owing the superimposition of adjacent anatomic structures over one another, magnification, and distortion. The advent of high-resolution CBCT now offers clinicians three-dimensional images that might overcome the limitations of two-dimensional images. In this section, we review the current literature regarding the use of CBCT as an adjunct to other techniques commonly used to diagnose periodontal disease. We conclude with a discussion of the benefits and pitfalls of this technology relative to conventional radiographs.

A number of studies have been done to determine whether CBCT provides additional information when used to evaluate alveolar bone loss relative to that obtained from periapical radiographs. These studies have been conducted on cadavers, dried skulls, models, and actual patient images. Considering the research done on patient images, de Faria Vasconcelos and colleagues[6] found the two to be equivalent when used to categorize the pattern of crestal bone loss (horizontal vs vertical). In the same study, it was reported that periapical radiographs and CBCT yielded statistically similar measurements of bone defect height and width. CBCT does have a clear advantage over conventional radiographs in that it provides cross-sectional views that allow clinicians to evaluate the pattern of bone loss on the buccal/facial and palatal/lingual aspects of teeth.[6,7]

Owing to the three-dimensional nature of the images provided by CBCT, it would be reasonable to speculate that this technique provides significantly more information regarding the morphology of infrabony defects when compared with periapical radiographs. This assumption has been verified in studies conducted on pig mandibles, human mandibles, dried human skulls, and actual patient images. As stated, the width (mesiodistal) and height (apicocoronal) dimensions of infrabony defects can be measured adequately with periapical radiographs. CBCT images provide additional information, including the buccopalatal/buccolingual dimensions of defects, the number of bony walls present at each level of a defect, and detection of the presence of dehiscences and/or fenestrations.[7–9] Taken together, such diagnostic information can be used for the purpose of more effectively providing a periodontal prognosis for a tooth as well as in determining the modality of surgical therapy (ie, respective vs regenerative therapy).

Another potential periodontal application of CBCT that has garnered research interest is the evaluation of furcations and interradicular bone. Periapical radiographs can show furcal bone loss, but provide limited information regarding the extent of the lesion (**Fig. 8**). High-resolution, selected field of view CBCT images not only demonstrate the presence of such defects, but also allow one to more accurately evaluate the number of roots involved as well as the shape and dimensions of the defects. This advantage has been confirmed in both in vitro experiments as well as in clinical practice. In a series of studies, Walter and colleagues[10,11] compared clinical, conventional intraoral radiographic, intraoperative, and CBCT techniques for assessing and classifying the extent of furcation involvement of maxillary molars in a cohort of patients. Comparisons were made considering the intraoperative measurements as the "gold standard." The authors found only a moderate level of agreement ($\kappa = 0.518$) between estimates of furcation involvement based on clinical versus CBCT evaluation. In contrast, there was a high level of agreement ($\kappa = 0.926$) between the intraoperative and CBCT assessments of furcation involvement. Furthermore, they reported significant discrepancies when the therapeutic approach was based on the clinical assessment as opposed to CBCT.[10] More recently, Qiao and colleagues[12] reported similar findings.

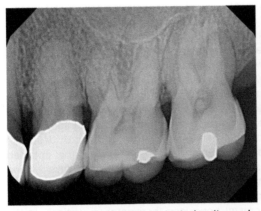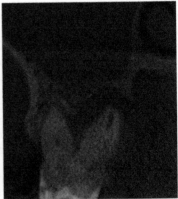

Fig. 8. A maxillary left molar periapical radiograph and the corresponding cone beam CT orthogonal section showing the limitation of two-dimensional imaging for demonstration of furcal defects. (*Courtesy of* David R. Silver, DMD, University of Pennsylvania School of Dental Medicine, Philadelphia, PA.)

These studies suggest that CBCT has significant potential for providing a more accurate assessment of furcation involvement compared with traditional clinical and radiographic criteria.

Currently, CBCT imaging is not used widely to diagnose periodontal disease. However, recent research suggests that the technology provides information that cannot be attained otherwise that could enable clinicians to better assess the extent of a patient's periodontal breakdown. In particular is the potential utility of CBCT images to assess infrabony defects and furcation involvement. With this capability, we may be more effective in developing a prognosis for a tooth, determining whether or not a tooth can be treated, and choosing the appropriate form of therapy. This being stated, additional research is needed to confirm and extend our current knowledge in well-designed clinical studies. There are also limitations to using CBCT on an everyday basis as an adjunct for periodontal evaluation. These cautions include but are not limited to masking of structures by scattering owing to the presence of metallic materials in a patient's mouth, the expense of CBCT scanners and the relatively high dose of radiation compared with that associated with conventional intraoral radiographs.[13] With the rapidly advancing technology and continuing clinical research, it is likely that these obstacles will be overcome such that CBCT become a component of the armamentarium used for periodontal evaluation, diagnosis and treatment planning.

RADIOGRAPHIC EVALUATION OF THE IMPLANT PATIENT

The treatment planning and placement of dental implants has become a routine component of periodontal practice. The ideal outcome is one in which[1] an implant maintains long-term osseointegration in the absence of inflammatory changes within the adjacent soft tissues,[2] supports a restoration without prosthetic complications such as abutment screw loosening or fractures among others, and[3] addresses the patient's functional, comfort, and esthetic needs. To achieve this, it is imperative that potential implant patients be evaluated carefully to develop the appropriate diagnosis and a team-oriented approach to treatment planning. Thus, the restorative dentist and surgeon must appraise the patient from the dental, esthetic, and radiographic perspectives. From a surgical standpoint, it is no longer acceptable to place an implant in the site of maximum volume. Owing to advances in bone regeneration technology, the implant should be located in the ideal position that allows the restorative dentist to deliver a functional, comfortable, and esthetic restoration.

In the course of evaluating the implant patient, the surgeon must determine the location, volume, and quality of bone available for implant placement in the context of the desired restorative outcome. To avoid surgical complications, it is also necessary to know the proximity of potential implant sites to vital structures such as adjacent teeth, the maxillary sinus, and inferior alveolar nerve canal. After a review of the medical, dental, and social histories, the patient is assessed clinically and via conventional radiographic approaches, including both periapical and panoramic images. The clinical and radiographic examinations provide the surgeon with an estimate of bone volume, bone quality, and location of relevant anatomic structures. However, this information can be extremely misleading. As shown in **Fig. 9**, two-dimensional radiographic evaluation alone of a patient who underwent replacement of the maxillary central incisor with an implant-supported crown could lead a clinician to believe that ample bone was present for the implant in both vertical and horizontal dimensions. The CBCT image of the same site clearly shows the absence of adequate buccal

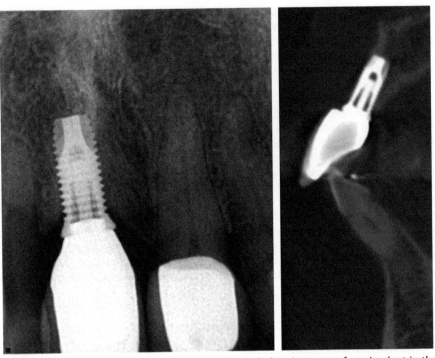

Fig. 9. A maxillary central incisor periapical radiograph showing a root form implant in the region of the right central incisor. Cone beam CT orthogonal reconstruction shows the absence of alveolar bone adjacent to the implant.

cortical bone. The information provided by the CBCT scan clearly demonstrated the horizontal osseous deficiency.

Relative to the clinical examination, conventional radiographs can be used for estimating the vertical dimension of available bone and proximity of potential implant sites to vital structures. It is critical that the limitations of these types of images be recognized. Foremost is the failure of periapical and panoramic radiographs to provide any information about the horizontal dimension of alveolar bone or the location of the residual ridge crest with respect to the opposing dentition. Owing to their inherent tendency to magnify structures, panoramic radiographs are also likely to lead to overestimates of ridge height while periapical images can overestimate or underestimate this measurement if not angulated properly.[14–16] Thus, in an overwhelming number of situations, even for experienced surgeons, it is recommended that CBCT imaging be used when evaluating an implant patient.

Current CBCT volumes provide a plethora of information that is not available with two-dimensional imaging. Furthermore, the technology has advanced to the point that CBCT scans can be done relatively inexpensively and at a radiation dose that in many instances is comparable with that of a panoramic radiograph when a limited volume is selected.[17,18] This topic is covered in great detail in a number of recent publications; we summarize herein what CBCT images provide in the context of evaluating and treatment planning an implant patient.[17,18] The three-dimensional images generated in CBCT scans allow clinicians to make specific measurements of the residual alveolar bone in a potential implant site in both the vertical and horizontal dimensions. A radiographic guide is used for this purpose (**Fig. 10**). The images are also extremely

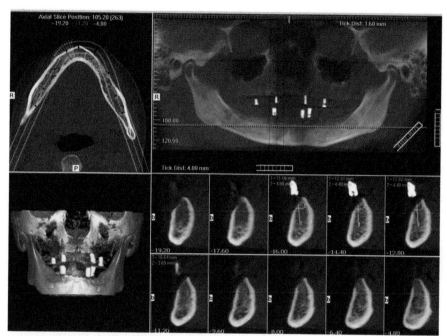

Fig. 10. Cone beam CT panoramic reconstruction and the cross-sectional views of the mandibular right canine–premolar region showing the available bone in the vicinity of a marker embedded in a mandibular radiographic guide. Similar reconstructions can be viewed for evaluation of other potential implant sites in the mandible and maxilla.

accurate in demonstrating the location of normal anatomic structures (ie, teeth, maxillary sinus, inferior alveolar nerve canal), alveolar deformities (ie, fenestrations and dehiscences), root resorption from erupting teeth (**Fig. 11**), and, equally important, pathologic abnormalities (**Fig. 12**).

With such information at hand, the feasibility of placing implants in their most desirable position can be accurately assessed while also determining the need for bone augmentation procedures before or at the time of fixture placement. For more complicated situations necessitating extremely precise positioning of implants, CBCT imaging can be used in conjunction with readily available software

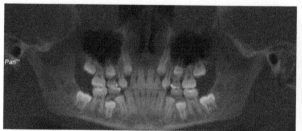
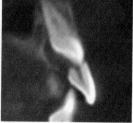

Fig. 11. Panoramic reconstruction from cone beam CT of an orthodontic patient who presented for evaluation of the maxillary lateral incisors. A cross-sectional reconstruction from the cone beam CT volume shows the resorption of the left lateral incisor resulting from the proximity of the erupting canine.

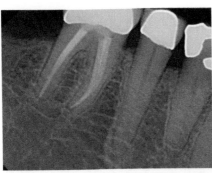
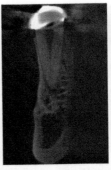
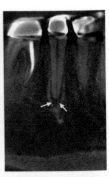

Fig. 12. Right mandibular second premolar periapical radiograph of a patient presenting with symptoms suggestive of endodontic origin that fails to demonstrate radiographic signs of apical pathoses. Cone beam CT cross-sectional and cropped panoramic reconstructions of the same tooth show definitive changes at the apical changes (*arrows*) that led to referral of the patient to an endodontist for root canal therapy.

to produce computer-generated surgical guides. Another aspect of implant dentistry in which CBCT imaging is proving invaluable to periodontists is in the diagnosis and treatment of periimplantitis. This term describes a relatively common group of clinical entities that manifest themselves as inflammatory-mediated bone resorption around dental implants. As with natural teeth, CBCT images provide views of the bone defects adjacent to implants that cannot be seen on conventional radiographs enabling clinicians to more effectively decide on a course of treatment ranging from exploration to attempting to regenerate the resorbed bone (**Figs. 13 and 14**). Taken together, the information provided by CBCT imaging is the gold standard by which other radiologic approaches to evaluating implant patients should be judged.

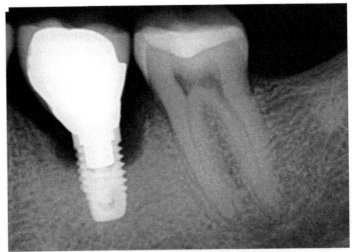

Fig. 13. Mandibular left molar periapical radiograph showing the restored root form implant in place of the first molar. The increasing size of the radiolucent crater and the clinical evaluation led to the diagnosis of periimplantitis.

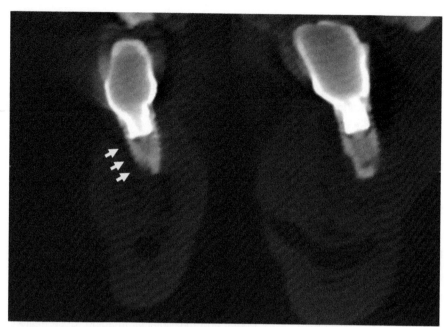

Fig. 14. Cone beam CT coronal and sagittal views of the same patient in **Fig. 13** with further evidence of periimplantitis. Note the absence of bone on the lingual aspect of the implant (*arrows*) and the presence of large lytic areas on the mesial and distal aspects of the fixture. These are radiographic findings consistent with a diagnosis of periimplantitis.

REFERENCES

1. Langland OE, Langlais RP, Preece JW. Principles of dental imaging. 2nd edition. Philadelphia, PA: Lippincott Williams & Wilkins; 2002. p. 57.
2. Koenig LJ, editor. Diagnostic imaging: oral and maxillofacial. 1st edition. Salt Lake City, UT: Amirsys, Inc; 2012. p. II-1–52.
3. du Bois AH, Kardachi B, Bartold P. Is there a role for the use of volumetric cone beam computed tomography in periodontics? Aust Dent J 2012;57:103–8.
4. Atchison KA, White SC, Flack VF, et al. Efficacy of the FDA selection criteria for radiographic assessment of the periodontium. J Dent Res 1995;74:1424–32.
5. Jeffcoat MK, Wang I-C, Reddy MS. Radiographic diagnosis in periodontics. Periodontol 2000 1995;7:54–68.
6. de Faria Vasconcelos K, Evangelista KM, Rodrigues CD, et al. Detection of periodontal bone loss using cone beam CT and intraoral radiography. Dentomaxillofac Radiol 2012;41:64–9.
7. Songa VM, Jampani ND, Babu V, et al. Accuracy of cone beam computed tomography in diagnosis and treatment planning of periodontal bone defects: a case report. J Clin Diagn Res 2014;8(12):ZD23–5.
8. Braun X, Ritter L, Jervøe-Storm PM, et al. Diagnostic accuracy of CBCT for periodontal lesions. Clin Oral Investig 2014;18(4):1229–36.
9. Leung CC, Palomo L, Griffith R, et al. Accuracy a reliability of cone-beam computed tomography for measuring alveolar bone height and detecting bony dehiscences and fenestrations. Am J Orthod Dentofacial Orthop 2010;137:S109–19.

10. Walter C, Kaner D, Berndt DC, et al. Three-dimensional imaging as a pre-operative tool in decision making for furcation surgery. J Clin Periodontol 2009; 26:250–7.

11. Walter C, Weiger R, Zitzmann NU. Accuracy of three-dimensional imaging in assessing maxillary molar furcation involvement. J Clin Periodontol 2010;7:436–41.

12. Qiao J, Wang S, Duan J, et al. The accuracy of cone-beam computed tomography in assessing maxillary molar furcation involvement. J Clin Periodontol 2014; 41(3):835–43.

13. Acar B, Kamburoğlu K. Use of cone beam computed tomography in periodontology. World J Radiol 2014;6(5):139–47.

14. Fortin T, Alik M, Isidori M, et al. Panoramic images versus three-dimensional planning software for oral implant planning in atrophied posterior maxillary: a clinical radiological study. Clin Implant Dent Relat Res 2013;15(2):198–204.

15. Guerroro ME, Noriega J, Castro C, et al. Does cone beam CT alter treatment plans? comparison of preoperative implant planning using panoramic versus cone-beam CT images. Imaging Sci Dent 2014;44(2):121–8.

16. Guerroro ME, Noriega J, Jacobs R. Preoperative implant planning considering alveolar bone grafting needs and complication prediction using panoramic versus CBCT images. Imaging Sci Dent 2014;44(3):213–20.

17. Pauwels R, Beinsberger J, Collaert B, et al. Effective dose range for dental cone beam computed tomography scanners. Eur J Radiol 2012;81:267–71.

18. Pauwels R. Cone beam CT for dental and maxillofacial Imaging: dose matters. Radiat Prot Dosimetery 2015;165(1–4):156–61.

Temporomandibular Joint Disorders and Orofacial Pain

Mansur Ahmad, BDS, PhD*, Eric L. Schiffman, DDS, MS

KEYWORDS

- TMJ • Degenerative joint disease • Orofacial pain • DC/TMD
- Synovial chondromatosis • Condylar fracture • Condylar hyperplasia and hypoplasia
- Diagnostic criteria

KEY POINTS

- Temporomandibular disorder is the second most common chronic musculoskeletal condition after chronic low back pain. As pain-related TMD can affect an individual's daily activities, psychosocial functioning, and quality of life, it is important to accurately diagnose these complex musculoskeletal disorders to provide the best clinical care.
- The new dual-axis diagnostic criteria for TMD offers an evidence-based assessment protocol for the clinician to use when screening patients for temporomandibular joint (TMJ) intra-articular disorders, but imaging is typically needed for a definite diagnosis.
- Both clinical history and examination, augmented as indicated with imaging, are needed to render proper TMJ intra-articular diagnoses. As several imaging modalities recommended in this article use ionizing radiation, careful clinical assessment with due consideration of the benefit to the patient must be carried out before ordering any imaging.

The temporomandibular joints (TMJs) play crucial roles in mastication and jaw mobility, and in verbal and emotional expression. Temporomandibular disorders (TMDs) include several disorders that can lead to orofacial pain symptoms. **Box 1** presents a TMD taxonomic classification adopted from a publication by a panel of experts developing the diagnostic criteria for TMD (DC/TMD) for the most common TMDs,[1] and the expanded TMD taxonomy for the more uncommon TMDs.[2] It has been reported that about 5% to 12% of the United States population is affected by TMD, and the annual cost of managing TMD, excluding cost related to imaging, is about $4 billion.[1] Plesh and colleagues[3] reported that in the 2000 to 2005 US National Health Interview Survey (NHIS) that included a total of 189,977 people, 4.6% (n = 8964) people had experienced temporomandibular joint and muscle disorder (TMJD).

University of Minnesota School of Dentistry, 515 Delaware Street Southeast, Minneapolis, MN 55455, USA
* Corresponding author. Diagnostic and Biological Sciences, University of Minnesota School of Dentistry, 7-536 Moos Tower, 515 Delaware Street Southeast, Minneapolis, MN 55455.
E-mail address: ahmad005@umn.edu

Dent Clin N Am 60 (2016) 105–124
http://dx.doi.org/10.1016/j.cden.2015.08.004
0011-8532/16/$ – see front matter © 2016 Elsevier Inc. All rights reserved.

dental.theclinics.com

Box 1
Taxonomy of temporomandibular joint disorders

I. Temporomandibular disorders
  a. Joint pain
  b. Joint disorders

    i. Disc disorders

    ii. Hypomobility disorders other than disc disorders

    iii. Hypermobility disorders
  c. Joint diseases

    i. Degenerative joint disease

    ii. Systemic arthritides

    iii. Condylysis/idiopathic condylar resorption

    iv. Osteochondritis dissecans

    v. Osteonecrosis

    vi. Neoplasm

    vii. Synovial chondromatosis
  d. Fractures
  e. Congenital/developmental disorders

II. Masticatory muscle disorders
  a. Muscle pain

    i. Myalgia

    ii. Tendonitis

    iii. Myositis

    iv. Spasm
  b. Contracture
  c. Hypertrophy
  d. Neoplasm
  e. Movement disorders
  f. Masticatory muscle pain attributed to systemic/central pain disorders

III. Headache
  a. Headache attributed to TMD

IV. Associated structures
  a. Coronoid hyperplasia

Progress in cross-sectional imaging using computed tomography (CT), MRI, and cone-beam CT (CBCT) has allowed better evaluation of the TMJ. Traditionally TMJ radiographic examinations included 2-dimensional images, such as transcranial, transmaxillary, and transpharyngeal projections, and submentovertex, lateral, and posteroanterior cephalometric radiographs.[4] Conventional and panoramic tomography has also been used in TMD diagnosis but has limited use in assessing the TMJs.[5]

The following sections provide a brief overview of the most common TMJ-related disorders and most appropriate imaging techniques. The latest recommendation from the panel of experts who developed the DC/TMD concluded that imaging should not be obtained routinely, but should be based on the clinical needs of the patient.[1]

DISC DISPLACEMENT

Disc displacement of the TMJ is a condition whereby the articular disc is displaced from its normal functional relationship with the condylar head and the articular fossa of the temporal bone (**Fig. 1**). Disc displacement is considered to have 4 clinical stages.[6]

- Stage I (disc displacement with reduction): the articular disc is displaced in closed-mouth position, and reduces to normal relationship, that is, the central narrow zone of the disc is in contact with the condylar head and articular eminence, in open-mouth position
- Stage II (disc displacement with reduction with intermittent locking): the disc is displaced in closed-mouth position, and intermittently locks in open-mouth position
- Stage III (disc displacement without reduction): the disc is displaced in closed-mouth position, and does not reduce to normal contact in open-mouth position (also referred to as closed lock)
- Stage IV (disc displacement without reduction): the disc is displaced and does not reduce, with perforation of the disc or posterior attachment tissues.

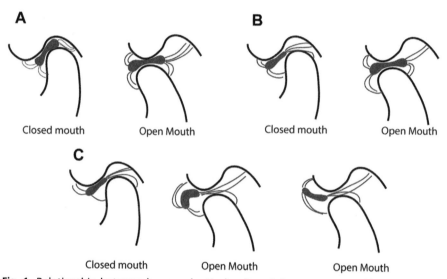

Fig. 1. Relationship between bone and articular disc of the temporomandibular joint. (*A*) Normal disc location in closed- and open-mouth position. In the closed-mouth position, the posterior band of the articular disc is located between 11:30 and 12:30 of a clock face. The central narrow zone of the disc is in contact with the condylar surface and the articular fossa. In the open-mouth position, the central narrow zone of the disc remains in contact with the condylar head and the articular eminence. (*B*) Disc displacement with reduction. In the closed-mouth position, the posterior band of the articular disc is displaced anterior to 11:30. The central narrow zone of the disc is not in contact with the condyle or the articular fossa. In the open-mouth position, the central narrow zone of the disc is in contact with the condylar head and articular eminence. (*C*) Disc displacement without reduction. In the closed-mouth position, the posterior band of the articular disc is displaced anterior to 11:30. The central narrow zone of the disc is not in contact with the condyle or the articular fossa. In the open-mouth position, the disc is anteriorly displaced, and may assume a normal biconcave shape or become deformed.

A commonly used classification of TMJ disc displacement, referred to as internal derangement, was described by Wilkes.[7] This classification (**Table 1**) described clinical and radiographic findings, the latter being based on MRI and tomography.

Individuals with disc displacement can be asymptomatic.[8] Persons who have disc displacement with reduction may have a normal range of jaw movement or limitations because of pain. Clinical examination may reveal joint sounds (eg, clicking and popping) during jaw movements. Individuals with disc displacement without reduction with limited opening may have deviation during opening toward the involved joint, and limited contralateral movements accompanied by pain and functional limitations, including compromised ability to eat.

Imaging

MRI of the TMJ in both closed and open positions is necessary for diagnosing stages of disc displacement (**Fig. 2**). Other radiographic examinations, such as panoramic radiography or CT, are not useful in determining the location of the disc. In some individuals with a history of trauma, fluid effusion may be present. Effusion can be identified with T2-weighted MRI, whereby effusion has high signal intensity (see **Fig. 2E2**, **Table 2**). The authors have updated the previous diagnostic criteria for disc displacement developed by their team (see **Table 2**).[5]

INFLAMMATORY DISTURBANCES OF THE TEMPOROMANDIBULAR JOINT

Arthralgia refers to joint pain, common causes of which include mechanical, metabolic, infectious, neuropathic, or inflammatory factors. When inflammation is present, this is referred to as arthritis,[2] one of the most prevalent chronic diseases. The TMJ may be affected by any form of arthritis. Tanaka and colleagues[9] classified arthritis as low-inflammatory or high-inflammatory disorder. Low-inflammatory arthritic disorders include degenerative joint disease or osteoarthritis, and posttraumatic arthritis. High-inflammatory arthritic disorders include infectious arthritis, adult and juvenile rheumatic arthritic conditions, and metabolic arthritic conditions, for example, gouty arthritis, psoriatic arthritis, lupus erythematosus, ankylosis spondylitis, Reiter syndrome, and arthritis associated with ulcerative colitis.

Table 1 Wilkes classification of disc displacement and degenerative joint disease	
Early stage (stage I)	Slight forward displacement and good anatomic contour of the disc. No osseous changes
Early/intermediate stage (stage II)	Slight forward displacement, and slight thickening of posterior edge or beginning anatomic deformity of disc. No osseous changes
Intermediate stage (stage III)	Anterior displacement with significant anatomic deformity/prolapse of disc (moderate to marked thickening of posterior edge). No osseous changes
Intermediate/late stage (stage IV)	Increase in severity over intermediate stage. Early to moderate degenerative osseous changes
Late stage (stage V)	Anterior disc displacement, nonreducing with perforation, gross anatomic deformity of the disc and hard tissues. Severe degenerative osseous changes

From Wilkes CH. Internal derangements of the temporomandibular joint. Pathological variations. Arch Otolaryngol Head Neck Surg 1989;115(4):470; with permission.

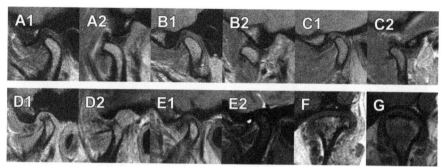

Fig. 2. MRI of the temporomandibular joints. *A1* and *A2* are from the same patient, in closed (*A1*) and open (*A2*) mouth position, showing normal disc relationship with the condylar head and articular fossa/eminence. *B1* and *B2* are from the same patient, in closed (*B1*) and open (*B2*) mouth position, showing anteriorly displaced intermediate zone of the disc (*B1*) and normal disc relationship with condylar head and articular eminence (*B2*). *C1* and *C2* are from the same patient, in closed (*C1*) and open (*C2*) mouth position, showing disc displacement with reduction. *D1* and *D2* are from the same patient, in closed (*D1*) and open (*D2*) mouth position, showing disc displacement without reduction. *E1* and *E2* are from the same patient in closed-mouth position. *E2*, which is a T2-weighted image, shows presence of effusion as a region of bright intensity. (*F, G*) Axially corrected coronal views from different patients, of (*F*) normal disc position and (*G*) laterally displaced disc. All images are proton density except *E2*.

DEGENERATIVE JOINT DISEASE

The terms degenerative joint disease (DJD), osteoarthritis, and osteoarthrosis are often used interchangeably.[1,5,9,10] Peck and colleagues[2] suggested that DJD be subdivided into osteoarthritis and osteoarthrosis, with both having the same diagnostic criteria but with the added feature of osteoarthritis denoting individuals with joint pain, whereas individuals with osteoarthrosis have DJD but no joint pain. Although its etiology is largely unknown, DJD is a disease often associated with trauma and the aging process. The joints first involved are those that bear the weight of the body and thus are subjected to continued stress and strain: the joints of the knees, hips, and spine. In the case of TMJs, primary DJD is by definition idiopathic. Secondary DJD is assumed to typically occur after the disc is displaced and bony contact exists between the condyle and articular fossa. However, there are reports that DJD can precede disc displacement. Clinical signs and symptoms of DJD are often remarkably absent even in the face of severe histologic or radiographic joint changes (i.e., osteoarthrosis).

RADIOGRAPHIC DIAGNOSTIC CRITERIA

DJD is diagnosed radiographically, as the clinical signs and symptoms have poor validity.[1] In an in-depth review, Larheim and colleagues[10] concluded that CBCT and CT are the reliable examinations to diagnose degenerative changes, and the diagnostic accuracy of CBCT for DJD is similar to that of CT. MRI and panoramic radiographs have limited value in diagnosing early degenerative changes.[5,11]

Three cardinal radiographic features that lead to a diagnosis of DJD are osteophyte, surface erosion, and subcortical pseudocyst.[5] These features are shown in **Fig. 3** and are defined as follows:

- An osteophyte is a marginal hypertrophy with sclerotic borders and exophytic angular formation of osseous tissue arising from the surface.

Table 2
Image analysis criteria for disc position based on MRI

Image Type	Mouth Position	Diagnosis	Posterior Band of the Disc	Intermediate Zone of the Disc
T1 or proton-density MRI, corrected sagittal view through the long axis of the condylar head	Closed mouth	Normal disc position	Relative to the superior aspect of the condyle, the border between the low signal of the disc and the high signal of the retrodiscal tissue is located between the 11:30 and 12:30 clock positions	Located between the anterior-superior aspect of the condyle and the posterior-inferior aspect of the articular eminence
		Indeterminant disc position	Relative to the superior aspect of the condyle, the low signal of the disc and the high signal of the retrodiscal tissue is located anterior to the 11:30 clock position	The condyle contacts the intermediate zone located between the anterior-superior aspect of the condyle and the posterior-inferior aspect of the articular eminence The intermediate zone of the disc is not in contact with the condyle
		Displaced disc	Relative to the superior aspect of the condyle, the low signal of the disc and the high signal of the retrodiscal tissue is located between the 11:30 and 12:30 clock positions	The intermediate zone of the disc is located anterior to the condyle
	Open mouth	Disc not visible	Neither signal intensity nor outlines make it possible to define a structure as the disc	
		Disc with reduction	Location of posterior band of the disc is not critical	The intermediate zone is located between the condyle and the articular eminence
		Disc without reduction		The intermediate zone is located anterior to the condylar head
T2 MRI, corrected sagittal view through the long axis of the condylar head	Closed mouth	Effusion present	A bright signal in either joint space that extends beyond the osseous contours of the fossa/articular eminence and/or condyle and has a convex configuration in the anterior or posterior recesses	
		Effusion absent	No bright signal in either joint space, or a bright signal in either joint space that conforms to the contours of the disc, fossa/articular eminence, and/or condyle	

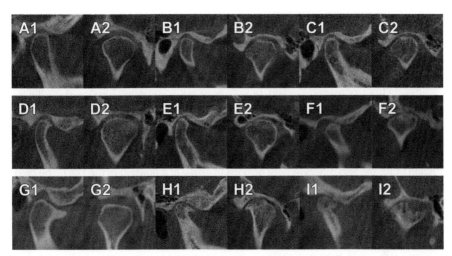

Fig. 3. CBCT findings of normal and different representations of degenerative joint disease. *A1* and *A2* are from the same patient, in corrected sagittal (*A1*) and corrected coronal (*A2*) orientations, showing a normal temporomandibular joint, which has smooth, rounded, and well-defined cortical margin of the condyle and the fossa. *B1* and *B2* are from the same patient, in corrected sagittal (*B1*) and corrected coronal (*B2*) orientations, showing flattening of the anterior and lateral slopes of the condylar head, indicating remodeling of the joint. *C1* and *C2* are from the same patient, in corrected sagittal (*C1*) and corrected coronal (*C2*) orientations, showing localized subcortical sclerosis of the condylar head, which indicates remodeling of the joint. The middle panel shows examples of grade 1 DJD. *D1* and *D2* are from the same patient, in corrected sagittal (*D1*) and corrected coronal (*D2*) orientations, showing an osteophyte at the anterior aspect of the condyle. *E1* and *E2* are from the same patient, in corrected sagittal (*E1*) and corrected coronal (*E2*) orientations, showing flattening and subcortical sclerosis of the anterior slope (*E1*) and localized erosion of the condyle (*E2*). *F1* and *F2* are from the same patient, in corrected sagittal (*F1*) and corrected coronal (*F2*) orientations, show the presence of a single subcortical pseudocyst. The lower panel shows examples of grade 2 DJD. *G1* and *G2* are from the same patient, in corrected sagittal (*G1*) and corrected coronal (*G2*) orientations, showing an anterior osteophyte larger than 2 mm (*G1*) and flattening of the superior and lateral slopes of the condyle (*G2*). *H1* and *H2* are from the same patient, in corrected sagittal (*H1*) and corrected coronal (*H2*) orientations, showing the presence of osteophytes and multiple subcortical pseudocysts. *I1* and *I2* are from the same patient, in corrected sagittal (*I1*) and corrected coronal (*I2*) orientations, showing the presence of osteophytes and multiple areas of erosion, one of which is wider than 2 mm.

- Surface erosion is loss of continuity of articular cortex of the condyle or the fossa.
- A subcortical pseudocyst is defined as a cavity below the articular surface that deviates from normal marrow pattern. It is not a true cyst but rather the loss of trabeculation.

Other radiographic findings related to possible osseous remodeling are articular surface flattening and subcortical sclerosis. Flattening and subcortical sclerosis may be indeterminate for degenerative joint disease as they may represent aging, functional remodeling of the joints, or a precursor to DJD.[10] Longitudinally, flattening and sclerosis may progress to DJD; as such it would represent regressive remodeling, whereas if it does not progress would represent adaptive remodeling.

- A surface flattening is defined as a loss of rounded contour of the surface of the condyle or the articular eminence; this can be present in normal joints and be a variation of normal.
- A subcortical sclerosis is defined as any increased thickness of the cortical plate in the load-bearing areas related to the adjacent non–load-bearing areas; this likely results from increased loading, or from normal loading when the disc is displaced.

In evaluating the TMJ, it is necessary to describe the extent of DJD. Although this is a diagnostic challenge, grading of DJD is important in evaluating progress or stability of the disorder.[10] Tanaka and colleagues[9] have developed a classification of the extent of DJD. In this classification the investigators have considered clinical signs, symptoms, imaging features, and management options to arrive at a grading of the DJD. The diagnostic criteria based on imaging are: stage I, early disease: mild to moderate erosive changes of the condyle/fossa/eminence; stage II, arrested disease: flattened condyle/eminence; and stage III, gross erosive changes, loss of condyle and eminence height, ankylosis, and/or hypertrophy of coronoid process. In another classification of the severity of the arthritis, Koos and colleagues[12] categorized the joints as class A (no form change), class B (deformation), and class C (destruction). The primary classes were subclassified as mild, moderate, and severe for flattening and erosion, and yes/no for osteophytes. These 2 classifications use the terminologies of mild, moderate, and gross/severe changes. Such terminologies are likely to be subjective during image interpretation. The reliability of these classification schemes is largely unknown.

To reduce the subjectivity of image interpretation, in unpublished work related to the DC/TMD Validation Project, the authors have developed the following image analysis criteria in grading the extent of DJD.[5] These diagnostic criteria can be used to interpret CT, CBCT, or MRI.

DJD is classified as grade 1 (see **Fig.** 3D1–F2) if the joint displays any 1 of the following features:

1. Osteophyte (the greatest length of the osteophyte is <2 mm when measured from tip of osteophyte to expected contour of condyle as viewed on the corrected sagittal section), or
2. Erosion (the greatest dimension of the erosion is <2 mm in depth and width), and the erosion is limited to a single occurrence only, or
3. Subcortical pseudocyst (the greatest dimension of the pseudocyst is <2 mm in depth and width) and the pseudocyst is limited to a single occurrence only

A DJD is classified as grade 2 (see **Fig.** 3G1–I2) if the joint displays 1 or more of the following features:

1. Osteophyte (the greatest length of the osteophyte is ≥2 mm measured from tip of osteophyte to expected contour of condyle as viewed on the corrected sagittal section), and/or
2. Erosion (the greatest dimension of the erosion is ≥2 mm in depth and width), or more than 1 erosion of any size, and/or
3. Subcortical pseudocyst (the greatest dimension of the pseudocyst is ≥), or more than 1 pseudocyst of any size, and/or
4. Two or more imaging signs of grade 1 DJD

For grading DJD, the authors adopted the following 2 principles:

1. Most advanced finding in all views will be used to arrive at the diagnosis of DJD. The most advanced finding should be visible in 2 image orientations.
2. If erosion and cyst are continuous, it is called erosion.

RHEUMATOID ARTHRITIS

Rheumatoid arthritis (RA) is a chronic inflammatory disease of unknown etiology, characterized by joint swelling, joint tenderness, and destruction of the synovial joints, leading to severe disability and premature mortality.[13] The distribution of joint involvement is nearly always polyarticular and frequently symmetrically bilateral. Patients usually manifest chronic episodic exacerbations and remissions. TMJ involvement in cases of RA is not particularly common despite this being a polyarticular disease.

Juvenile idiopathic arthritis (JIA) (juvenile RA or Still disease) is a pediatric rheumatic disease. TMJ involvement in JIA patients may be as high as 87%. Some studies indicate that TMJ can be the only joint involved with JIA. The patient may be asymptomatic, without any clinical signs and symptoms. The first clinical signs may be limited range of motion and asymmetry of the mandible, and class II malocclusion attributable to irreversible condylar resorption.

Imaging

Radiographic examination (**Fig. 4**) of RA of the TMJ includes panoramic radiography,[14] CT,[15] and MRI.[16] Erosion of the condylar head is the most common finding

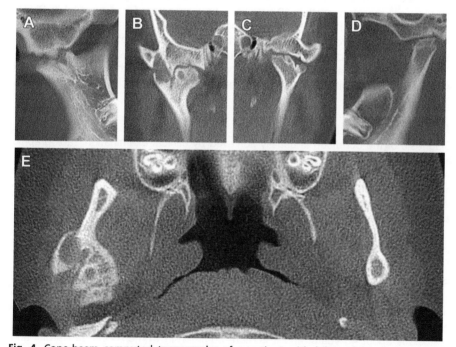

Fig. 4. Cone-beam computed tomography of a patient with bilateral involvement with rheumatoid arthritis. (*A*) Corrected sagittal view of the right joint. Superior margin of the condylar head is irregular. (*B*) Axially corrected coronal view of the right joint, which shows interdigitation of bony projections that lead to ankylosis of the joint. A subcortical pseudocyst is present in the condylar head. (*C, D*) Sagittal and coronal sections of the left joint. Superior margin of the left condylar head is irregularly flat and has prominent notching. The articular fossa is also flat. (*E*) Axial section of the same patient at the level of the right condylar head. Note the excessive enlargement of the right condylar head with subcortical pseudocysts and irregular margins.

of RA on a panoramic radiograph.[14] Goupille and colleagues[15] reported that characteristic findings of RA in CT are erosion, subcortical pseudocyst, flattening of the articular eminence, erosion of the glenoid fossa, and decreased joint space. Using MRI, Kretapirom and colleagues[16] classified 4 types of osseous changes in the condyle: type I, abnormal signal intensity of the condylar bone marrow without erosion or resorption; type II, surface erosion of the condylar cortex; type III, bone resorption extending within half of the condylar head; and type IV, bone resorption involving more than half of the condylar head. Unlike the findings in DJD, the disc in RA can be in the normal position despite significant osseous changes. Disc displacement may be a late phenomenon in RA. In contrast to DJD, in RA osteophyte formation is not a frequent finding. Effusion is significantly more frequent in RA patients than in patients with DJD.

SEPTIC (INFECTIOUS) ARTHRITIS

The incidence of arthritis resulting from a specific infection is low when compared with the occurrence of DJD and RA. Until recently, about 40 cases had been reported in the English literature. Leighty and colleagues[17] reviewed the existing literature, which showed that most common organism is *Staphylococcus aureus*. The spread of infection is either directly from a penetrating wound or from hematogenous origin. Cai and colleagues[18] reported another 40 patients who were treated in a hospital in China, most of whom had a hematogenous source of infection.

Patients suffering from acute septic arthritis complain chiefly of sudden severe TMJ pain with extreme tenderness on palpation over the joint area or with jaw manipulation. The severe pain typically restricts the motion of the jaw. During the healing process of septic arthritis the joint may undergo osseous or fibrous ankylosis, resulting in severe limitation of motion.

Imaging

Diagnosis of the condition is usually achieved by clinical examination, radiographic evaluation, and aspiration of the fluid in the joint area. A recent study by Gayle and colleagues[19] suggested that MRI and contrast-enhanced CT should be acquired to assess for joint effusion, cortical destruction, signs of inflammatory changes, and ankylosis of the joint. These investigators also recommend that a contrast-enhanced CT scan be acquired before joint aspiration.

LOOSE JOINT BODIES
Synovial Chondromatosis

Synovial chondromatosis (**Fig. 5**) is a rare benign condition whereby nodular cartilaginous or osteocartilaginous entities proliferate in the joint synovium. These entities may become loose from the synovium and continue to grow in size in the joint space. Bilateral synovial chondromatosis is rare. The mean age of patients with synovial chondromatosis is about 45 years, and it is more common in women. Guarda-Nardini and colleagues[20] have reported 3 clinical cardinal signs and symptoms of synovial chondromatosis:

- Pain in the preauricular area
- Swelling, facial asymmetry, and joint deformity
- Limited joint function

Additional signs and symptoms include occlusal changes, ipsilateral posterior open bite, headache, and joint sounds.

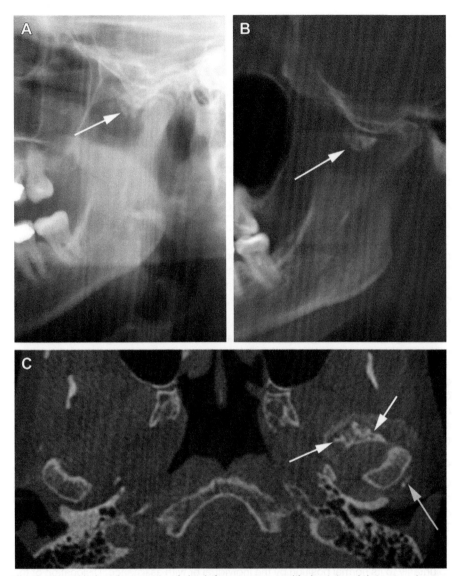

Fig. 5. Synovial chondromatosis of the left temporomandibular joint. (*A*) Sectional panoramic radiograph shows synovial chondromatosis (*arrow*) associated with the left temporomandibular joint. (*B*) Section of a reconstructed panoramic view of a CBCT of the same patient, showing presence of synovial chondromatosis (*arrow*) at the anterior aspect of the left condylar head. (*C*) Axial view at the level of the TMJs of the left TMJ. Synovial chondromatosis (*arrows*) is present at the anterior and posterior margins of the condylar head.

Imaging

Panoramic radiographs can demonstrate signs of synovial chondromatosis when the cartilage ossifies. CT and MRI are useful imaging examinations for diagnosis and treatment planning.[2,21] MRI displays multiple nodular entities (cartilaginous or osseous), joint effusion, and isointense signal tissues within the joint spaces and capsule.[22]

Noyek and colleagues[23] provided the following radiographic diagnostic criteria for synovial chondromatosis:

- Widening of the joint space
- Limitation of motion
- Irregularity of joint surfaces
- Presence of calcified loose bodies (cartilage)
- Sclerosis of the glenoid fossa and mandibular condyle

TRAUMATIC DISTURBANCES OF TEMPOROMANDIBULAR JOINTS

Traumatic injuries to the TMJs can be broadly categorized into 3 types: (1) fracture of the TMJ complex, (2) dislocation of the condyle, and (3) ankylosis of the joint.

Fracture of the Temporomandibular Joint Complex

About 17% to 52% of mandibular fractures involve condylar fracture (**Fig. 6**).[24] Condylar fractures may be classified according to the anatomic location: the condylar head (intracapsular), the condylar neck (extracapsular), and the subcondylar region. Condylar fractures may also be classified as nondisplaced, deviated, displaced (typically anterior, medial, or lateral), and dislocated. Another classification is based on the orientation of the fracture line, for example, horizontal, vertical, or compression type.

Imaging

Initial imaging for screening a suspected trauma to the condylar region should be performed with panoramic radiography.[25] A fractured condyle, which is not displaced, may be difficult to detect on a panoramic radiograph. Plain radiographs, such as open-mouth Towne or transorbital views, can provide limited information on the condylar fracture. Cross-sectional imaging with CT or CBCT and 3-dimensional (3D) reconstruction of the fractured region is the imaging modality of choice. To evaluate acute condylar trauma, bilateral sagittal and coronal MR images can provide additional information on disc position, capsular tear, and hemarthrosis.[26]

Dislocation of the Condyles

Condylar dislocation is primarily of 2 types: anterior or cranial dislocations. Cranial dislocation, whereby the condylar head is dislocated into the cranial fossa because of trauma, is rare. The causative trauma is typically motor vehicle or sports related. Trauma may also dislocate the condylar head posteriorly. Anterior dislocation of the TMJ, which is more common than cranial dislocation, when the head of the condyle moves anteriorly over the articular eminence into such a position that may be returned voluntarily to its normal position by the individual or with assistance. Dislocation of the condyle can be categorized as follows:

A. Cranial
B. Anterior
    a. Subluxation (self-reducing by the patient)
    b. Luxation (non–self-reducing by the patient; requires assistance)
    c. Habitual
    d. Fracture

Imaging

Panoramic radiography or CT/CBCT has limited diagnostic value for the hypermobility disorders of subluxation, luxation, or individual dislocation of the condylar

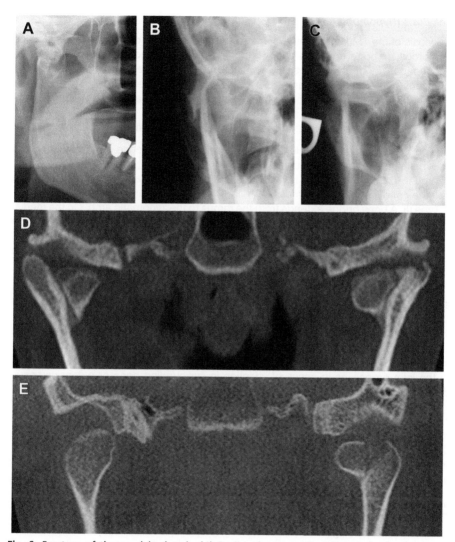

Fig. 6. Fracture of the condylar heads. (*A*) Sectional panoramic radiograph of a fractured condylar head superimposed over the neck of the condyle. The displaced fractured fragment is either on the lateral or medial aspect of the neck. (*B*) Open-mouth Towne projection showing an example of horizontal fracture of the neck of the condyle that is displaced laterally. (*C*) Open-mouth Towne projection showing an example of horizontal fracture of the neck of the condyle that is displaced medially. (*D*) Coronal section from a CBCT, showing bilateral vertical fractures of the condylar heads. (*E*) Coronal section from a CBCT, showing a vertical and medially displaced fracture of the left condylar head.

head, except to identify the location of the condylar head.[2] If the patient has chronic pain related to subluxation or luxation, MRI can be acquired to evaluate the status of the disc and the capsule. Cranial or anterior dislocation related to fracture requires CT or CBCT with 3D reconstruction. In addition, MRI should be obtained to evaluate the extent of injury to the brain tissues.

Ankylosis (Hypomobility)

Ankylosis of the TMJ is a disorder whereby adhesion of joint components takes place by fibrous or bony union, resulting in loss of function and movement. The most frequent causes of ankylosis of the TMJ are traumatic injuries, and local or systemic infections. Other causes of ankylosis include systemic disease such as ankylosing spondylitis, RA, psoriasis, or previous TMJ surgery. Bilateral ankylosis is often a result of RA.

In 1986 Sawheny classified ankylosis of the TMJ into 4 different types[27]:

Type I. The condylar head is flattened or deformed. Presence of fibrous adhesion makes movement impossible.

Type II. The condylar head is deformed and a small bony adhesion exists between the condyle and articular fossa. The articular surfaces are mostly well defined.

Type III. A bony bridge extends from the ramus to the zygomatic arch. On the medial aspect, atrophic and displaced condylar head is still present. The articular surface of the fossa is intact. The articular disc is also probably intact.

Type IV. The architecture of the joint is lost because of a bony bridge extending from the ramus to the temporal bone.

A simpler classification of TMJ ankylosis identifies 2 types: intra-articular ankylosis and extra-articular ankylosis. In intra-articular ankylosis, the joint undergoes progressive destruction of the meniscus with flattening of the mandibular fossa, thickening of the head of the condyle, and narrowing of the joint space. This type of ankylosis is basically fibrous, although ossification in the scar may result in a bony union. Extra-articular ankylosis results in a "splinting" of the TMJ by a fibrous or bony mass external to the joint proper, as in cases of infection in surrounding bone or extensive tissue destruction and scarring.

Ankylosis of the joint occurs at any age, but most cases occur before the age of 10 years. Distribution is approximately equal between the genders. The individual may or may not be able to open the mouth to any appreciable extent, depending on the type of ankylosis. In complete ankylosis, bony fusions will absolutely limit movement. There is usually somewhat greater motion in fibrous ankylosis than in bony ankylosis.

Imaging

Panoramic radiography has a limited role in detecting ankylosis. Fibrous ankylosis is better evaluated using MRI. In fibrous ankylosis, the joint space is often limited. The articulating surfaces of the condyle and the fossa may be irregular. Irregular surfaces appear to interdigitate in a locking fashion. In bony ankylosis, a bony bridge exists from the condylar head to the articular fossa. CT or CBCT is the imaging modality of choice in detecting osseous ankylosis.[2]

DEVELOPMENT DISTURBANCES OF TEMPOROMANDIBULAR JOINT

At the time of birth, the TMJs are incompletely formed. Therefore, developmental disturbance to the TMJ can occur either before or after birth. Kaneyama and colleagues[28] have classified developmental disturbances as follows:

1. Hypoplasia or aplasia of the condyle
   a. Congenital or primary hypoplasia or aplasia
   b. Acquired or secondary hypoplasia or aplasia
2. Condylar hyperplasia
3. Bifid condyle

Condylar Hypoplasia or Aplasia

Condylar aplasia is failure of development of the mandibular condyle, and condylar hypoplasia is underdevelopment of the condyle. Aplasia or hypoplasia may be congenital or acquired, and may occur unilaterally or bilaterally (**Fig. 7**).

Congenital, or primary, hypoplasia or aplasia is characterized by unilateral or bilateral underdevelopment or absence of the condyle, usually caused by disturbances in the first or second branchial arches. Conditions that show congenital hypoplasia or aplasia include Treacher-Collins syndrome, oculo-auriculo-vertebral syndrome, hemifacial macrosomia, Pierre-Robin sequence, and Hurler syndrome. In congenital variety, both the joints are usually affected but the primary clinical finding may be unilateral.

The acquired or secondary form of hypoplasia may be due to any agent that interferes with the normal development of the condyle. Local causes that may initiate condylar hypoplasia include trauma, infection of the mandible or middle ear, and therapeutic doses of radiation.

Imaging

Initial imaging may be limited to plain films and panoramic radiography. Xi and colleagues[29] demonstrated that CBCT and 3D reconstruction of the CBCT data provide an invaluable diagnostic advantage over conventional radiography for treatment planning and follow-up. A series of lateral cephalometric radiographs

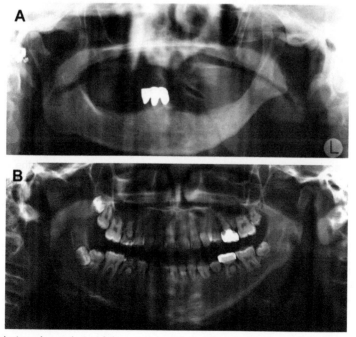

Fig. 7. Aplasia or hypoplasia of the condyle. (*A*) An 85-year-old woman whose left condylar head and ramus are aplastic because of an osteomyelitis that had affected her left mandible when she was 10 years old. (*B*) Example of hypoplasia of the left condyle and ramus caused by childhood treatment with radiation therapy. Note multiple teeth with stunted roots as a result from the radiation therapy.

acquired over a period of time also provides information on the progression of the disease.[2]

Hyperplasia of Mandibular Condyle

Condylar hyperplasia or hyperactivity is a rare unilateral enlargement of the condyle. Although the cause of this condition is unknown, it has been suggested that mild chronic inflammation, resulting in a condition analogous to a proliferative osteomyelitis, stimulates the growth of the condyle or adjacent tissues. The unilateral occurrence strongly suggests a local phenomenon. Obewegeser and Makek[30] have classified condylar hyperplasia into 3 categories.

- Type A is hemimandibular hyperplasia, causing asymmetry in the vertical plane. In this type the growth is unilateral in the vertical plane, with minimal deviation of the chin. Typically the maxilla shows compensatory growth. In the absence of maxillary growth, an open bite may be present on the same side.
- Type B is hemimandibular elongation causing asymmetry in the transverse plane. In this type the chin is deviated toward the contralateral side with no vertical asymmetry. Cross-bite may be present.
- Type C is a combination of types A and B, and exhibits hyperplastic features unilaterally or bilaterally.

Imaging

Diagnosis of condylar hyperplasia is made by a combination of clinical and radiographic findings. The patients usually exhibit a unilateral, slowly progressive elongation of the face with deviation of the chin away from the affected side. The enlarged condyle may be clinically evident or, at least, palpated. Condylar hyperplasia presents a striking radiographic appearance in both coronal and sagittal views. Panoramic radiography[31] may be used as an initial imaging method for identifying condylar hyperplasia, but for quantitative evaluation and follow-up, 3D imaging using CT or CBCT is necessary (**Fig. 8**).[32] Differential diagnosis includes osteochondroma.

Bifid Condyle

Bifid condyle, which is usually an incidental finding on radiographic examination, is characterized by a varying depth of a groove or depression around the midline of the condylar head. A deep groove may result in an appearance of duplicity of the condylar head. Usually bifidity is unilateral, although bilateral bifid condyles, a rare condition that affects less than 1% of the population, have been reported.[28] However, Miloglu and colleagues[33] suspect that the incidence of bifid condyles is underreported. Even rarer are trifid condyles. The etiology of bifidity is controversial, although several theories have been proposed.[34] One theory speculates that bifidity may originate in the embryo, where blood supply to the condylar head is limited. Another theory suggests microtrauma or trauma being the cause of bifidity, due to either birth trauma or transcoronal fracture of the condylar head. Others have suggested that radiotherapy, infection, or systemic factors such as endocrine disorders and genetic factors play a role in bifidity of the condyle.

Imaging

Although panoramic radiographs may be used to evaluate the presence of bifid condyle,[33] such depression is better detected on CT coronal or sagittal orientation of a cross-sectional imaging and 3D reconstruction (**Fig. 9**).[35]

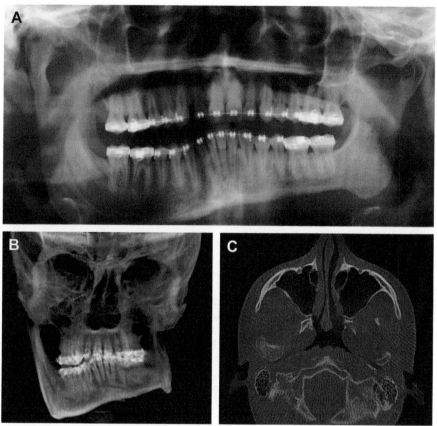

Fig. 8. (*A*) Panoramic radiograph showing unilateral hyperplasia of the right condyle and right ramus. (*B*) Three-dimensional reconstruction of CBCT data of the same patient, showing significant facial asymmetry and right-sided posterior open bite. (*C*) Axial section of the same patient, showing significant hyperplasia of the right condyle in comparison with the left.

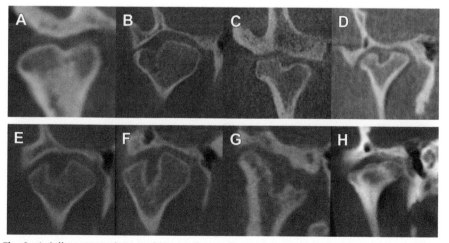

Fig. 9. Axially corrected coronal views of condyles showing examples of bifidity. (*A–G*) Bifid condyles may have slight midline depression to almost a duplication of the condylar head. (*H*) Mild trifid appearance of the condylar head.

SUMMARY

TMD is the second most common chronic musculoskeletal condition after chronic low back pain.[1] As pain-related TMD can affect an individual's daily activities, psychosocial functioning, and quality of life, it is important to accurately diagnose these complex musculoskeletal disorders to provide the best clinical care. The new dual-axis DC/TMD offers an evidence-based assessment protocol for the clinician to use when screening patients for TMJ intra-articular disorders, although imaging is typically needed for a definitive diagnosis. Both clinical history and examination, augmented as indicated with imaging, are needed to render proper TMJ intra-articular diagnoses. As several imaging modalities recommended in this article use ionizing radiation, careful clinical assessment with due consideration of the benefit to the patient must be carried out before ordering any imaging.

REFERENCES

1. Schiffman E, Ohrbach R, Truelove E, et al. Diagnostic criteria for temporomandibular disorders (DC/TMD) for clinical and research applications: recommendations of the International RDC/TMD Consortium Network* and orofacial pain special interest group†. J Oral Facial Pain Headache 2014;28(1):6–27.
2. Peck CC, Goulet JP, Lobbezoo F, et al. Expanding the taxonomy of the diagnostic criteria for temporomandibular disorders. J Oral Rehabil 2014;41(1):2–23.
3. Plesh O, Adams SH, Gansky SA. Temporomandibular joint and muscle disorder-type pain and comorbid pains in a national US sample. J Orofac Pain 2011;25(3):190–8.
4. Hunter A, Kalathingal S. Diagnostic imaging for temporomandibular disorders and orofacial pain. Dent Clin North Am 2013;57(3):405–18.
5. Ahmad M, Hollender L, Anderson Q, et al. Research diagnostic criteria for temporomandibular disorders (RDC/TMD): development of image analysis criteria and examiner reliability for image analysis. Oral Surg Oral Med Oral Pathol Oral Radiol Endod 2009;107(6):844–60.
6. Barkin S, Weinberg S. Internal derangements of the temporomandibular joint: the role of arthroscopic surgery and arthrocentesis. J Can Dent Assoc 2000;66(4):199–203.
7. Wilkes CH. Internal derangements of the temporomandibular joint. Pathological variations. Arch Otolaryngol Head Neck Surg 1989;115(4):469–77.
8. Haiter-Neto F, Hollender L, Barclay P, et al. Disk position and the bilaminar zone of the temporomandibular joint in asymptomatic young individuals by magnetic resonance imaging. Oral Surg Oral Med Oral Pathol Oral Radiol Endod 2002;94(3):372–8.
9. Tanaka E, Detamore MS, Mercuri LG. Degenerative disorders of the temporomandibular joint: etiology, diagnosis, and treatment. J Dent Res 2008;87(4):296–307.
10. Larheim TA, Abrahamsson AK, Kristensen M, et al. Temporomandibular joint diagnostics using CBCT. Dentomaxillofac Radiol 2015;44(1):20140235.
11. Alkhader M, Ohbayashi N, Tetsumura A, et al. Diagnostic performance of magnetic resonance imaging for detecting osseous abnormalities of the temporomandibular joint and its correlation with cone beam computed tomography. Dentomaxillofac Radiol 2010;39(5):270–6.
12. Koos B, Tzaribachev N, Bott S, et al. Classification of temporomandibular joint erosion, arthritis, and inflammation in patients with juvenile idiopathic arthritis. J Orofac Orthop 2013;74(6):506–19.

13. Aletaha D, Neogi T, Silman AJ, et al. 2010 Rheumatoid arthritis classification criteria: an American College of Rheumatology/European League Against Rheumatism collaborative initiative. Arthritis Rheum 2010;62(9):2569–81.
14. Helenius LM, Hallikainen D, Helenius I, et al. Clinical and radiographic findings of the temporomandibular joint in patients with various rheumatic diseases. A case-control study. Oral Surg Oral Med Oral Pathol Oral Radiol Endod 2005;99(4):455–63.
15. Goupille P, Fouquet B, Valat JP. Computed tomography of the temporomandibular joint in rheumatoid arthritis. J Rheumatol 1992;19(8):1315–6.
16. Kretapirom K, Okochi K, Nakamura S, et al. MRI characteristics of rheumatoid arthritis in the temporomandibular joint. Dentomaxillofac Radiol 2013;42(4): 31627230.
17. Leighty SM, Spach DH, Myall RW, et al. Septic arthritis of the temporomandibular joint: review of the literature and report of two cases in children. Int J Oral Maxillofac Surg 1993;22(5):292–7.
18. Cai XY, Yang C, Zhang ZY, et al. Septic arthritis of the temporomandibular joint: a retrospective review of 40 cases. J Oral Maxillofac Surg 2010;68(4):731–8.
19. Gayle EA, Young SM, McKenna SJ, et al. Septic arthritis of the temporomandibular joint: case reports and review of the literature. J Emerg Med 2013;45(5):674–8.
20. Guarda-Nardini L, Piccotti F, Ferronato G, et al. Synovial chondromatosis of the temporomandibular joint: a case description with systematic literature review. Int J Oral Maxillofac Surg 2010;39(8):745–55.
21. Miyamoto H, Sakashita H, Wilson DF, et al. Synovial chondromatosis of the temporomandibular joint. Br J Oral Maxillofac Surg 2000;38(3):205–8.
22. Wang P, Tian Z, Yang J, et al. Synovial chondromatosis of the temporomandibular joint: MRI findings with pathological comparison. Dentomaxillofac Radiol 2012; 41(2):110–6.
23. Noyek AM, Holgate RC, Fireman SM, et al. The radiologic findings in synovial chondromatosis (chondrometaplasia) of the temporomandibular joint. J Otolaryngol Suppl 1977;3:45–8.
24. Zachariades N, Mezitis M, Mourouzis C, et al. Fractures of the mandibular condyle: a review of 466 cases. Literature review, reflections on treatment and proposals. J Craniomaxillofac Surg 2006;34(7):421–32.
25. Chrcanovic BR. Open versus closed reduction: diacapitular fractures of the mandibular condyle. Oral Maxillofac Surg 2012;16(3):257–65.
26. Gerhard S, Ennemoser T, Rudisch A, et al. Condylar injury: magnetic resonance imaging findings of temporomandibular joint soft-tissue changes. Int J Oral Maxillofac Surg 2007;36(3):214–8.
27. Sawhney CP. Bony ankylosis of the temporomandibular joint: follow-up of 70 patients treated with arthroplasty and acrylic spacer interposition. Plast Reconstr Surg 1986;77(1):29–40.
28. Kaneyama K, Segami N, Hatta T. Congenital deformities and developmental abnormalities of the mandibular condyle in the temporomandibular joint. Congenit Anom (Kyoto) 2008;48(3):118–25.
29. Xi T, Schreurs R, van Loon B, et al. 3D analysis of condylar remodelling and skeletal relapse following bilateral sagittal split advancement osteotomies. J Craniomaxillofac Surg 2015;43(4):462–8.
30. Obwegeser HL, Makek MS. Hemimandibular hyperplasia-hemimandibular elongation. J Maxillofac Surg 1986;14(4):183–208.
31. Kjellberg H, Ekestubbe A, Kiliaridis S, et al. Condylar height on panoramic radiographs. A methodologic study with a clinical application. Acta Odontol Scand 1994;52(1):43–50.

32. Nolte JW, Karssemakers LH, Grootendorst DC, et al. Panoramic imaging is not suitable for quantitative evaluation, classification, and follow up in unilateral condylar hyperplasia. Br J Oral Maxillofac Surg 2015;53(5):446–50.
33. Miloglu O, Yalcin E, Buyukkurt M, et al. The frequency of bifid mandibular condyle in a Turkish patient population. Dentomaxillofac Radiol 2010;39(1):42–6.
34. Sala-Perez S, Vazquez-Delgado E, Rodriguez-Baeza A, et al. Bifid mandibular condyle: a disorder in its own right? J Am Dent Assoc 2010;141(9):1076–85.
35. Tanner JM, Friedlander AH, Chang TI. Bilateral bifid mandibular condyles diagnosed with three-dimensional reconstruction. Dentomaxillofac Radiol 2012; 41(8):691–5.

Benign Jaw Lesions

Anita Gohel, BDS, PhD[a],*, Alessandro Villa, DDS, PhD, MPH[b],
Osamu Sakai, MD, PhD[c,d,e]

KEYWORDS

- Benign odontogenic cyst • Benign odontogenic tumor • Cystic lesions • Mandible
- Maxilla

KEY POINTS

- Benign lesions of the jaws can be either odontogenic or nonodontogenic and have a variety of cystic and solid appearances.
- The radiographic features of plain films in conjunction with advanced imaging can help the clinician in the differential diagnosis, presurgical planning, and management of the lesion.
- Both intraoral and panoramic radiographs and advanced imaging features are useful in assessing the benign lesions of the jaws.
- The location, margins, internal contents, and effects of the lesions on adjacent structures are important features in diagnosing the lesions.

INTRODUCTION

Benign lesions can develop from both odontogenic and nonodontogenic tissues in the maxilla and mandible. Odontogenic lesions can arise from tooth-forming epithelium, mesenchymal tissue, or both.[1] In the mandible, odontogenic lesions originate superior to the mandibular canal. Neural and vascular lesions often originate within the mandibular canal, whereas lesions with epicenter inferior to the inferior alveolar canal are usually nonodontogenic in origin.

Disclosure Statement: The authors have nothing to disclose.
[a] Oral & Maxillofacial Radiology, Department of General Dentistry, Henry M. Goldman School of Dental Medicine, Boston University, 100 East Newton Street, G118, Boston, MA 02118, USA;
[b] Division of Oral Medicine and Dentistry, Department of Oral Medicine, Infection and Immunity, Dana Farber Cancer Institute, Brigham and Women's Hospital, Harvard School of Dental Medicine, 1620 Tremont Street, Suite BC-3-028, Boston, MA 02120, USA; [c] Department of Radiology, Boston Medical Center, Boston University School of Medicine, 820 Harrison Avenue, Boston, MA 02118, USA; [d] Department of Otolaryngology – Head and Neck Surgery, Boston Medical Center, Boston University School of Medicine, 820 Harrison Avenue, Boston, MA 02118, USA; [e] Department of Radiation Oncology, Boston Medical Center, Boston University School of Medicine, 820 Harrison Avenue, Boston, MA 02118, USA
* Corresponding author.
E-mail address: agohel@bu.edu

Benign odontogenic lesions are characterized by well-defined margins with regular borders causing expansion, displacement of adjacent structures, and directional root resorption. Intraoral and panoramic radiographs can show the superior-inferior and antero-posterior extent of the lesion. However, additional imaging, including cone beam computed tomography (CBCT), multidetector-row CT (MDCT), and MRI, is needed to effectively diagnose the extent of the lesion in all 3 planes. CBCT and MDCT imaging are highly useful for showing the extent of the lesion, expansion, and any ossifications/calcifications. MDCT has a better soft tissue resolution compared with CBCT. MRI is effective in differentiating cysts and tumors, evaluating the infiltration in the jawbone and surrounding soft tissue and detecting bone marrow changes of the jaw.[2] Combining radiography with advanced imaging techniques, including CT and MRI, can improve the accuracy of diagnosing the benign lesions in the jaws.

ODONTOGENIC CYSTS

A cyst contains fluid and is lined by an epithelium and is surrounded by a connective tissue. The fluid in the cyst is secreted by the lining cells or is derived from surrounding tissues. The fluid in the cyst exerts equal pressure in all directions so the cysts appear round or oval on radiographs. Cysts are broadly classified as odontogenic cysts and nonodontogenic cysts.

Odontogenic cysts are 2.25 times more frequently seen than odontogenic tumors.[3] Radiographically, they appear as lytic round or hydraulic-shaped lesions, with well-defined corticated margins (**Table 1**). Long-standing cysts may have dystrophic calcifications within them.

Radicular (Periapical) Cysts

Radicular (periapical) cysts are the most common odontogenic cysts found at the apices of a nonvital tooth resulting from inflammation of the periapical tissues secondary to caries or trauma.[3,4] These lesions appear radiolucent with well-defined and corticated margins. Large periapical cyst may cause root resorption, displacement of adjacent structures, and expansion (**Fig. 1**). CBCT images may be superior compared with periapical radiographs in detecting a periapical lesion.[5] There are 25% to 60% more periapical lesions detected by CBCT compared with intraoral periapical radiographs.[6,7] A radicular cyst remaining after the extraction of the tooth is a residual cyst.

Dentigerous Cysts

Dentigerous cysts appear as a pericoronal radiolucency associated with an unerupted or impacted tooth (**Fig. 2**). These cysts are caused by expansion of dental follicles resulting from accumulation of fluid between the tooth crown and epithelial components[8] often affecting the maxillary canine and mandibular third molar.[9] Dentigerous cysts are known to cause considerable displacement of the teeth with which it is associated. Maxillary teeth may be pushed into the antrum,[8] and mandibular third molars may be displaced into the ramus or inferior border of the mandible.[10,11]

Lateral Periodontal Cysts

Lateral periodontal cysts arise from the epithelial rests lateral to the tooth root. It appears as a well-defined, lytic lesion with a corticated boundary. The botryoid variety may appear multilocular.[12]

Table 1 Salient imaging features of jaw cysts			
Cysts	Radiographic Findings	CBCT/MDCT Findings	MRI Findings
Radicular cyst	Round radiolucent lesions with sclerotic borders at the apices of nonvital teeth.	Better demonstrate the extent of the cyst, expansion in all dimensions.	High T2 (high fluid content) and variable T1 signal intensity. Contrast-enhanced MR images show rim enhancement consistent with inflammation.
Residual cyst	Well-defined radiolucency with sclerotic borders apical to an extraction site.	Better demonstrate the extent of the cyst, expansion in bucco-lingual direction.	High T2 (high fluid content) and variable T1 signal intensity. Contrast-enhanced MR images show rim enhancement consistent with inflammation.
Dentigerous cyst	Well-defined pericoronal radiolucency with corticated borders causing substantial displacement. Expansion and root resorption may be present. Cortical boundaries are usually preserved.	Better demonstrate the extent of the cyst, expansion in bucco-lingual direction.	Low-to-intermediate signal T1 and high signal on T2-weighted mages with signal void representing the crown. Can help recognize mural ameloblastomas forming within the cyst lining.
Nasopalatine cysts	Well-defined radiolucency in the anterior maxillary region in midline. Can displace roots of adjacent teeth. The lesion is usually palatal to the teeth.	Better demonstrate the extent of the cyst, expansion in all 3 dimensions.	Water density/signal, may have increased density or T1 signal due to high protein concentration.
Simple bone cyst	Usually seen in the posterior mandible as a radiolucency scalloping between the roots of the teeth. Well-defined superiorly, but the inferior borders may not be well defined.	Better demonstrate the extent of the cyst, expansion in all 3 dimensions.	Variable signal depending on protein concentration within the cyst.

NONODONTOGENIC CYSTS
Nasopalatine Duct/Incisive Canal Cysts

Nasopalatine duct/incisive canal cysts are the most common nonodontogenic cysts in the maxilla.[13,14] These cysts are thought to arise from proliferation of epithelial remnants of the embryologic nasopalatine duct.[15] Most of the cysts are found in the incisive foramen or the canal in the anterior maxilla. The cysts may appear as a periapical radiolucency in association with the maxillary anterior teeth, but the associated teeth are vital (**Fig. 3**). On CBCT scan, the average diameter of these cysts was reported to be around 14 mm with a tendency to be larger in men.[14,16]

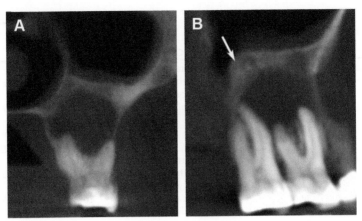

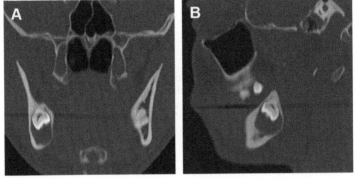

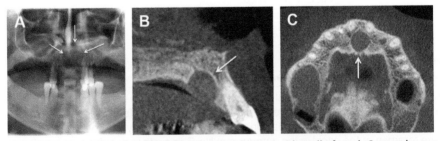

Fig. 1. Radicular cyst in a 54-year-old woman. Coronal (*A*) and Sagittal (*B*) CBCT images show a circular shape lucent lesion around the tooth root. The sclerotic margin (*arrow*) is most likely in response to secondary infection.

Fig. 2. Dentigerous cyst in a 28-year-old man incidentally found at a routine dental checkup. Coronal (*A*) and sagittal (*B*) CT images show a lucent lesion associated with the crown of the right mandibular third molar. Although there is mild expansile change and cortical erosion, there is no aggressive destruction of the mandible.

Fig. 3. (*A*) Nasopalatine duct cyst in a 38-year-old man incidentally found. Cropped panoramic radiograph shows a cyst (*arrows*) in the midline in the maxilla displacing the roots of incisors. (*B, C*) Nasopalatine duct cyst in a 37-year-old woman. Sagittal (*B*) and axial (*C*) CBCT images show a cyst palatal to the maxillary central incisors.

Simple Bone Cyst

Simple bone cyst is not a true cyst but a cavity within the jaws lined by connective tissue. Mainly seen in the mandibular posterior region, usually in the second decade of life, these lesions appear to scallop between the roots of the teeth giving it a multilocular appearance (**Fig. 4**).[17] Theses cysts are usually asymptomatic and rarely cause expansion.[18]

BENIGN ODONTOGENIC TUMORS

Benign odontogenic tumors grow slowly and appear well defined with smooth and sometimes corticated borders.[19] Unlike the cysts, these lesions may be radiolucent, mixed density, or radiopaque depending on the tissue of origin. They do exert pressure on surrounding tissues and can cause displacement, expansion, and root resorption (**Table 2**).

Keratocystic Odontogenic Tumors

Keratocystic odontogenic tumors (KOT) are most commonly located in the posterior mandible, with a male predilection, often in association with an impacted tooth. KOTs may have scalloped borders with mainly unilocular interior,[20] and are sometimes multilocular. In the body of the mandible, KOTs are noted to grow with minimal expansion, and significant expansion may occur in the ramus. KOTs can resorb roots of teeth and displace adjacent structures but at a lesser frequency than dentigerous cysts (**Fig. 5**).[21] There may be daughter cysts that extend into the surrounding bone and, thus, there is a high recurrence rate—as much as 28%.[22] Multiple KOTS in a young patient should raise the possibility of basal cell nevus syndrome (**Fig. 6**). Gorlin & Goltz[23] described the syndrome with multiple basal cell carcinoma, keratocystic odontogenic tumors, and bifid ribs. Additionally, calcification of the falx cerebri, palmar and plantar epidermal pits, spine and rib anomalies, relative macrocephaly, frontal bossing, medulloblastomas, cleft lip or palate, and developmental malformations may also be present. Multiple KOTs may be the first manifestation of this syndrome, occurring as early as the first decade of life.[24]

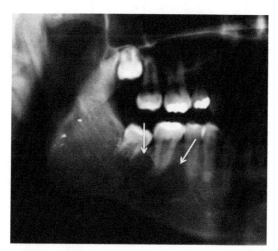

Fig. 4. Simple bone cyst in a 16-year-old boy. Cropped panoramic radiograph shows the lesion the right mandibular body (*arrows*). Notice the lesion scalloping between the roots of mandibular premolar and molars.

Table 2
Salient imaging features of benign odontogenic tumors

Benign Odontogenic Tumor	Radiographic Findings	CBCT/MDCT Findings	MRI Findings
KOT	Unilocular/multilocular lesions with scalloped margins. May appear as a pericoronal radiolucency. Expansion more prominent in the ramus. Root resorption and displacement to a lesser extent. If multiple, consider the possibility of basal cell nevus syndrome.	Better demonstrate the extent of the cyst, presence of daughter cyst especially with MDCT.	Higher signal on T1-weighted and lower signal on T2-weighted images compared with ameloblastoma Slight contrast enhancement Malignant transformation into squamous cell carcinoma may occur
Ameloblastoma	Well-defined unilocular/multilocular radiolucency. May appear as a pericoronal radiolucency. Extensive root resorption.	Better demonstrate the extent of the lesion and osseous destruction. Better able to delineate the cortical destruction.	Heterogeneous intermediate signal on T1-weighted images with heterogeneous enhancement after intravenous contrast administration.
Calcifying epithelial odontogenic tumor	Well-defined radiolucency with calcifications. May appear as pericoronal radiolucency with calcifications close to the crown.	Better demonstrate the extent of the lesion, expansion in bucco-lingual direction, and calcifications.	Predominantly hypointense on T1-weighted and mixed hyperintensity on T2-weighted images with heterogeneous enhancement.
Odontoma	Well-defined mixed density (teethlike) with a thin radiolucent capsule. Compound odontoma have toothlike structures, whereas complex odontoma appears as an irregular mass of calcified tissue. May interfere with the eruption if associated with a tooth.	Can demonstrate the extent of the lesion, expansion in all 3 dimensions.	Signal void, possibly with rim of fluid signal.

Ameloblastic Fibro-Odontoma	Well-defined radiolucent/mixed density lesion occlusal to a developing teeth.	Can demonstrate the extent of the lesion, expansion in all 3 dimensions. Can better depict areas of calcifications.	Signal void, possibly with rim of fluid signal.
Adenomatoid Odontogenic Tumor	Well-defined radiolucent/mixed density lesion usually in the anterior maxillary region. If associated with an impacted tooth, the lesions are found more apically on the root than are dentigerous cysts.	Better demonstrate the extent of the lesion, expansion in all 3 dimensions. Better depict areas of calcifications	Intermediate to low signal on T1 and high signal on T2-weighted images.
Odontogenic myxoma	Well-defined to poorly defined, unilocular or multilocular radiolucent lesion. Scalloped margins with fine straight septa may be noted. Expansion, root resorption, and tooth displacement also seen.	Better demonstrate the extent of the lesion, expansion. Better reveal the extension of the lesion into adjacent soft tissue.	Mixed signal on T1 and heterogeneous hyperintense signal on T2-weighted images with varying patterns of enhancement, often with lobulated appearance.
Cementoblastoma	Well-defined mixed density lesion at the apices of mandibular posterior teeth. Radiolucent rim surrounding the lesion. Can cause root resorption and expansion.	Better demonstrate the extent of the lesion, expansion.	Signal void.

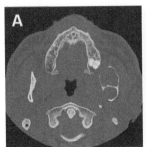
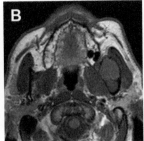
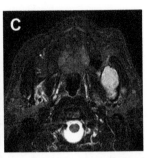

Fig. 5. Keratocystic odontogenic tumor in a 64-year-old man presented with left cheek swelling. Axial CT (*A*) shows a multiloculated cystic lesion that shows significant expansile change and cortical erosion in the left mandibular ramus. Axial T1- (*B*) and T2-weighted (*C*) MR image shows low-to-intermediate T1 signal and intermediate-to-high T2 signal within the lesion, reflecting proteinaceous contents within the cavity.

Odontoma

Odontoma is the most common odontogenic tumor of the mandible. The lesion consists of various tooth components, including dentin and enamel, that have developed abnormally (**Fig. 7**). A compound odontoma forms an agglomeration of small structures resembling teeth, whereas a complex odontoma forms an amorphous calcified mass in a disorderly pattern.[25] Nearly 50% of odontomas are associated with an impacted tooth and may prevent the eruption of the teeth.[26]

Ameloblastoma

Ameloblastoma most commonly occurs in the posterior mandible, typically in the third molar region, with associated follicular cysts or impacted teeth. The slow growth of the tumor can lead to significant expansion of the mandible. The expansile, radiolucent tumor can be unilocular or multilocular, with a characteristic "soap bubble–like" appearance. CT findings include cystic areas of low attenuation with scattered isoattenuating regions representative of soft tissue components.[2] The lesion can also erode through the cortex with extension into the surrounding oral soft tissues (**Fig. 8**).[27] Ameloblastomas can cause significant resorption of the roots of adjacent teeth.[28]

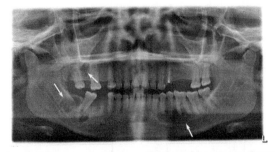

Fig. 6. Keratocystic odontogenic tumor in a 42-year-old woman. Panoramic radiograph shows a KOT in the right maxillary molar region (*arrow*), another KOT in the mandibular right posterior region (*arrow*), and another KOT in the left mandibular body (*arrow*). Multiple KOTs are seen in a patient with basal cell nevus syndrome.

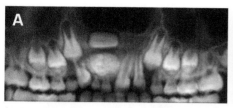
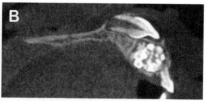

Fig. 7. Odontoma in an 8-year-old girl presented for orthodontic consult. Panoramic (*A*) and sagittal (*B*) reformatted CBCT images show a compound odontoma in the anterior maxilla preventing the eruption of the right permanent maxillary central incisor.

Odontogenic Myxoma

Odontogenic myxoma is seen more in females and more frequently in the mandible. The margins can range from well defined to poorly defined and may perforate the cortical boundaries to extend into the soft tissue.[29] The lesions are usually multilocular with straight thin and wispy septation (**Fig. 9**). Odontogenic myxoma may cause displacement of teeth, although root resorption may be rarely noted.[30]

Calcifying Epithelial Odontogenic Tumor

Calcifying epithelial odontogenic tumor (Pindborg tumor) is composed of epithelial cells in a fibrous stroma. Most tumors are located in the premolar or molar region of the mandible, and about half of them are associated with the crown of an impacted tooth.[31,32] The tumor typically appears radiolucent with scattered calcified components[33] close to the crown of the impacted teeth.

Cementoblastoma

Cementoblastoma is a neoplasm of cementum that typically occurs in patients younger than 25 years. Usually found in association with the apex of the first molars, the lesion appears as a round, well-defined, mixed density/radiopaque mass with a thin radiolucent rim (**Fig. 10**).[34,35]

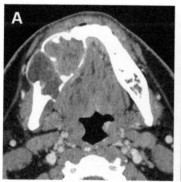
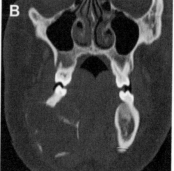

Fig. 8. Ameloblastoma in a 28-year-old man presenting with a right jaw swelling. Axial contrast-enhanced CT (*A*) shows a multiloculated lesion with significant expansile change and cortical erosion and destruction. Note a solid component shows heterogeneous enhancement, whereas a cystic component shows water density. Coronal CT with bone algorithm reconstruction (*B*) better shows significant expansile change and cortical erosion and destruction. Note erosion of a root of the right mandibular premolar indicating aggressiveness of the lesion.

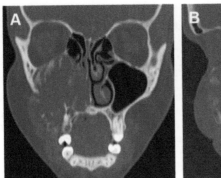
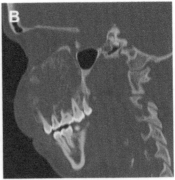

Fig. 9. Odontogenic myxoma in a 20-year-old man presenting with right cheek swelling. Coronal (*A*) and sagittal (*B*) CT images show a large expansile mixed density lesion in the right maxilla occupying the maxillary sinus. Note displacement and erosion of roots of multiple right maxillary teeth, reflecting aggressiveness of the lesion.

Ameloblastic Fibro-Odontoma

Ameloblastic fibro-odontoma typically appears as a well-defined, pericoronal radiolucent lesion with calcifications in the posterior mandible or maxilla. These lesions may be unilocular or multilocular and can be associated with impacted teeth.[36] They can also appear superficial to a crown of an impacted tooth and may prevent the eruption of the associated tooth.[37]

Adenomatoid Odontogenic Tumors

Adenomatoid odontogenic tumors are seen mainly in females in the anterior maxillary region. The tumors appear as well-defined radiolucent lesions with varying amounts of calcifications and can displace or prevent the eruption of teeth (**Fig. 11**). If attached to a tooth, the lesions are found more apically on the root than are dentigerous cysts.[2,38]

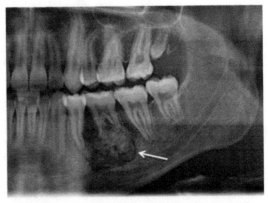

Fig. 10. Cementoblastoma in a 17-year-old boy. Cropped panoramic radiograph shows a mixed density lesion with a radiolucent border (*arrow*) at the apices of the mandibular first molar causing root resorption.

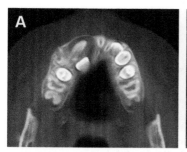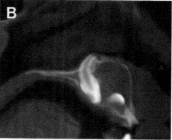

Fig. 11. Adenomatoid odontogenic tumor in a 10-year-old boy. Axial (*A*) and sagittal (*B*) CBCT images show an expansile lucent lesion associated with an unerupted lateral incisor in the anterior maxillary region displacing the incisors and canine.

BENIGN NONODONTOGENIC TUMORS
Neural Lesions

Neural lesions such as schwannomas and neurofibromas may appear as well-defined radiolucent lesions and can cause fusiform enlargement of the canal (**Table 3**).[39] Neurofibromas can expand and perforate the cortical boundaries.

Table 3
Salient imaging features of benign nonodontogenic tumors

Nonodontogenic Tumors	Radiographic Findings	CBCT/MDCT Findings	MRI Findings
Neurofibroma	Well-defined causing fusiform enlargement of the mandibular canal.	Better demonstrate the extent of the lesion.	Low signal on T1 and intermediate to high signal intensity on T2-weighted images.
Osteoma	Well-defined radiopaque. May be exophytic. If multiple osteomas, consider the possibility of Gardner's syndrome.	Better demonstrate the extent of the lesion.	Signal void.
Central hemangioma	Well defined to poorly defined. May appear multilocular with large marrow spaces. If within the canal, the entire canal may appear wider.	Can demonstrate the extent of the lesion.	Intermediate signal on T1 and hyperintense signal intensity on T2-weighted images. Marked contrast enhancement.
Arteriovenous malformation	Well defined to poorly defined. May appear multilocular. Mandibular canal maybe enlarged and appear tortuous.	Regional osteolytic changes, cortical erosion/resorption. Avid enhancement with tortuous and dilated feeding arteries and draining veins.	Abnormal flow void within the jawbone and surrounding soft tissues. Marked enhancement with dynamic contrast enhanced studies.

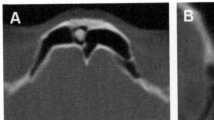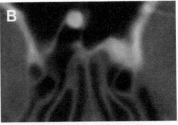

Fig. 12. Osteoma in a 53-year-old man found incidentally. Axial (*A*) and coronal (*B*) CBCT images show a homogenous radiopaque lesion in the frontal sinus.

Osteoma

Osteoma appears as a well-defined uniform radiopacity and also can be exophytic. Osteomas can also be noted in the sinuses (**Fig. 12**). Multiple osteomas may indicate the possibility of Gardner's syndrome, which is characterized by multiple osteomas, epidermoid cysts, and polyps of the intestine, which have strong predilection to become malignant. The osteomas may precede the asymptomatic intestinal polyps.[40]

Vascular lesions such as *central hemangioma* and *arteriovenous malformation* are usually seen in the posterior mandible as a unilocular or multilocular lesion[41] with large marrow space and coarse trabeculation. When the epicenter is within the canal, the canal can be enlarged throughout its course, and the mental foramen may be enlarged. These lesions may erode the surrounding bone (**Fig. 13**). Calcifications (phleboliths) are often seen in venous malformation in the surrounding soft tissue.[42]

OTHER LESIONS
Central Giant Cell Granuloma

Central giant cell granuloma is an aggressive benign lesion seen in adolescents and young adults (**Table 4**). The lesion is often seen in the anterior mandible as a well-defined noncorticated unilocular or multilocular radiolucency.[43] Some lesions may have faint granular calcifications. The granular bone can form thin septa, which are

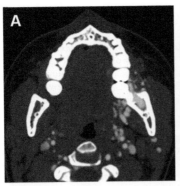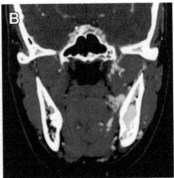

Fig. 13. Arteriovenous malformation in a 24-year-old woman presenting with uncontrolled hemorrhage from the gum. Axial (*A*) and coronal (*B*) contrast-enhanced CT images show numerous tortuous vessels around the left mandibular ramus, and within the medial pterygoid and masseter muscles, in addition to abnormal enhancement within the marrow space of the ramus.

Table 4
Salient imaging features of cystlike jaw lesions

Other Cystlike Lesions	Plain Radiography Findings	CBCT/MDCT Findings	MRI Findings
Central Giant Cell Granuloma	Well-defined borders in mandible. Maxillary lesions may be poorly defined. Radiolucent with granular calcifications. Wispy septation perpendicular to the periphery of the lesion. Can displace teeth and resorb roots. May destroy the cortical plates and extend to surrounding soft tissue.	Better delineate the extent of the lesion. Better reveal the extension of the lesion into adjacent soft tissue.	Low-to-intermediate signal intensity at T1- and T2-weighted images. Avid heterogeneous enhancement.
Ossifying fibroma	Well defined with a lucent/mixed density/radiopaque interior. May have a radiolucent border. Can cause expansion and displacement of adjacent structures.	Better demonstrate the extent of the lesion and expansion.	Low signal on T1- and low to intermediate signal intensity on T2-weighted images Variable degree of contrast enhancement
Aneurysmal bone cyst	Well-defined circular or spherical radiolucency. Maybe unilocular or multilocular with thin wispy septation perpendicular to the periphery of the lesion. Can cause a lot of expansion. Can displace teeth and resorb roots.	Better demonstrate the extent of the lesion. Multiloculated/septated expansile lesion with fluid-fluid levels.	Multiloculated/septated expansile lesion with variable internal signal and low signal rim. Better demonstrate the fluid-fluid levels and identify the solid component. Avis enhancement of cyst wall and septations with contrast.
Lingual salivary gland depression/Stafne defect	Well-defined radiolucent lingual cortical defect with a sclerotic margin near inferior to the mandibular canal.	Not needed, but can demonstrate the lingual cortical defect	Not required.

perpendicular to the edge of the lesion. These lesions can displace adjacent structures (**Fig. 14**) and cause root resorption. In nearly half the cases, cortical perforation may be noted.[44]

Ossifying Fibroma, Cemento-Ossifying Fibroma, or Cementifying Fibroma

Ossifying fibroma, cemento-ossifying fibroma, or cementifying fibroma are typically seen in the third and fourth decades of life, mainly in the posterior mandibular region. The lesions are well defined and can appear radiolucent, radiopaque, or with mixed opacity depending on the degree of calcification. As the lesions mature, they become more radiopaque.[45] Juvenile ossifying fibroma is an aggressively growing variant of

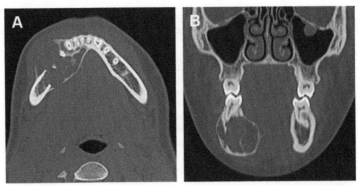

Fig. 14. Central giant cell granuloma in an 18-year-old woman presenting with a mandibular swelling. Axial (*A*) and coronal (*B*) CT images show expansile lucent lesion in the right mandibular body with displacement of a tooth root and significant cortical erosion.

the tumor, typically occurring in boys younger than 15 years of age. The lesion has been reported to arise within both the mandible and paranasal sinus regions and grow quite rapidly.[2]

Lingual Salivary Gland Depression

Lingual salivary gland depression appears as a well-defined radiolucency generally below the mandibular canal usually in the posterior mandible. Defects in the mandibular posterior region are related to submandibular gland defect (**Fig. 15**) and in the mandibular canine and premolar regions are related to the sublingual gland (**Fig. 16**). These defects maybe the result of salivary gland growth, and the cavity is usually filled with fat and salivary gland tissue.[1]

Aneurysmal Bone Cyst

Aneurysmal bone cyst is seen mainly in young people in the posterior mandibular region. These lesions may appear with unilocular or multilocular radiolucency with expansion of cortical boundaries.[46] On CT, an expansile hypoattenuating lesion with numerous fluid-fluid levels can be seen. MRI shows multiloculated lesions with fluid-fluid level, contrast enhancement of the wall, and septi.[1]

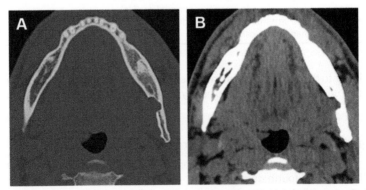

Fig. 15. Lingual salivary gland defect in a 47-year-old man. Axial bone (*A*) and soft tissue (*B*) reconstructed CT images show a well-defined cortical defect on the lingual surface of the angle of the left mandible. Note soft tissue density extending into the defect (*B*).

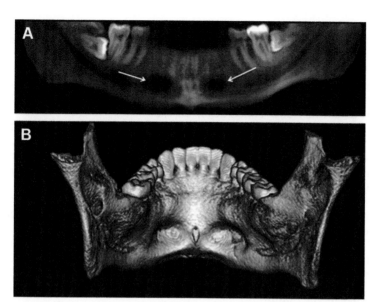

Fig. 16. Lingual salivary gland defect in a 19-year-old man. Reformatted panoramic (*A*) and volume-rendered 3-dimensional (*B*) CBCT images show well-defined cortical defects on the lingual surfaces of the anterior mandible.

SUMMARY

Benign lesions of the jaws can be either odontogenic or nonodontogenic and have a variety of cystic and solid appearances. The radiographic features of plain radiographs in conjunction with advanced imaging can help the clinician in the differential diagnosis, presurgical planning, and management of the lesion.

REFERENCES

1. Devenney-Cakir B, Subramaniam RM, Reddy SM, et al. Cystic and cystic-appearing lesions of the mandible: review. AJR Am J Roentgenol 2011; 196(Suppl 6):WS66–77.
2. Dunfee BL, Sakai O, Pistey R, et al. Radiologic and pathologic characteristics of benign and malignant lesions of the mandible. Radiographics 2006;26(6): 1751–68.
3. Johnson NR, Gannon OM, Savage NW, et al. Frequency of odontogenic cysts and tumors: a systematic review. J Investig Clin Dent 2014;5(1):9–14.
4. Chapman MN, Nadgir RN, Akman AS, et al. Periapical lucency around the tooth: radiologic evaluation and differential diagnosis. Radiographics 2013;33(1): E15–32.
5. Tyndall DA, Rathore S. Cone-beam CT diagnostic applications: caries, bone assessment, and endodontic applications. Dent Clin North Am 2008;52(4): 825–41.
6. Patel S, Wilson R, Dawood A, et al. The detection of periapical pathosis using periapical radiography and cone beam computed tomography – Part 1: pre-operative status. Int Endod J 2012;45(8):702–10.
7. Lofthag-Hansen S, Huumonen S, Gröndahl S, et al. Limited cone-beam CT and intraoral radiography for the diagnosis of periapical pathology. Oral Surg Oral Med Oral Pathol Oral Radiol Endod 2007;103(1):114–9.

8. Edamatsu M, Kumamoto H, Ooya K, et al. Apoptosis-related factors in the epithelial components of dental follicles and dentigerous cysts associated with impacted third molars of the mandible. Oral Surg Oral Med Oral Pathol Oral Radiol Endod 2005;99(1):17–23.

9. Buyukkurt MC, Omezli MM, Miloglu O. Dentigerous cyst associated with an tooth in the maxillary sinus: a report of 3 cases and review of the. Oral Surg Oral Med Oral Pathol Oral Radiol Endod 2010;109(1):67–71.

10. Bux P, Lisco V. Ectopic third molar associated with a dentigerous cyst in the subcondylar region: report of case. J Oral Maxillofac Surg 1994;52(6):630–2.

11. Tümer C, Eset AE, Atabek A. Ectopic impacted mandibular third molar in the region associated with a dentigerous cyst: a case report. Quintessence Int 2002; 33(3):231–3.

12. Siponen M, Neville BW, Damm DD, et al. Multifocal lateral periodontal: a report of 4 cases and review of the literature. Oral Surg Oral Med Oral Pathol Oral Radiol Endod 2011;111(2):225–33.

13. Ely N, Sheehy EC, McDonald F. Nasopalatine duct cyst: a case report. Int J Paediatr Dent 2001;11(2):135–7.

14. Escoda Francolí J, Almendros Marqués N, Berini Aytés L, et al. Nasopalatine duct cyst: report of 22 cases and review of the literature. Med Oral Pathol Oral Cir Bucal 2008;13(7):E438–43.

15. Anneroth HG, Stuge U. Nasopalatine duct cyst. Int J Oral Maxillofac Surg 1986; 15(5):572–80.

16. Suter VG, Sendi P, Reichart PA, et al. The nasopalatine duct cyst: an of the relation between clinical symptoms, cyst dimensions, and of neighboring anatomical structures using cone beam computed. J Oral Maxillofac Surg 2011;69(10): 2595–603.

17. An SY, Lee JS, Benavides E, et al. Multiple simple bone cysts of the jaws:review of the literature and report of three cases. Oral Surg Oral Med Oral Pathol Oral Radiol 2014;117(6):e458–69.

18. Forssell K, Forssell H, Happonen RP, et al. Simple bone cyst. Review of literature and analysis of 23 cases. Int J Oral Maxillofac Surg 1988;17(1):21–4.

19. Kaneda T, Minami M, Kurabayashi T. Benign odontogenic tumors of the mandible maxilla [review]. Neuroimaging Clin N Am 2003;13(3):495–507.

20. Sansare K, Raghav M, Mupparapu M, et al. Keratocystic odontogenic tumor: systematic review with analysis of 72 additional cases from Mumbai, India. Oral Surg Oral Med Oral Pathol Oral Radiol 2013;115(1):128–39.

21. Titinchi F, Nortje CJ. Keratocystic odontogenic tumor: a recurrence analysis clinical and radiographic parameters. Oral Surg Oral Med Oral Pathol Oral Radiol 2012;114(1):136–42.

22. MacDonald-Jankowski DS. Keratocystic odontogenic tumour: systematic review. Dentomaxillofac Radiol 2011;40(1):1–23.

23. Gorlin RJ, Goltz RW. Multiple nevoid basal cell epithelioma, jaw cysts and bifid rib: a syndrome. N Engl J Med 1960;262:908–12.

24. Casaroto AR, Loures DC, Moreschi E, et al. Early diagnosis of Gorlin-Goltz syndrome: case report. Head Face Med 2011;25(7):2.

25. Budnick SD. Compound and complex odontomas. Oral Surg Oral Med Oral Pathol 1976;42(4):501–6.

26. Kaugars GE, Miller ME, Abbey LM. Odontomas. Oral Surg Oral Med Oral Pathol 1989;67(2):172–6.

27. Scholl RJ, Kellett HM, Neumann DP, et al. Cysts and cystic lesions of the: clinical and radiologic-histopathologic review. Radiographics 1999;19(5):1107–24.

28. Kim SG, Jang HS. Ameloblastoma: a clinical, radiographic and histopathologic analysis of 71 cases. Oral Surg Oral Med Oral Pathol Oral Radiol Endod 2001; 91:649–53.
29. Noffke CE, Raubenheimer EJ, Chabikuli NJ, et al. Odontogenic myxoma: of the literature and report of 30 cases from South Africa. Oral Surg Oral Med Oral Pathol Oral Radiol Endod 2007;104(1):101–9.
30. Peltola J, Magnusson B, Happonen RP, et al. Odontogenic myxoma radiographic study of 21 tumours. Br J Oral Maxillofac Surg 1994;32(5):298–302.
31. Pindborg JJ. A calcifying epithelial odontogenic tumor. Cancer 1958;11:838–43.
32. Ching AS, Pak MW, Kew J, et al. CT and MR imaging appearances of an extra-osseous calcifying epithelial odontogenic tumor (Pindborg tumor). AJNR Am J Neuroradiol 2000;21(2):343–5.
33. Hada MS, Sable M, Kane SV, et al. Calcifying epithelial tumor: a clinico-radio-pathological dilemma. J Cancer Res Ther 2014;10(1):194–6.
34. Sharma N. Benign cementoblastoma: a rare case report with review of. Contemp Clin Dent 2014;5(1):92–4.
35. Lemberg K, Hagström J, Rihtniemi J, et al. Benign cementoblastoma in a primary lower molar, a rarity. Dentomaxillofac Radiol 2007;36:364–6.
36. Zouhary KJ, Said-Al-Naief N, Waite PD. Ameloblastic fibro-odontoma: expansile mixed radiolucent lesion in the posterior maxilla: a case report. Oral Surg Oral Med Oral Pathol Oral Radiol Endod 2008;106(4):e15–21.
37. Soares RC, Godoy GP, Neto JC, et al. Ameloblastic fibro-odontoma: report of a case presenting an unusual clinical course. Int J Pediatr Otorhinolaryngol 2006; 1(3):200–3.
38. Chindasombatjaroen J, Poomsawat S, Kakimoto N, et al. Calcifying cystic odon-togenic tumor and adenomatoid odontogenic tumor: radiographic evaluation. Oral Surg Oral Med Oral Pathol Oral Radiol 2012;114(6):796–803.
39. Suga K, Ogane S, Muramatsu K, et al. Intraosseous schwannoma originating in alveolar nerve: a case report. Bull Tokyo Dent Coll 2013;54(1):19–25.
40. Panjwani S, Bagewadi A, Keluskar V, et al. Gardner's Syndrome. J Clin Sci 2011; 1:65.
41. Zlotogorski A, Buchner A, Kaffe I, et al. Radiological features of haemangioma of the jaws. Dentomaxillofac Radiol 2005;34(5):292–6.
42. Mandel L, Perrino MA. Phleboliths and the vascular maxillofacial lesion. J Maxillofac Surg 2010;68(8):1973–6.
43. Kruse-Lösler B, Diallo R, Gaertner C, et al. giant cell granuloma of the jaws: a clin-ical, radiologic, and study of 26 cases. Oral Surg Oral Med Oral Pathol Oral Ra-diol 2006;101(3):346–54.
44. Stavropoulos F, Katz J. Central giant cell granulomas: a systematic review of the radiographic characteristics with the addition of 20 new cases. Dentomaxillofac Radiol 2002;31(4):213–7.
45. Gondivkar SM, Gadbail AR, Chole R, et al. Ossifying fibroma of jaws: report of two cases and literature review. Oral Oncol 2011;47(9):804–9.
46. Motamedi MH. Aneurysmal bone cysts of the jaws: clinicopathological features, radiographic evaluation and treatment analysis of 17 cases. J Craniomaxillofac Surg 1998;26:56–62.

Diagnostic Imaging of Malignant Tumors in the Orofacial Region

Steven R. Singer, DDS*, Adriana G. Creanga, BDS, MS, DABOMR

KEYWORDS

- Malignancy • Diagnosis • Clinical correlations • Radiographic features • Tumors

KEY POINTS

- Malignancies often have serious consequences, including disfigurement and death.
- All radiographs should be examined for signs of malignant lesions.
- Characteristic appearances of malignant lesions include ill-defined borders, asymmetric appearance, destruction of adjacent bone and cortical borders, and radiolucency with pieces of trapped bone.
- All bony lesions should be visualized completely and, where possible, in 3 dimensions.
- Histopathologic examination is generally the gold standard for final diagnosis of malignant lesions.

INTRODUCTION

This article highlights the radiographic features of malignant lesions and presents the clinical correlations that may aid in the initial diagnosis of orofacial malignancies.

The word "malignant" comes from the Latin *malignare*, meaning "to act wickedly" (*mal* = "bad"). Cancer appears when a stimulus triggers abnormal changes to the chromosomes within cells. The initial stage that can be detected by histopathologic examination is called dysplasia (abnormality) and there are multiple evolutionary stages known, such as carcinoma in situ, primary neoplasm, and secondary or metastatic neoplasm. Most changes take place at the subcellular level and manifest themselves as uncontrolled multiple cell divisions and persistence of old cells while young cells do not mature and differentiate. The clinically visible aspect is usually a late one,

Financial Disclosures: The investigators of this article have no financial conflicts to disclose.
Department of Diagnostic Sciences, Division of Oral and Maxillofacial Radiology, Rutgers School of Dental Medicine, 110 Bergen Street, Newark, NJ 07101, USA
* Corresponding author. Rutgers School of Dental Medicine, Room D-860, 110 Bergen Street, Newark, NJ 07101.
E-mail address: steven.singer@sdm.rutgers.edu

Dent Clin N Am 60 (2016) 143–165
http://dx.doi.org/10.1016/j.cden.2015.08.006
0011-8532/16/$ – see front matter © 2016 Elsevier Inc. All rights reserved.

dental.theclinics.com

illustrated by the cancerous growth, tumor, or mass. It may be at this point that radiographically evident changes also occur.

In contrast to a benign lesion, a malignant tumor is characterized by uncontrolled growth potential, an aggressive and invasive nature, and the ability to metastasize. If a tumor arises de novo it is called a primary tumor, and if it originates from a distant tumor it is referred to as secondary or metastatic. Metastases share the tissues of the primary tumor, but they occur in a different and, frequently, distant location. Metastases illustrate the spread of cancer cells, usually traveling through the blood or lymph vessels, and can invade and develop in any other anatomic region. Often, the first site of neoplastic invasion is the nearby lymph nodes.

According to the National Cancer Institute, "head and neck cancers, which include cancers of the oral cavity, larynx, pharynx, salivary glands and nose/nasal passages, account for 3% of all malignancies in the US." Cancers of the oral cavity represent 85% of all head and neck cancers,[1] the eighth most common malignancy in males and 15th most common in females. Estimates for 2015 are far from gratifying. The Oral Cancer Foundation and American Cancer Society estimate in 2015 that 43,000 to 45,000 new cases of oral and oropharyngeal cancers with 8000 to 8650 deaths (approximately 1 per hour) will occur in the United States.[2] An estimated 1 in 92 adults will be diagnosed with oral or pharyngeal cancer in their lifetime.[3]

There are multiple and varied risk factors involved in the development of head and neck cancerous lesions. For example, the use of tobacco and alcohol is strongly related to oral cancer. According to the American Cancer Society, "3 out of 4 people with oral cancer have used tobacco, alcohol or both." It is said that combining the use of tobacco and alcohol will increase the risk of a malignancy by 15 times.[4]

Viruses have been also implicated in the development of oral and oropharyngeal cancer and, of these, human papillomavirus (HPV) types 16 and 18 are strongly associated and are thought to cause about half of all oropharyngeal cancer cases. HPV is a common virus, and in most instances the person's immune system will clear the HPV infection. Only 1% of those infected will display a lack of immune response.[2,4,5]

Sun exposure is also a risk factor for developing skin cancers, manifesting itself in the orofacial region as lip cancer. Furthermore, diets that lack vegetables and fruits, personal history of cancer, betel nut chewing, and other unspecific or minor risk factors are researched, known, and cited.[4] At one time a controversy regarding the relationship between mouthwash use and increased risk for developing oral cancer arose, but proved to have no scientific evidence.[6]

Demographic characteristics have changed over the years. Historically, cancer usually affected older people and, with respect to oral cancers, mostly male smokers or heavy drinkers. The newly recognized HPV16 association with oropharyngeal cancer should eventually shed some light on the more recent reports of changes in age, gender, and race of persons with oral cancer.

Radiology can be a valuable tool in the detection and diagnosis of malignant disease, as intraosseous malignancies, in addition to those that start peripherally but later invade bone, can cause detectable changes in the calcified structures of the teeth and bone. Many of the changes to bone brought about by malignancies either tend to be lytic or cause alterations to the normal trabecular pattern. The characteristic irregular and spike patterns of resorption of the roots of teeth are other changes to calcified structures that may originate from a malignancy.

Although malignancies represent a small fraction of both the common and uncommon lesions of the jaws, early detection is of constant and significant concern to practicing dentists. Along with regular oral cancer screenings, clinical surveillance for suspicious lesions, routine intraoral dental imaging, and panoramic radiographs often provide the ability to effectively visualize osseous lesions of malignant disease.

Initial discovery of oral and maxillofacial malignancies may result from complaints of pathognomonic symptoms, discovery of soft-tissue components of lesions during intraoral and extraoral examinations, or, rarely, radiographic findings. Most lesions are discovered late, after invasion of the regional lymph nodes, which may have become enlarged and sometimes painful. At present there is no specific tool or test in widespread use by dentists that could aid in oral and maxillofacial cancer screening and detection, other than meticulous clinical examination of the hard and soft tissues of the orofacial regions in addition to follow-up of suspected lesions with further testing, including appropriate radiographic examinations. The final and definitive diagnosis is generally the histopathology report, supplemented with clinical and radiographic findings.

The National Institute of Dental and Craniofacial Research describe one method of clinical examination.[3,7] The American Cancer Society and American Dental Association recommend that primary care clinicians and dentists initiate periodic examinations of the oral cavity and throat as part of routine cancer-related screenings.[2,3,8,9] The high-risk areas for oral cancer are the lateral borders of the tongue, the floor of the mouth and ventral side of tongue, the soft palate, and the tonsils. These and all of the other visible structures should be carefully examined during an oral cancer screening.

Oral cancer screening is an extremely important and sensitive topic, but despite the attention that cancer receives in both professional and lay publications, most oral cancers go unnoticed in their initial detectable stages. Dentists are trained to search for white or red patches, in addition to ulcers, during clinical examinations. Radiographic signs are also emphasized. This approach should be expanded to include HPV-related malignancies, which typically do not display discolored patches and, therefore, may go undetected for longer periods. Nevertheless, early detection, even if sometimes difficult, is the goal and currently is the main factor that might provide an improved prognosis. These recommended oral cancer screenings take place every 3 years for persons older than 20 and annually for those older than 40 years.[2,3,8,9]

Tables 1–4 show the pertinent details of benign and malignant lesions, and their differentiation from inflammatory lesions.

Table 1			
Frequently used and encountered terms in radiographic analysis			
Appearance	**2D Radiographs**	**CBCT/MDCT**	**MRI**
White	Radiopaque	High density (bone)	High-intensity signal (fluid, fat)
	Contrast agents: enhancement		
Black	Radiolucent	Low density (air, fluid)	Low-intensity signal (cortical bone)
Gray	Gray appearance is extremely relative to surroundings; can appear Radiopaque (sinusitis) or Radiolucent (intraosseous tumor)	Soft-tissue density	Isointense to muscle

Table 2
Radiographic features of malignant tumors

Features	Common to All	Unique to Some
Location and size	Almost anywhere; invade bone from soft tissues in risk areas; various sizes	Posterior mandible: sarcomas and metastases
Shape and borders	Irregular, ill-defined and noncorticated borders, finger-like projections, permeative pattern	Well-defined: some SCCs, IMC
Internal structure and density	Radiolucent: destructive, permeative pattern; remnant trabeculae	Radiopaque: osteosarcomas, breast and prostate metastases
Effects on surrounding structures	Irregular widening of the periodontal ligament space with floating-teeth appearance, resorption of cortical outlines, invasion of adjacent structures, no periosteal reaction	Root resorption: sarcomas and multiple myeloma. Periosteal reaction with sunray/hair-on-end appearance: osteosarcomas and prostate metastases

CLASSIFICATION

Once there is an initial diagnosis, advanced functional and anatomic imaging allows the cancer to be classified according to TNM staging. T is used to describe the primary tumor (size, aggressiveness), N addresses involved nearby lymph nodes, and M describes distant metastases. It is internationally accepted and used, but of importance

Table 3
Radiographic features of benign and malignant tumors to aid in making a differential diagnosis

Features	Benign	Malignant
Location	Almost anywhere (intraosseous or arising in soft tissue or cartilage)	Almost anywhere, depending on tissue of origin
Shape	Regular	Irregular
Borders	Corticated, well-defined; if inflamed can become poorly defined or punched-out, noncorticated; narrow transition zone	Mostly ill-defined; moth-eaten, permeative/infiltrative; wide transition zone
Density	Radiolucent, mixed, or radiopaque	Mostly radiolucent, with remnant trabeculae
Size	Varying sizes: from very small to extremely large	Same
Internal structure	Various degrees of homogeneity and different trabecular patterns: "honeycomb," "soap bubble," "tennis racket," etc. Uni- or multilocular	Heterogeneous, usually no discernible trabecular pattern. Remnant trabeculation
Effects on surrounding structures	Thinning and displacement of roots, cortical plates, sinus floor, mandibular canal. Rarely interruption/effacement	Rare displacement, mostly interruption with invasion of adjacent structures/spaces

Table 4
Radiographic features that differentiate malignancies from inflammatory lesion

Features	Inflammation	Malignancy
Location	Invades bone from adjacent structures (maxillary sinuses, teeth, soft tissues)	Same
Shape	Irregular	Same
Borders	Ill-defined, permeative, rarely corticated; wide transition zone	Same
Density	Depending on stage, varies from radiolucent to opaque and also mixed; sequestrum formation	Mostly radiolucent; remnant trabeculation may mimic sequestra
Size	Any size	Any size
Internal structure	Altered/resorbed trabecular pattern	Same
Effects on surrounding structures	Resorptive and/or stimulating new bone formation effects on adjacent cortices/medullar bone Root resorption Interruption/perforation of cortices Periosteal reaction ("onion skin")	No effect in surrounding trabecular bone No periosteal reaction (exception osteosarcoma: "sunburst") Most frequently no root resorption Perforation, pathologic fracture, invasion present

only when solid tumors are considered or assessed. It is of no use for staging a diffuse malignancy such as leukemia.

There are other classifications, depending on:

Tissue of Origin
- Carcinomas: epithelial origin
- Sarcomas, mesenchymal
- Hematopoietic malignancies: blood and lymph
- Metastases

Location of Head and Neck Cancers
- Oral
- Lips
- Nasal and nasopharyngeal
- Paranasal sinuses
- Oropharyngeal
- Larynx, thyroid, middle ear, salivary glands

Point of Origin
- Intraosseous/bony
- Soft tissue

1. Carcinomas are malignant tumors of epithelial origin that can arise in either soft tissue or bone.
   a. Squamous cell carcinoma (SCC) arises in the epithelium of the mucous membranes and skin. It is the second most common cancer of the skin after basal cell carcinoma, and is usually found in areas exposed to sunlight. It seems to affect males more than females (2:1) and more so in the sixth and seventh decades.
   SCC is also the most common head and neck malignancy and best portrays the term "oral cancer." Almost 90% of all head and neck cancers are SCCs. It

should be noted that 25% of oral malignancies are HPV-related and may not provide the typical presentation. SCC is also the most common malignancy of the oral cavity. When it occurs in the oral cavity, it most frequently involves the keratinized mucosa of the posterior mandible. SCC lesions can be easily confused with a benign growth when they are represented by a nontender soft-tissue mass or a nonhealing ulcer that eventually will cause resorption of the underlying bone (see **Figs. 3–5**). In addition to the mucosa, SCC can originate in other soft tissues, including the salivary glands, tongue (**Fig. 1**), floor of the mouth, and tonsillar area (Waldeyer ring).

b. SCC may also originate in bone (**Figs. 2–4**). It is then referred to as primary intraosseous SCC.[10–12] Primary intraosseous SCCs are thought to arise from trapped odontogenic epithelial remnants (rests of Malassez). It is a rare malignancy, more frequently affecting males than females. Primary intraosseous SCC most commonly arises in the posterior mandible (retromolar pad).

c. Another type of intraosseous epithelial malignancy is central (intraosseous) mucoepidermoid carcinoma (IMC). The mucoepidermoid carcinoma (MC) is the most common intraosseous salivary malignancy, and only 2% to 4% of all MC occur in the jaws, especially posterior mandible areas (mandible/maxilla ratio = 3:1 or 4:1).

d. Other sites of origin of intraosseous epithelial malignancies are the epithelial layers of an originally benign entity, such as an odontogenic cyst[13,14] (residual,[15] dentigerous) or tumor (keratocystic odontogenic tumor,[16] ameloblastoma[17]). These lesions are a variant of the intraosseous type, characterized by the malignant transformation of the epithelial lining, most likely as a result of a long-standing chronic inflammation within the benign tumor or cyst. The terminology for the ameloblastic type is ameloblastic carcinoma, which can develop de novo (most frequently) or from malignant transformation of the epithelial layer of a benign ameloblastoma. This lesion should be differentiated from malignant ameloblastoma, which is an aggressive form of ameloblastoma, histologically a well-differentiated, benign tumor that can still cause distant metastases (lungs).[18]

e. Malignancies of the paranasal sinuses are rare entities represented by SCC, adenocarcinoma, or adenoid cystic carcinoma (ACC) developing from the

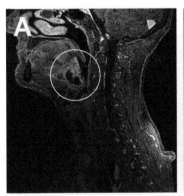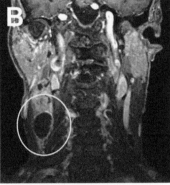

Fig. 1. Contrast-enhanced MR image of squamous cell carcinoma of the base of the tongue (*A*-sagittal slice) with invasion of lymph nodes (*B*-coronal). *Circles* indicate region of interest. (*Courtesy of* Dr Adrian T. Creanga, Ovidius University, Constanta, Romania.)

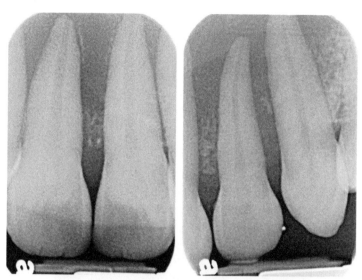

Fig. 2. Periapical radiographs of squamous cell carcinoma in the anterior maxilla: partially effaced lamina dura, and bone destruction with remnant trabeculation.

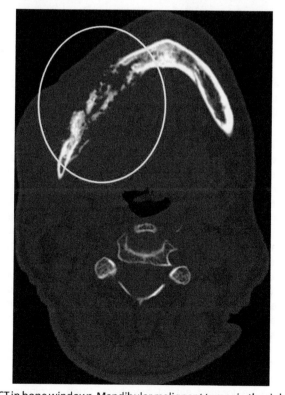

Fig. 3. Axial MDCT in bone windows. Mandibular malignant tumor in the right body, irregular moth-eaten appearance, permeative pattern, and cortical bone destruction with trabecular remnants. *Circle* indicate region of interest. (*Courtesy of* Dr Adrian T. Creanga, Ovidius University, Constanta, Romania.)

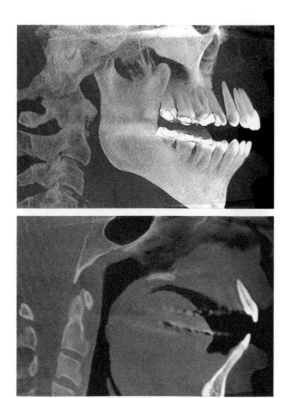

Fig. 4. CBCT sagittal slice and reconstructed cephalometric image showing bone destruction in the anterior maxilla with appearance of "floating teeth." (*Courtesy of* Dr Lois Levine, Wantagh, New York.)

mucosal lining (Schneiderian membrane).[19] SCC of the paranasal sinuses represents only 3% of all head and neck cancers, with the maxillary sinuses being affected most. SCC of the paranasal sinuses also affects males more, as opposed to ACC, which affects females twice as often and is more aggressive, with higher recurrence rates and higher incidence of distant metastases. Adenocarcinomas occur more in the ethmoid sinuses and seem to be related to hardwood dust exposure. The long-standing, mostly asymptomatic evolution of these lesions makes them difficult to be discovered in incipient phases. Therefore they are most frequently found in later stages, when the exact origin is difficult to establish. In fact, a lesion in the paranasal sinuses could have arisen in the maxilla (intraosseous, minor salivary gland of palatal mucosa, gingiva) and then invaded the maxillary sinus, or may have actually originated within the sinus, in the Schneiderian membrane.

f. Other types of carcinomas seen in the orofacial structures include salivary adenocarcinomas (polymorphous low grade, acinic cell), ACCs, MCs, and carcinomas arising in a benign pleomorphic adenoma (carcinoma ex benign mixed tumor). These lesions can affect any salivary gland, both major and minor, and therefore can be located almost anywhere. Such carcinomas can be slow-growing or fast-growing, and can evolve asymptomatically or be associated with pain and paresthesia. Besides these characteristic salivary malignancies, the salivary glands can be also affected by sarcomas, lymphomas, or metastases.

2. Sarcomas are malignancies of mesenchymal origin, originating from, and also producing, various types of abnormal tissues.[20] In comparison with previously described carcinomas, sarcomas tend to affect younger male patients. Their most characteristic clinical presentation is painful swelling. The most commonly found types are as follows.

   a. Osteosarcoma[21] is an uncommon malignant bone tumor, representing only 20% of all sarcomas. The jaw type represents about 6% to 8% of all osteosarcomas, and both intraosseous and extraosseous forms occur. The extraosseous types include parosteal and periosteal osteosarcomas. This tumor is also known as osteogenic sarcoma because of its ability to produce immature or abnormal bone (osteoid). It usually evolves asymptomatically until it becomes clinically evident as an intraoral or extraoral swelling that usually extends beyond the lower border of the mandible. The lesions are typically tender on palpation, diffuse and immobile, and possibly associated with lip/chin paresthesia, with and without trismus (**Figs. 5** and **6**).

   b. Chondrosarcomas[22] are only half as common as osteosarcomas. One percent to 3% of all chondrosarcomas appear in the head and neck area, with the most common site being the maxilla, followed by mandible, ramus, nasal septum, and paranasal sinuses.

   c. Fibrosarcoma is a malignant tumor of fibroblasts, producing collagen and elastin. Fibrosarcoma is very common in the extremities, with only 10% of all lesions occurring in the head and neck area. These tumors are known to be found in the nose and sinuses of young adults and children.

   d. Ewing sarcoma[23] is an extremely rare malignancy of neuroectodermal origin, more common in long bones (only 1%–2% in the craniofacial area) and affecting mostly young Caucasian males (approximately 80% are younger than 20 years). It represents the third most common bone malignancy of childhood, after osteosarcomas and chondrosarcomas. The clinical examination reveals local pain (most frequent symptom) and an associated palpable soft-tissue mass. Radiography reveals large poorly defined radiolucencies with adjacent soft-tissue invasion (**Fig. 7**).

   e. Other sarcomas found in the jaws include rhabdomyosarcoma, leiomyosarcoma, angiosarcoma, and liposarcoma, among others.

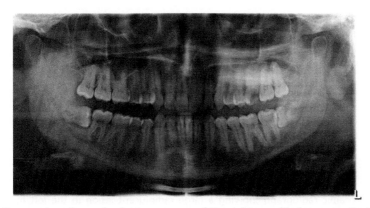

Fig. 5. Panoramic radiograph of osteosarcoma of the right mandibular ramus. Radiopaque entity with sunray appearance of the periosteal reaction. (*Courtesy of* Dr Frederico Prates, Porto Alegre, Brazil.)

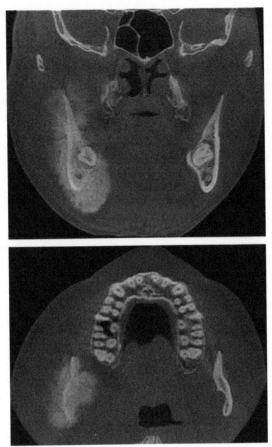

Fig. 6. CBCT coronal, sagittal, and axial slices. Osteogenic osteosarcoma, high-density area, and periosteal reaction. (*Courtesy of* Dr Frederico Prates, Porto Alegre, Brazil.)

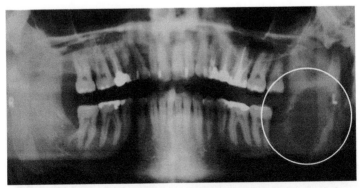

Fig. 7. Panoramic radiograph showing a large radiolucent lesion in the left mandibular ramus with pathologic fracture. The final diagnosis was Ewing sarcoma. *Circle* indicate region of interest. (*Courtesy of* Dr Joseph Rinaggio, Rutgers School of Dental Medicine, Newark, NJ, USA.)

3. Hematopoietic malignancies are uncommon in the head and neck area, and include the following.

   a. Multiple myeloma (plasma cell myeloma or plasmacytoma) is a hematopoietic malignancy originating in the medullar portion of bone. It represents 1% of all malignancies and 10% of all hematologic neoplasms, affecting jaws in 30% of cases. Multiple myeloma affects older black males more frequently, and its characteristic feature is pain in the lumbar spine with or without pathologic fracture. When occurring in the skull, it produces characteristic radiographic appearances referred to as "pepper-pot" or "raindrops" skull with multiple, well-defined, punched-out lesions of varying sizes, involving the skull vault.

   b. Non-Hodgkin lymphoma (malignant lymphoma, lymphosarcoma) is diagnosed annually in approximately 60,000 persons in the United States. Most frequently it arises in lymph nodes and grows as a nonpainful soft-tissue mass. When occurring in the oral cavity (posterior hard palate, gingiva, and mandible), it may arise and develop within bone or soft tissues and is considered an extranodal lesion, most frequently as part of a multifocal disease.

   c. Burkitt lymphoma[24] is an aggressive B-cell lymphoma that is considered to be a type of non-Hodgkin lymphoma; it mostly affects children, with 2 known main subtypes. The African endemic affects the jaws of African young male children (mean age 8 years), and is strongly related to Epstein-Barr virus and malaria. The sporadic or American subtype is not seen in jaws, as it mostly affects abdominal organs. A third subtype is the form associated with human immunodeficiency virus.

   d. Leukemia is a generic term that represents a vast number of hematopoietic malignancies (acute or chronic, myelogenous or lymphoblastic, and lymphocytic) that affect both adults and children. The clinical signs are mostly systemic, represented by frequent infections, easy bleeding, and bruising and fever. When occurring in the orofacial area, clinical signs are related to the marked incapacity to fight bacteria: inflammation (gingivitis/marginal periodontitis) and nonhealing ulcers. The radiographic signs are minimal (widened periodontal ligament space) or absent (**Figs. 8** and **9**).

4. Metastases[25–27] are known as secondary malignancies, and represent the spread of a primary tumor through the bloodstream from a distant site. Metastases often originate from breast, lung, prostate, colon and rectum, thyroid, or ovaries, and are most frequently of carcinomatous origin. In fact, metastatic carcinoma is the most frequent bone cancer, with more than 80% of all cases affecting the mandible. Their radiographic appearance is extremely variable, from radiolucent, to mixed, to completely radiopaque (**Fig. 10**). Most metastases, however, are characterized by a radiolucent appearance (**Fig. 11**).

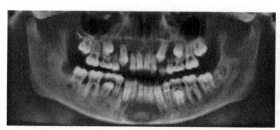 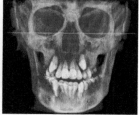

Fig. 8. CBCT panoramic reconstruction and 3D reconstruction in a patient with leukemia.

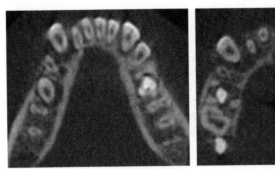

Fig. 9. Leukemia. Axial CBCT slices of maxilla and mandible showing widened periodontal ligament spaces and alveolar bone destruction.

The common clinical appearance indicating the existence of a malignancy is made up of 1 or more of the following features: mobile, displaced teeth; intraoral white or red patches; nonhealing ulceration with indurated or rolled borders; affected local or regional nerve functions, including anesthesia, paresthesia, hypotonia or atonia; effects of compression or invasion of blood vessels (eg, soft-tissue or bone necrosis, intraoral bone exposure); and locoregional lymphadenopathy (nonpainful, indurated, nonmobile nodes).

Patient complaints may include disgeusia, hypogeusia, or ageusia (distorted, limited, or absent taste), unexplained hemorrhage, epistaxis, foul taste and smell, lack of normal healing after surgery or trauma, unexplained or rapidly growing swelling or pain, trouble swallowing, sore throat that will not go away, earache, weight loss, anesthesia, paresthesia, hypotonia, or atonia. All these are nonspecific findings that may or may not directly indicate a malignancy, but must be pursued.

Based on patient history, complaint, and clinical findings, radiographs are prescribed. Certainly all lesions with underlying bone, even when the suspicion of malignancy is low, should be imaged (**Fig. 12**). Often, plain film (periapical or panoramic) imaging, with a second (occlusal) projection at 90° to the initial view, will allow visualization of changes to bone in the area. An understanding of the common paths of travel for malignancies may dictate imaging of certain regions, even when the detected

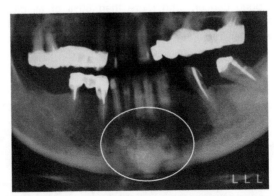

Fig. 10. Cropped panoramic radiograph showing a noncorticated and well-defined radiopacity in the anterior mandible (metastasis from breast cancer). *Circle* indicate region of interest. (*Courtesy of* Dr Adrian T. Creanga, Ovidius University, Constanta, Romania.)

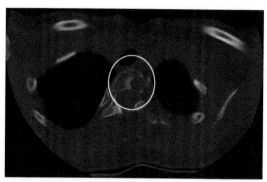

Fig. 11. Vertebral metastasis. Well-defined, punched-out, noncorticated radiolucency. *Circle* indicate region of interest. (*Courtesy of* Dr Adrian T. Creanga, Ovidius University, Constanta, Romania.)

lesion may not overlie bone. An example of this might be a lesion on the lateral border of the tongue, which may ultimately invade the bone of the posterior mandible.

All clinical findings should be correlated with radiographic features and vice versa. It should be noted that a 50% to 60% change in bone demineralization must occur for the osseous change to be radiographically visible. Therefore, a clinically apparent lesion may not yet be radiographically evident, even though there is some invasion of the bone. The final diagnosis is always made by the histopathologic examination.

Although the sequelae of undetected malignancy can be devastating, radiographic screening for detection of malignancies is seldom productive. Furthermore, it is certainly not cost effective to provide radiographic screenings for the purpose of detecting malignancies. Although radiographs are not prescribed for the purpose of detecting occult malignant lesions, it is imperative to examine all radiographs for signs of malignancy, regardless of clinical suspicion. Most of the radiographically visible malignant lesions are incidental findings.

RADIOGRAPHIC DIAGNOSIS

Diagnostic imaging is involved at many and different levels in the detection, evaluation, and management of malignant lesions.

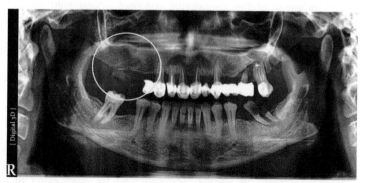

Fig. 12. Malignant tumor located in the right edentulous maxilla. Ill-defined, noncorticated radiolucency with interruption of the cortex and associated soft-tissue mass. *Circle* indicate region of interest. (*Courtesy of* Dr Adrian T. Creanga, Ovidius University, Constanta, Romania.)

1. Initial diagnosis
2. Accurate staging
3. Establishing the presence of invasion and spread, to better plan surgery and radiation therapy
4. Assessment of bony and lymph node involvement
5. Aid in determining an accurate biopsy site and/or excision, and so forth

Radiographic Examination

Radiographs of the jaws must be examined in a consistent and organized fashion. Because most lesions tend to be on one side of the jaws or the other, a general check for asymmetries should be made. Cortical borders are checked for effacement, expansion, thinning, scalloping, erosion, and other changes. Destruction of cortical borders indicates more aggressive lesions, whereas evidence of remodeling processes favors a diagnosis of less aggressive lesions. The lamina dura of the teeth, and crestal cortication, are part of the cortical boundaries of the maxilla and mandible, and should be included in the examination of cortices. Alterations in these structures include effacement, loss of distinct boundaries, replacement with new remodeled bone, and widening of the periodontal ligament space. Normal trabecular patterns demonstrate a response to physiologic stress. Alterations in these patterns indicate a response to nonphysiologic stressors.

Imaging Protocols

Although malignancies can be detected effectively on routine intraoral imaging (see **Fig. 7**), including periapical, bitewing, and occlusal radiographs, follow-up imaging is generally required. It should be stated that the entire lesion must be visible on the radiograph, along with a surrounding border of unaffected bone. Visualization of the third dimension (z axis) is also essential. Although follow-up imaging studies will almost undoubtedly included advanced imaging, an occlusal radiograph taken at 90° to the initial view can provide knowledge as to the full extent of the lesion, in addition to effects on adjacent structures.

Imaging Modalities

1. Conventional (intraoral and panoramic radiographs; scintigraphy). Possible findings of radiographic signs of malignancy include:
   a. Irregular widening of the periodontal ligament space with "floating-tooth" appearance mimicking periodontal disease. Displacement or resorption of the teeth is rare
   b. Poorly defined, noncorticated lesions, with a moth-eaten or punched-out appearance
   c. Irregularly shaped, heterogeneous internal structure, radiolucent, radiopaque, or mixed density area ± trabecular remnants.
   d. Destruction of cortical borders (floor of the maxillary sinus, nasal fossa, hard palate, alveolar ridge), enlargement of the mandibular canal and/or mental foramen, periosteal reaction
   e. Soft-tissue growth/mass (gingiva), invasion of adjacent structures (sinuses, mandibular canal, and so forth)
   f. Overall rapid growth of lesions, accompanied by destruction of adjacent anatomic structures

2. Advanced imaging, which includes 2 major types:
   a. Anatomic imaging (or structural), for example, dental computed tomography (CT) (cone-beam CT [CBCT]), medical CT (Multidetector CT [MDCT]) with or without contrast, and MRI.
   b. Functional imaging records metabolic activity, blood flow, and chemical composition. Positron emission tomography (PET) or PET-fused MDCT, single-photon emission CT (SPECT), and functional MRI (fMRI, eg, diffusion MRI) all offer an advanced 3-dimensional (3D) view and analysis of all maxillofacial structures (bone and soft tissue). These modalities are used to establish an accurate location and the full extent of a lesion (destruction and invasion of adjacent structures) based on metabolic activity. PET is capable of identifying very early lesions, owing to its ability to detect cellular metabolic activity related to malignancy. Functional imaging is used for diagnosing, staging, and even follow-up of different types of cancers. MRI offers the best soft-tissue contrast and therefore is used to diagnose soft-tissue conditions, such as temporomandibular joint–related conditions, soft-tissue neoplasia, and lymph node or perineural invasion.

Nuclear medicine is a medical specialty that uses internal sources of radiation (radioactive substances: technetium-99m, gallium-67, iodine-123 and -131, and so forth) for both diagnosis and treatment of certain conditions. Scintigraphy is a 2-dimensional (2D) nuclear medicine functional imaging modality. For the diagnostic imaging part, external detectors (gamma cameras) capture and record images from the internally emitted radiation, as opposed to conventional radiographs for which external x-ray sources are used. The 3D aspect of nuclear medicine is represented mainly by SPECT imaging, which uses gamma rays and is based on monitoring tissue biological activity in the area scanned.

Panoramic radiographs are useful for examining a large area of the jaws and adjacent structures. Although the resolution of a panoramic radiograph is lower than that of direct films or digital imaging, it is often adequate for initial identification of potentially malignant lesions, and is certainly higher than the resolution of advanced imaging modalities, such as CBCT, MDCT, and MRI.

Where available, CBCT can provide visualization of the third dimension in both multiplanar projections and oblique views. It is limited by its capacity to image only the hard tissues, with soft-tissue imaging confined to outlines. An important point is that, in general, oral and maxillofacial imaging can be confined to visualization of the lesion in 3 dimensions, as advanced functional and anatomic imaging will be prescribed as part of a workup to determine the staging of the malignancy. Although the resolution of CBCT is about half of that of panoramic radiographs, it is often adequate to determine the defining radiographic features of malignant lesions. Furthermore, CBCT permits multiplanar and oblique reconstructions, allowing the viewer to identify changes in complex hard-tissue structures including the maxilla, ethmoid and sphenoid bones, osteomeatal complex, and temporal bone.

MRI is an imaging technique that relies on the interaction of various components of the body with a strong magnetic field. The magnetic field creates a temporary realignment of the hydrogen atoms in the structure. Based on molecular structure of the anatomic component, a different signal will be transmitted to the detector when a radiofrequency (RF) pulse is applied perpendicular to the magnetic field. It must be emphasized that this technique does not rely on ionizing radiation.

MRI accurately images both hard and soft tissues; however, it is most useful for soft-tissue imaging, as it produces images that discriminate between soft-tissue components (fat, nerve, and connective tissue), fluid, and tumors.

MRI is used in dentistry for imaging of the soft-tissue components of the temporo-mandibular joint. It is also useful in imaging tumors, as the tumor can often be distinguished from the surrounding normal tissues and structures on MR images.

A peculiar feature of MRI is the appearance of calcified structures. Because calcified structures, such as bone and teeth, are low in water content and, therefore, low in hydrogen atoms, they reflect the RF signal poorly, leaving a dark area on the resultant image. This effect is termed nonenhancing or low signal intensity. Soft-tissue structures typically have higher water content and, therefore, produce images of varying shades of gray.

Different scanning protocols are used, based on the anticipated findings. T1-weighted images are used for demonstration of anatomic structures; characteristically fat will appear bright (enhancing), whereas water takes on a dark appearance.

When a tumor is known or suspected, T2-weighted images are generally preferred. In these images water appears bright, whereas fat appears darker. Lesions (both benign and malignant) tend to have higher water content than normal tissue and, therefore, will appear brighter than the surrounding tissues. In addition, benign lesions may have a cystic component with high water content. Moreover, benign and malignant tumors may cause liquefaction from tissue necrosis, producing an enhancing signal. Perineural invasion and, thus, tumor spread are best seen on contrast-enhanced T1-weighted MRI. In this case, MRI is preferred to CT because of reduced metallic artifacts and better soft-tissue contrast. The same enhanced soft-tissue contrast is extremely useful in assessing regional lymph node invasion. In these cases, CT will mostly show indirect signs of nerve invasion, such as enlargement or displacement of foramina and, in later stages, bone erosion. Contrast-enhanced protocols are preferred for both modalities because of the inherent ability to assess the vascular component.

Initial Detection of Lesions

Detection of malignancies of the jaws takes several different paths. The most straightforward diagnosis can often be made from patients' complaints that include obvious clinical signs of malignancies, including paresthesia, dysesthesia, swelling, ulceration, and bleeding. Detection of suspicious lesions during routine oral cancer screening also can begin the diagnostic process. Radiographs are indicated when a clinically suspicious lesion overlies bone.

For radiographic assessment, it is always important to remember that interpretation of radiographs is mainly a subjective process. The radiographic appearance of anatomic structures is based on the interactions of x-ray photons with the components of the oral cavity and surrounding structures. The energy levels of the photons are based on the type of x-ray machine and the strings used, and the x-ray detector. Some notions are clear and straightforward: air appears black, bone appears white, and soft tissues appear in various shades of gray. Depending on surrounding structures, fluid or soft tissue may appear opaque. This appearance can be illustrated with lesions seen developing within the paranasal sinuses, in contrast to the radiolucent appearance it has when located within bone (see **Table 1**).

Specific radiographic features of malignancies include radiolucent (hypodense) internal architecture with indistinct borders, projections of the lesion into normal bone, effacement of medullary bone, and destruction of adjacent cortical borders. Although most intraosseous lesions do not produce bone, it is not uncommon for pieces of nonvital bone to be entrapped in the soft tissue of the lesion, yielding a mixed-density appearance (**Fig. 13**).

Pathologic fractures are frequently seen as a by-product of the bony destruction. Once a cortical border has been breached and expansion of the lesion is unchecked

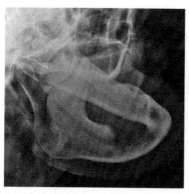
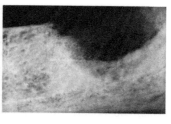

Fig. 13. Mandibular malignant tumor-gingival carcinoma with invasion of underlying bone. Irregularly shaped, ill-defined, noncorticated radiolucency with slight evidence of trabecular remnants within (right) and wide of area of transition (left). (*Courtesy of* Dr Adrian T. Creanga, Ovidius University, Constanta, Romania.)

by adjacent structures, lesions tend to grow as masses with smooth soft-tissue borders (**Fig. 14**); this holds especially true when lesions in the posterior maxilla expand through the sinus floor into the lumen of the maxillary sinus. Effects of malignancies on adjacent teeth include displacement mimicking premature eruption and root resorption. The appearance of root resorption caused by malignancy differs from the blunted appearance generated by inflammation, benign cysts or tumors, and orthodontic tooth movement. Resorption caused by malignancy gives the root a spiked and irregular appearance. A pathognomonic feature of malignant lesions is the lack of surrounding reactive bone, giving malignant lesions a punched-out appearance usually associated with multiple myeloma, but is also seen in other lesions. A typical feature of sarcomas that have expanded through the periosteum of the primary bone is a sunray appearance found within a soft-tissue mass (see **Figs. 5** and **6**).

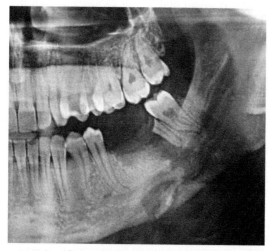

Fig. 14. Cropped panoramic radiograph showing osteomyelitis with sequestrum formation close to the inferior border of the left mandible.

Radiographic Appearance

When describing and assessing a radiographic image, there are certain features to follow.

1. Size. Although a characteristic of malignancy is rapid and uncontrolled growth, it should be remembered that all lesions do start out small. Therefore, the following radiographic features may also apply to small lesions. If a lesion is suspicious it should be followed up, regardless of size.
2. Location. Both primary and metastatic tumors may be found anywhere in the maxillofacial region. Tumors can originate in either bone (primary intraosseous tumor) or soft tissue, secondarily invade bone (gingival carcinoma) or nearby structures, or travel from distant originating sites (eg, prostate, breast, kidney) through blood or lymph and metastasize at maxillofacial level. Primary carcinomas are most frequently seen in the high-risk areas mentioned earlier (eg, floor of the mouth, tonsils, Waldeyer ring, soft palate, tongue), whereas sarcomas mostly affect the posterior mandible. Metastases are more common in the posterior regions of both jaws.
3. Shape and borders. Characteristically, most malignancies have irregular shapes and poorly defined, noncorticated margins, appearing to blend in with surrounding normal bone (permeative or infiltrative patterns). When assessing an osteolytic lesion, a wide zone of transition may indicate an aggressive and infiltrative process. A narrow zone of transition with well-defined borders favors a benign lesion. Rarely, if it is slow-growing and invading bone from surrounding soft-tissue structures, a malignant lesion could exhibit defined and somewhat corticated outlines. Asymmetrical shapes of lesions, in both 2D and 3D imaging, should be considered suspicious (see **Fig. 12**). A significant exception is the IMC, which can exhibit well-defined sclerotic borders.
4. Density and internal structure/architecture. Most malignancies appear as unilocular or multilocular radiolucencies, as they tend to cause bone destruction without inducing reactive bone formation. Sometimes, because of their rapid advancement, malignancies may display remnant sparse trabeculation. Other tumors either produce abnormal bone (osteogenic sarcomas) or induce abnormal reactive bone formation (metastatic prostate and breast cancers) so that their appearance, at least in part, is radiopaque. Rapidly growing lesions may entrap pieces of trabecular bone, yielding a radiolucent appearance with some radiopaque foci, or display ill-defined, thick, coarse bony septa with an overall multilocular, multicystic appearance, as is sometimes seen in IMC. This tumor also exhibits a mixed radiopaque-radiolucent appearance.
5. Effects on surrounding structures. Malignant lesions are usually aggressive, rapidly evolving, and generally destructive and invasive. Owing to their rapid evolution, roots of teeth are usually unaffected, appearing to be "floating in air" because of the destruction of the alveolar support and effacement of the lamina dura (see **Figs. 1**B, **2**, and **8**). Sarcomas and multiple myelomas may cause root resorption. When root resorption is present, it usually follows a "spiked" pattern, as opposed to the regular horizontal resorption or displacement seen in benign tumors (ameloblastoma, Pindborg tumor), inflammatory lesions, or cysts. Destruction of cortical outlines and invasion of adjacent spaces or structures through the path of least resistance (eg, maxillary sinus, nasal fossa, carotid space, mandibular canal) is common. If outer cortical plates are destroyed or interrupted, there is usually no periosteal reaction. An exception would be sarcomas, whereby unusual patterns of reactive new bone formation are noted when the lesion has expanded beyond

the periosteum of the primary site. Descriptive terms of these bony growth include "sunray," "sunburst," "hair-on-end," and even "onion skin" if secondarily infected or inflamed. Another characteristic appearance of the periosteal reaction is the Codman triangle, seen in aggressive lesions such as Ewing sarcomas or, rarely, osteosarcomas. Aggressive lesions have an extremely rapid evolution that will not allow the periosteal new layers to ossify completely, so only the edges will have a bony appearance (see **Table 2**).

Management

If a suspicious lesion is observed clinically it should be radiographed, especially when there is underlying bone. The first step in imaging small lesions should always be conventional radiographs. In some cases a simple intraoral periapical radiograph would suffice. If size or location indicates, panoramic radiographs will offer a comprehensive overview of the entire oral and maxillofacial complex.

Even if the clinical diagnosis is reasonably certain, advanced imaging should be considered to obtain more information such as exact location, full extent, and lymph node or perineural invasion. MDCT with contrast, MRI, or PET scans are huge aids in diagnosis, localization of lesions, planning, staging, surgical excision, radiation, and chemotherapy. Advanced functional and anatomic imaging is usually performed on prescription of the oncologist, and may be based on the diagnosis of tissue type and the genetic typing of the tumor.

The usual course of treatment involves a multidisciplinary approach and is usually represented by a combination of surgical excision (for tumor removal) with usually wide clearance margins (1.5–2 cm) with or without radical neck resection (stage depending), followed by radiation therapy with or without chemotherapy (to destroy any remaining malignant cell).

Radiographic follow-up of patients with cancer is mandatory: radiographs are generally indicated every 3 months in the first year, every 6 months in the second year, and once a year from the third year onward. However, protocols for radiographic follow-up change based on evidence.

Essential considerations for postradiation therapy are the potential sequelae of xerostomia, radiation caries, and osteoradionecrosis. In cases of multiple myeloma and other bone conditions, bisphosphonate medication is administered and, therefore, medication-related osteonecrosis of the jaws (MRONJ) is a distinct possibility.[28] The risk of MRONJ among patients with cancer depends on the type of drug and dose administered, and is about 1%. MRONJ is similar clinically and radiographically to osteoradionecrosis and osteomyelitis. Radiographic features of osteonecrotic conditions include sequestrum formation, a mixed hyperdense and hypodense appearance of the medullary bone, with a moth-eaten appearance, and erosion of cortical borders of both the surfaces of the bone and internal structures, such as canals. In the mandible, the inferior alveolar canal may appear widened, with poorly defined borders. Diagnosis may often be made from the careful examination of the patient's dental and medical history. Osteonecrotic conditions require an initial triggering stimulus, which is almost always an invasive dental procedure: extraction, endodontic or periodontal treatment, or other procedures whereby oral bacteria may be introduced into the bone. Therefore, careful examination and treatment of a patient undergoing either radiation therapy or bisphosphonate medication is essential and should be prioritized. Teeth with poor prognoses should be extracted and any anticipated invasive procedure should be completed before administration of radiation therapy or bisphosphonates. It is also significant that osteonecrotic conditions may mimic metastatic or primary lesions of malignancies, so biopsy may be indicated (**Figs. 15** and **16**).

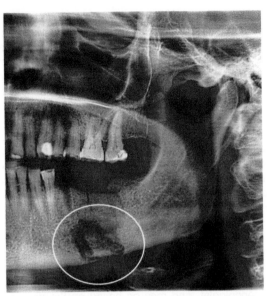

Fig. 15. MRONJ with sequestrum formation. Well-defined, noncorticated, mixed-density lesion located at the level of the inferior border of the mandible. *Circle* indicate region of interest. (*Courtesy of* Dr Adrian T. Creanga, Ovidius University, Constanta, Romania.)

Differential Diagnoses

In general, it is difficult differentiate one malignant tumor from another based solely on the radiographic appearance. Malignancies have many common radiographic features. Furthermore, different stages of development of some tumors may produce different effects (see **Tables 3** and **4**).

1. Carcinomas are usually well discernible from other malignancies, especially if there is a correlating clinical appearance and histologic features. Diagnostic difficulties are presented by lesions that may have similar radiographic features, such as inflammation, including apical inflammatory lesions, marginal periodontitis, and osteomyelitis (see **Fig. 10**). Even though the radiographic appearance of carcinomas tends to be

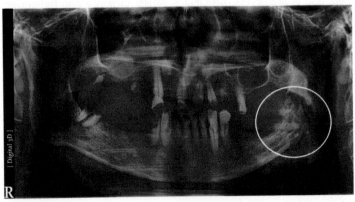

Fig. 16. Osteoradionecrosis of left mandible. *Circle* indicate region of interest. (*Courtesy of* Dr Adrian T. Creanga, Ovidius University, Constanta, Romania.)

similar to that of inflammatory lesions, involving mostly bone destruction, there is usually no periosteal reaction in malignant lesions. The remnant trabeculation mentioned earlier can sometimes mimic the sequestra found in osteomyelitis. If the tumor becomes secondarily infected, differentiation would be almost impossible and final diagnosis would require a more thorough, advanced imaging modality (CT with contrast, MRI, PET, nuclear medicine imaging). When originating in bone, malignancy can sometimes mimic periapical cysts or granulomas. When odontogenic cysts become infected they tend to lose cortication and become less well defined, a common malignant feature that may easily be misread. Other benign entities should be considered, especially when assessing a slow-growing, low-grade malignancy such as IMC, ameloblastoma, keratocystic odontogenic tumor, or glandular odontogenic cyst.

2. Metastatic disease should be considered first if the existence of the primary tumor is known. Other entities to consider are primary malignancies and marginal periodontal disease.

3. Regarding sarcomas, entities to consider are other sarcomas, benign fibro-osseous lesions, and metastases, depending on the internal structure and overall appearance. Diagnostic features to remember are the characteristic patterns of the periosteal reaction, especially "sunray" and Codman triangles (see **Figs. 3** and **4**). Sometimes the result of a histopathologic analysis of a chondrosarcoma slice may be identical to that of fibrous dysplasia, so a final diagnosis will rely mostly on the radiographic features.

SUMMARY

Although malignancies in the orofacial structures are rare, early diagnosis and treatment may have a significant impact on the long-term survival and quality of life of patients. Along with a thorough medical and surgical history, considerations of habits such as alcohol and tobacco use, and meticulous clinical examination, radiographs play a valuable role in the diagnosis of malignant lesions. All practitioners should be familiar with radiographic prescribing guidelines and the radiographic characteristics of malignancies to ensure the earliest diagnosis possible. Also important is that early-stage malignant lesions, as viewed on a radiograph, may not yield enough information to yield an exact diagnosis. The goal for practitioners should be to identify suspicious lesions and make the appropriate referrals, so that a diagnosis and treatment can be obtained rapidly.

All long-standing, nonhealing clinically visible lesions overlying bone should be imaged.
Irregular borders, destructive patterns, and invasion of surrounding structures are most suggestive of malignancy.
Radiographic appearance is relative and subjective, and perception depends on surrounding structures and contrast. Soft tissue appears opaque in the maxillary sinus and lucent when within bone.
Most frequently, malignancy does not cause a periosteal reaction, a fact that helps to differentiate it from inflammatory lesions.
Risk areas for oropharyngeal cancer are lateral borders of the tongue, the floor of the mouth and ventral side of tongue, the soft palate, and the tonsils.
Although radiographs are not taken for the sole purpose of cancer screening, all radiographs acquired are carefully and thoroughly examined.
Cortical bone appears white on radiographic images (conventional or CT) and black on MRI. The fat content of trabecular bone marrow will make it appear bright on T1-weighted images.
The final and definitive diagnosis is almost always based on the histopathologic examination of the biopsy specimen, but the "road" to there is always paved with correlations made between clinical and radiographic findings.

REFERENCES

1. Available at: http://www.cancer.gov/researchandfunding/progress/snapshots/headandneck.
2. Available at: http://www.oralcancerfoundation.org/.
3. Available at: http://www.ada.org/en/member-center/oral-health-topics/cancer-oral.
4. Available at: http://www.cancer.gov/publications/patient-education/WYNTK_oral.pdf.
5. Tomar S, Graves CA, Altomare D, et al. Human papillomavirus status and gene expression profiles of oropharyngeal and oral cancers from European American and African American patients. Head Neck 2015. http://dx.doi.org/10.1002/hed.24072.
6. Gandini S, Negri E, Boffetta P, et al. Mouthwash and oral cancer risk quantitative meta-analysis of epidemiologic studies. Ann Agric Environ Med 2012;19(2):173–80.
7. Available at: http://www.nidcr.nih.gov/oralhealth/Topics/OralCancer/DetectingOralCancer.htm#TheExam.
8. Omar E. Current concepts and future of noninvasive procedures for diagnosing oral squamous cell carcinoma—a systematic review. Head Face Med 2015;11(1):6.
9. Brocklehurst P, Kujan O, O'Malley LA, et al. Screening programmes for the early detection and prevention of oral cancer. Cochrane Database Syst Rev 2013;(11):CD004150.
10. Tiwari M. Primary intraosseous carcinoma of the mandible: a case report with literature review. J Oral Maxillofac Pathol 2011;15(2):205–10.
11. Lugakingira M, Pytynia K, Kolokythas A, et al. Primary intraosseous carcinoma of the mandible: case report and review of the literature. Oral Maxillofac Surg 2010;68(10):2623–9.
12. Chan KC, Pharoah M, Lee L, et al. Intraosseous mucoepidermoid carcinoma: a review of the diagnostic imaging features of four jaw cases. Dentomaxillofac Radiol 2013;42(4):20110162.
13. Jain M, Mittal S, Gupta DK. Primary intraosseous squamous cell carcinoma arising in odontogenic cysts: an insight in pathogenesis. J Oral Maxillofac Surg 2013;71(1):e7–14.
14. Araújo JP, Kowalski LP, Rodrigues ML, et al. Malignant transformation of an odontogenic cyst in a period of 10 years. Case Rep Dent 2014;2014:762969.
15. Muglali M, Sumer AP. Squamous cell carcinoma arising in a residual cyst: a case report. J Contemp Dent Pract 2008;9(6):115–21.
16. Park HK, Kim TS, Geum DH, et al. Mandibular intraosseous squamous cell carcinoma lesion associated with odontogenic keratocyst: a case report. J Korean Assoc Oral Maxillofac Surg 2015;41(2):78–83.
17. Kallianpur S, Jadwani S, Misra B, et al. Ameloblastic carcinoma of the mandible: report of a case and review. J Oral Maxillofac Pathol 2014;18(Suppl 1):S96–102.
18. Slootweg PJ, Müller H. Malignant ameloblastoma or ameloblastic carcinoma. Oral Surg Oral Med Oral Pathol 1984;57(2):168–76.
19. Das S, Kirsch CF. Imaging of lumps and bumps in the nose: a review of sinonasal tumours. Cancer Imaging 2005;5:167–77.
20. Yamaguchi S, Nagasawa H, Suzuki T, et al. Sarcomas of the oral and maxillofacial region: a review of 32 cases in 25 years. Clin Oral Investig 2004;8(2):52–5.
21. Chittaranjan B, Tejasvi MA, Babu BB, et al. Intramedullary osteosarcoma of the mandible: a clinicoradiologic perspective. J Clin Imaging Sci 2014;4(Suppl 2):6.

22. Pontes HA, Pontes FS, de Abreu MC, et al. Clinicopathological analysis of head and neck chondrosarcoma: three case reports and literature review. Int J Oral Maxillofac Surg 2012;41(2):203–10.

23. Rao BH, Rai G, Hassan S, et al. Ewing's sarcoma of the mandible. Natl J Maxillofac Surg 2011;2(2):184–8.

24. Ugar DA, Bozkaya S, Karaca I, et al. Childhood craniofacial Burkitt's lymphoma presenting as maxillary swelling: report of a case and review of literature. J Dent Child (Chic) 2006;73(1):45–50.

25. Hirshberg A, Shnaiderman-Shapiro A, Kaplan I, et al. Metastatic tumours to the oral cavity—pathogenesis and analysis of 673 cases. Oral Oncol 2008;44(8): 743–52.

26. Hirshberg A, Buchner A. Metastatic tumours to the oral region. An overview. Eur J Cancer B Oral Oncol 1995;31B(6):355–60.

27. Varghese G, Singh SP, Sreela LS. A rare case of breast carcinoma metastasis to mandible and vertebrae. Natl J Maxillofac Surg 2014;5(2):184–7.

28. Ruggiero SL, Dodson TB, Fantasia J, et al, American Association of Oral and Maxillofacial Surgeons. American Association of Oral and Maxillofacial Surgeons position paper on medication-related osteonecrosis of the jaw—2014 update. J Oral Maxillofac Surg 2014;72(10):1938–56.

Benign Fibro-Osseous Lesions of the Jaws

Kenneth Abramovitch, DDS, MS[a,b],*, Dwight D. Rice, DDS[a]

KEYWORDS

- Benign cementoblastoma • Juvenile ossifying fibroma
- Craniofacial fibrous dysplasia • McCune Albright syndrome • Ossifying fibroma
- Florid osseous dysplasia • Periapical osseous dysplasia

KEY POINTS

- Fibro-osseous lesions share a common histology of benign fibrous connective tissue with varying degrees of mineralization such that histologic information alone is inadequate for a diagnosis. Variations in the location of the lesions, age and gender of the patient affect the behaviors that range from insidious to aggressive neoplasias, hamartomas and dyspalsias. Specific radiographic presentations become major findings in establishing a diagnosis.
- Osseous dysplasia in the jaws have multiple presentations that range from periapical osseous dysplasia (POD), focal osseous dysplasia (Fo OD) to florid osseous dysplasia (Fl OD). The histologic patterns are similar but the location and degree of extension are the variables that differentiate these types.
- Odontogenic neoplasms that fit into the category of benign fibro-osseous lesions include the ossifying fibroma and the benign cementoblastoma.
- Monostotic and polyostitic fibrous dysplasias affect larger areas in the craniofacial complex. The size and extent of the lesions are the major determinants of their degrees of morbidity.

INTRODUCTION

Some of the earliest discussions on fibro-osseous lesions of the jaws have been presented by Waldron and Giansanti.[1–3] These lesions are grouped together because histologically they show replacement of bone with benign connective tissue along with varying degrees of mineralization. In the jaws, these mineralization patterns vary in

[a] Department of Radiologic and Imaging Sciences, School of Dentistry, Loma Linda University, 11092 Anderson Street, Prince Hall 4409, Loma Linda, CA 92350, USA; [b] Department of Radiology, School of Medicine, Loma Linda University, 11030 Anderson Street, Prince Hall 4409, Loma Linda, CA 92350, USA
* Corresponding author. School of Dentistry, Loma Linda University, 11092 Anderson Street, Prince Hall 4409, Loma Linda, CA 92350.
E-mail address: kabramovitch@llu.edu

Dent Clin N Am 60 (2016) 167–193
http://dx.doi.org/10.1016/j.cden.2015.08.010
0011-8532/16/$ – see front matter © 2016 Elsevier Inc. All rights reserved.

appearance between patterns of woven bone and acellular cementum. However, the distinctions between woven bone and acellular cementum have often been difficult to determine. Because of the similarity, a detailed description of the histologic differences between cementum and bone is not included in this discussion. In general, early-stage lesions demonstrate fibroblast-like cells in proliferating fibrous connective tissue with interspersed areas of mineralization. As the lesions increase in size and become more mature, the degree of mineralization increases to dense, sclerotic, acellular, avascular mineralized tissue.[4,5] The histologic patterns are frequently so ubiquitous that the histologic information alone is often inadequate to commit to a definitive diagnosis.[6]

Despite the histologic ubiquity, their behaviors vary significantly. Variations occur due to their location, and the age and gender of the patient. Some exhibit an insidious presence, whereas others are extensive and aggressive. Some lesions are neoplastic, whereas others are hamartomas or dysplastic. Because of the broad range of morbidity among them, the range of treatments varies depending on the diagnosis. Therefore, it is important to be able to differentiate between them in the preliminary diagnostic process.

The radiographic presentations, along with the location of the bony changes, are often extremely critical diagnostic features to help render a differential or working diagnosis in lieu of an automatic biopsy procedure. Therefore the unique and specific radiographic presentations may be one of the main criteria for preliminary diagnosis. Hence, it is of utmost significance that clinicians be familiar with their range of presentation, and be able to develop a differential diagnosis.

OSSEOUS DYSPLASIA IN THE JAWS

Osseous dysplasias in the jaws are the most common of the fibro-osseous lesions. These lesions are more commonly referred to as cemental dysplasias, cemento-osseous dysplasias or cementomas. However, recent publications suggest that references to the term cementum should be discontinued.[7,8] The rational is that cementum cannot really be identified in histologic specimens nor can it be identified with any certainty on radiographic images. Various references have in the past also reported that a histologic identification of cementum is difficult to establish or confirm. The mineralized masses are more comfortably referred to as amorphous woven bone patterns.

Three different types of distribution patterns have been described; periapical, focal, and florid. The periapical pattern is described when the lesions occur adjacent to the periapices of teeth, or in the vicinity of teeth in edentate cases. It affects multiple teeth and multiple quadrants of the maxilla and mandible, but it is more common in the mandible.

The focal pattern is used to describe situations when the lesion is only identified in one area of a single tooth or even multiple adjacent teeth. The possibility that a focal dysplasia may eventually occur in other parts of the jaws develops over time.

The florid description is a more widespread or extensive distribution of the periapical form. A clear delineation between the periapical and the florid patterns has not been reported and is often subjective. If the periapical pattern is present in 3 or 4 quadrants, or is extensive in the jaws, the term florid is often applied. Although there is no distinct delineation between alveolar bone and basal bone in the maxilla or mandible, we are of the opinion that when periapical osseous dysplasia (POD) apically extends to a recognizable area of the basal bone, then the term florid becomes more appropriate.

Demographic indices of gender, age, and race, the location of the lesion, the lack of symptoms, and the radiographic findings all support a diagnosis of osseous dysplasia in the jaws.

Periapical Osseous Dysplasia

General comments

These lesions occur when fibrous connective tissues replace the mineralized pattern of alveolar bone. When these changes in the periapical regions of the dentition occur, the term POD is used. As previously alluded to, other names used in the past include periapical cemental dysplasia, periapical cemento-osseous dysplasia, and periapical cementoma.

Clinical presentation

POD presents in young and middle-aged adults. The median age has been reported at 39 years. There is a high gender prominence with more than 90% of cases occurring in women. There is also a racial predominance. Most cases occur in blacks. Asians are also affected but to a lesser extent. A minority of cases occur in whites.

There are few clinical signs noted in POD. The dentition and the overlying mucosa remain unaffected by the bone changes. There are no symptoms and teeth remain vital despite the changes in the supporting bone. As the changes in POD become more extensive, expansion of the buccal and lingual cortices may occur. Only in these instances may changes may be noted clinically. Tooth displacement does not occur.

Radiographic features

There are variable appearances to these lesions that are primarily a function of time. In the earliest stages, radiolucent patterns are identified in the periapical regions of the alveolar bone, which changes the radiographic appearance of the typical attachment pattern of the adjacent teeth to the alveolar bone. The resultant radiolucent lesions closely resemble the periapical radiolucent patterns seen in a chronic dentoalveolar abscess. However, in these early POD cases, there are usually no signs of pulpal necrosis and there is no associated history of trauma (**Figs. 1** and **2A–C**). Another interesting finding is that these lesions are not always centered adjacent to the anatomic apices of the adjacent teeth. The advent of cone beam computed tomography (CBCT) has permitted better localization of these lesions, demonstrating the lack of centricity at the anatomic root apices. In such cases, these lesions may be more buccal or lingual, or occur along the lateral aspects of the anatomic apex. **Fig. 2D–H** shows a case where the radiolucent patterns are not epicentered around the anatomic apices of the teeth.

With time, mineralization begins to occur within the fibrous tissue and radiopaque areas appear within the matrix (**Figs. 3–5**). The description of this particular pattern is that of mixed radiolucent-radiopaque pattern.

As the condition continues to mature, the radiolucent areas diminish and a denser and more homogeneous radiopaque pattern can be seen (refer to **Figs. 6–8** for examples of this more advanced phase).

Management

POD may be considered a self-limiting condition. The changes in bone over a lifetime are not expected to require treatment from overgrowth of bone as in a true neoplasm. However, POD may predispose patients to potential problems with bone sequestration and low-grade osteomyelitis from any concurrent periapical or periodontal disease or trauma from a surgical procedure, such as end osseous root-form implant placement. These problems arise because of the reduced blood supply in relation to the dense acellular woven bony matrix. As mentioned previously, with time, POD can be expected to increase in size because of the radiolucent rim, which is usually osteoid in nature. As this occurs and the blood supply is further diminished in relation

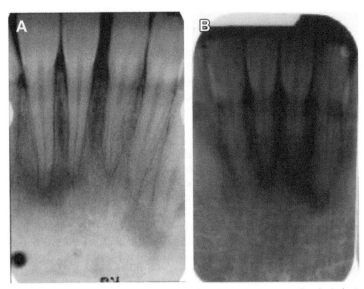

Fig. 1. (*A*, *B*) Periapical radiographic examples of early-stage osseous dysplasia lesions in the anterior mandible of black women less than 35 years of age. The lesions are in the periapical region changing the radiographic appearance of the typical attachment pattern of the adjacent dentition to the alveolar bone. In these cases, the alveolar bone pattern changes as bone is replaced by fibrous tissue. This presents a pattern where the periodontal ligament and lamina dura are lost and there is an appearance of radiolucency at the apices of the affected teeth.

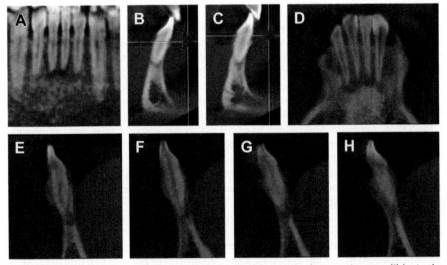

Fig. 2. CBCT imaging of early-stage osseous dysplasia lesions in the anterior mandible. In the first case, the coronal (*A*) and related cross-sections (*B*, *C*) show the irregular pattern of fibrous connective tissue replacement of the mandibular central incisor periapical tissues. In the second case, the coronal (*D*) and related cross-sections (*E–H*) show how the dysplastic changes and the radiolucent patterns are not centered at the anatomic apices, quite unlike the periapical changes noted with dentoalveolar abscess formation. These changes are similar to **Fig. 1** where the periodontal ligament and lamina dura are lost and there is an appearance of radiolucency at the apices of the affected teeth. (*Courtesy of* Dr Douglas Snider, Chico, CA.)

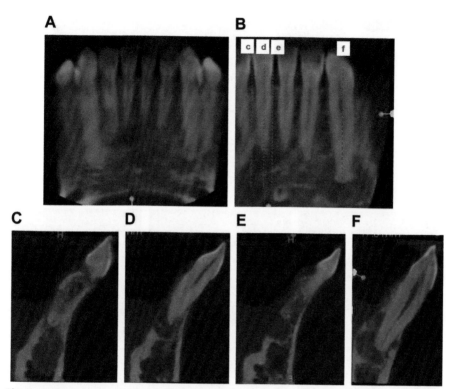

Fig. 3. CBCT Findings of POD in a 35-year-old black woman. On tooth #22, there is a well-demarcated, noncorticated periapical mixed radiolucent-radiopaque lesion. This area is at the anatomic tooth apex and extends to the mid-root level along the lingual aspect of the root. Mild lingual expansion is also noted. It has an ovoid shape ~9 × 10 mm in greatest dimensions. A 2-mm diameter radiolucency is also present along the facial periodontal ligament. These patterns lack the circumferential epicentered pattern of radiolucency related to chronic dentoalveolar abscess. At tooth #25, the well-demarcated, noncorticated periapical radiolucent lesion extends to but does not alter the apices of the adjacent teeth #24 and #26. It has a small ~2-mm diameter radiopacity within the lumen. It also extends to and thins the lingual cortical outline. This area is not expansive. A similar ovoid area is noted inferior to #25 and #26. It is not near the apices but has a similar pattern to the #25 and #22 lesions. (*A*) Coronal reconstruction of the anterior mandible. (*B*) Coronal reconstruction of the anterior mandible with the locations of the cross-sectional images (*C–F*). (*C*) Cross-section of #25/#26 inter-radicular area. (*D*) Cross-section of #25. (*E*) Cross-section of #25 near midline. (*F*) Cross-section of #22. The alphabets and dotted lines in **Fig. 3**B identify the locations of **Fig. 3**C–F.

to the mass of bone, adjacent periapical or periodontal infections may become more difficult to manage.

A frequent restorative question often arises in situations where there is an edentulous alveolar ridge and dental implants are being considered as a treatment option. Although dental implant placement is not specifically contraindicated, the compromised blood supply to the anterior mandible compromises the prognosis of prosthodontic implant treatment. The risk of implant failure may be higher because, as the radiopaque pattern in the area of osseointegration becomes denser, the less likely it is that osseointegration can occur. However, a definitive prognosis is not possible and each case must be considered on an individual basis. Using contemporary standards of informed consent, patients must be informed and cautioned that there is a

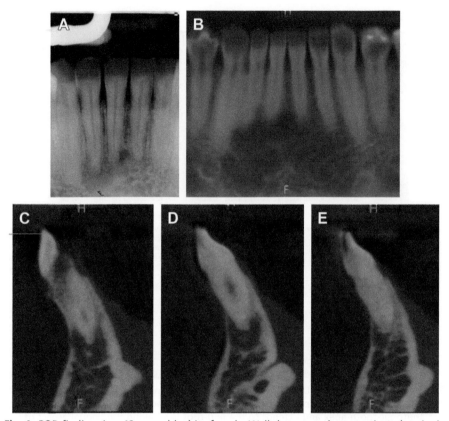

Fig. 4. POD findings in a 48-year-old white female. Well-demarcated, noncorticated periapical mixed radiolucent-radiopaque lesions. They all extend to the buccal cortex but do not cause expansion. At the apex of #24, the lesion has more buccal orientation and lacks the epicentricity of lesions associated with a chronic pulp. All teeth in the anterior mandible were vital to pulp vitality testing. Although more common in middle-aged African American women, these periapical dysplasias have a 15–20% incidence in white women. (*A*) Periapical radiograph. (*B*) Reconstructed coronal CBCT multiplanar image. (*C*) Reconstructed cross-sectional multiplanar CBCT image of tooth #26. (*D*) Reconstructed cross-sectional multiplanar CBCT image of tooth #25. (*E*) Reconstructed cross-sectional multiplanar CBCT image of tooth #24.

greater risk of peri-implantitis and implant failure. Patients must be informed of this and be willing to accept this risk.

Focal Osseous Dysplasia

General comments

The designation of this focal variant is historical as the clinical and radiographic features are similar to POD.[9,10] Many cases of this focal variant are predominantly posterior or early cases of POD where multiple sites have not yet been identified. However, when these focal cases mature and become more mineralized, ie, mixed radiolucent-radiopaque to more radiopaque and are still at a single site, then the term focal osseous dysplasia (ie, Fo OD) is appropriate. Race differences between the focal and periapical variant have been speculated, but the current consensus is that there should not be a racial distinction between the focal and the periapical variant and that they are synonymous.[7,8,11]

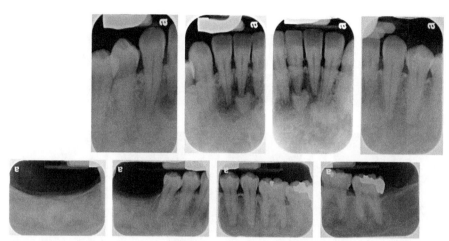

Fig. 5. Moderate mandibular POD. There is a mixed density pattern with dense periapical mineralization in the anterior and posterior areas. These images also show the dense patterns of mineralization that remain separate from the root outlines.

Radiographic features

The features are similar to POD. In the cases of the focal variant Fo OD illustrated, they have a more localized pattern, which is clearly not typical of the generalized pattern of POD. **Figs. 9–11** show large early patterns of mixed radiolucent-radiopaque density that extend to the basal bone. These patterns are present in both the anterior and posterior locations.

Figs. 12 and **13** are examples of more densely mineralized lesions. The denser mineralized patterns are to be expected in older female patients. The associated panoramic image in **Fig. 12** confirms the unifocal presentation.

Management

The management of Fo OD is similar to POD. Biopsy is rarely indicated to establish a histologic diagnosis as the radiographic features differ from the other fibro-osseous lesions discussed in this article.

Florid Osseous Dysplasia

General comments

Florid osseous dysplasia (Fl OD) was first described by Melrose and colleagues,[4] and they referred to it as florid cemento-osseous dysplasia. The lesions are generally extensive as the term "florid" implies. The exact incidence is difficult to establish as it is thought that many cases are not reported because of the variable presentations and lack of symptomatology in many unreported or undocumented cases.[12,13]

Clinical presentation

In general, Fl OD predominates in female black populations, but to a lesser extent, it is also found in Asian and white female populations. A hereditary pattern has also been described and this may, in fact, be a different type of Fl OD with a unique autosomal dominant inheritance pattern.[12,13]

Radiographic features

Because these lesions develop with time, there is a variable range of presentation dependent on the chronicity of the pattern. Early patterns of Fl OD have radiolucent

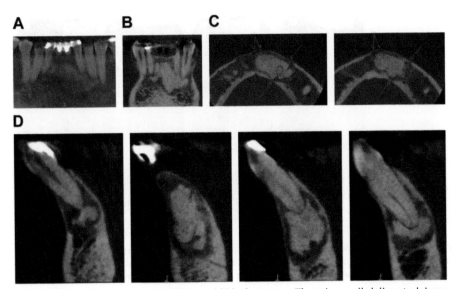

Fig. 6. Mature POD findings in a 67-year-old black woman. There is a well-delineated, irregularly outlined homogeneous radiopaque density with a radiolucent rim of 1 to 2 mm in thickness. The superior margin follows the outline of the anterior dentition apices from #22 to #27, but maintains separation from the dentin root outlines. The periphery has a radiolucent rim adjacent trabecular bone of varying density. The adjacent bone is sclerotic in many areas but not consistently. The inferior margin extends to the mid-height of the anterior mandibular basal bone. The buccal and lingual margins extend to and actually thin the buccal and lingual mandibular cortices. There is also expansion in the vicinity of the midline. The lingual canal and foramen on the lingual midline are not affected. (*A*) CBCT panoramic reconstruction showing the degree of mineralization, the degree of inferior extension and the mediolateral extent of mature POD. (*B*) Reconstructed coronal multiplanar CBCT image also showing the degree of mineralization, the degree of inferior extension and the mediolateral extent of mature POD. (*C*) Reconstructed axial multiplanar CBCT images showing the degree of mineralization, and the degree of buccolingual extension in the lower third of the lesion. The right image is the more inferior or the axial sections. Thinning of the buccal and lingual cortices (*broken line arrows*) and buccal cortical expansion (*solid arrows*) are noted in cases of mature POD. (*D*) From left to right, consecutive reconstructed parasagittal (cross-sectional) multiplanar CBCT images through tooth #26, mid-pontic area, tooth #23, and tooth #22. Features in the axial and coronal reconstructions are further demonstrated in these sections. These images also demonstrate that the lesion remains separate from the root structures of the adjacent teeth and also maintains a radiolucent periphery. (*Courtesy of* Dr Luke H. Iwata, Loma Linda, CA.)

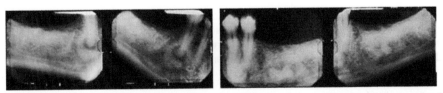

Fig. 7. Mature POD findings in the posterior mandible. The lesions affect multiple areas and demonstrate the well-delineated dense patterns with irregular outlines. The patterns remain in the periapical areas of extracted teeth, particularly on the left side.

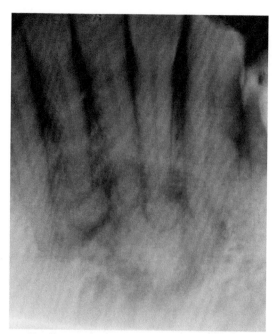

Fig. 8. Mature POD findings in the anterior mandible. This single periapical image shows the dense pattern of mineralization with an enlarging radiolucent periphery. The areas remain separate from the root outlines.

patterns that are not well demarcated in the alveolar bone of tooth bearing areas. With time, the outlines increase and the mineralizations gradually opacify, with varying patterns of mixed radiolucency-radiopacity. As these lesions enlarge, they extend to the basal bone of the maxilla and mandible. The shapes of the mineralizing patterns vary

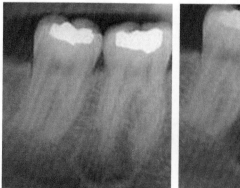
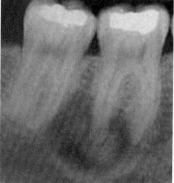

Fig. 9. A case of Fo OD at the distal apex of #30. These images demonstrate the progression of the lesion over a span of nearly 4 years (45 months). The patient did not develop any other similar areas of osseous dysplasia. The increase in size and mineralization are noted in this timespan. The mineralization remains separate from the root outline.

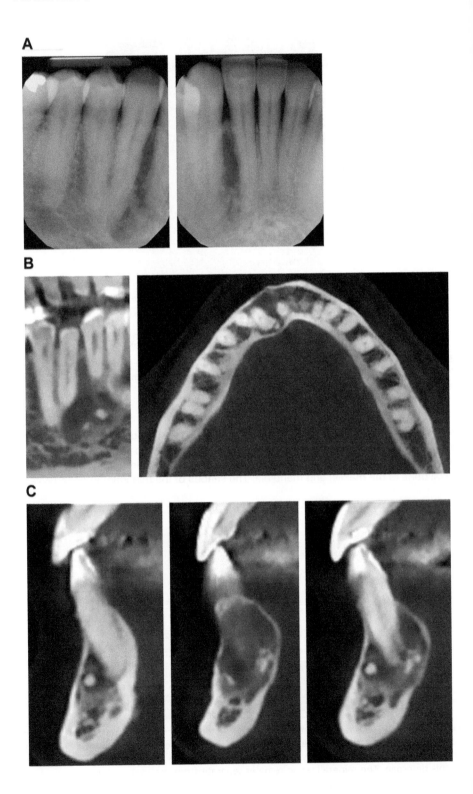

from diffuse and lobular outlines that either gradually enlarge or coalesce to form larger mineralized patterns (**Figs. 14** and **15**).

It has been reported that the enlarging pattern of avascular mineralization may account for the tendency to form the simple bone cysts often seen in FI OD (**Fig. 16**). Enlargement is also associated with expansion. Because these enlargements occur in a benign fashion, they can attain demonstrable proportions before being documented as incidental findings at clinical or radiographic examination.

Management

These lesions are generally considered self-limiting. However, because of their propensity to expand and possibly develop simple bone cysts, osteoplasty and biopsy are often indicated. Another indication for management similarly occurs in the presence of trauma; this is either due to a chronic ill-fitting appliance or an acute event which initiates inflammation and infection as a result of the poor vascularity of the mineralized matrix. Extension of dental infection also exacerbates, and surgical debridement may then be indicated if nonsurgical management is not effective. In some cases, the debridement of necrotic infected tissue may be extensive, creating surgical defects that lead to challenging surgical and prosthodontic management. Bone grafting and implants have been successful in challenging cases.[14]

Benign Cementoblastoma

General comments

Benign cementoblastoma is considered a true neoplasm of odontogenic connective tissue origin. Although a slow growing neoplasm, it maintains potential for uncontrolled, unlimited growth. It occurs predominately in younger individuals, in the second and third decades but may also be seen later in life. It is also a predominately mandibular lesion affecting posterior teeth. There is a 78% incidence in the mandible and 90% occurrence on molars.[7] Occurrences in the maxilla are rare. There have also been a few reports of benign cementoblastoma in the primary dentition.[15,16] The occurrence of multiple benign cementoblastomas is rare but has been reported.[17,18] It does not have a strong gender predilection, although in some cases a male predilection has been noted. The lesion originates on the root surface and displaces the periodontal ligament as it develops a circumferential growth pattern from the root surface.

Clinical presentation

Cementoblastoma is an asymptomatic lesion which is first noticed as an asymptomatic unilateral facial swelling. Because it often has an innocuous presence, it may often be noticed first either clinically by altered facial contours or from a radiographic examination.

◀——

Fig. 10. A case of Fo OD in the anterior mandible between teeth #26 and #28. These images demonstrate the alveolar and basal bone mixed radiolucent-radiopaque buccolingual expansion. It measures ~20 × 12 × 10 mm in greatest dimensions. The expansion is primarily toward the lingual with thinning of both the buccal and lingual cortices. Few but prominent, well-delineated amorphous radiopaque foci are noted in the lumen. From the biopsy, the histologic examination demonstrated segments of moderately cellular dense fibrous connective tissue with osteoblast-rich trabeculae of woven bone; and scattered acellular globular deposits of woven bone. (*A*) Periapical images. (*B*) Reconstructed paracoronal and axial multiplanar CBCT images. (*C*) Reconstructed parasagittal multiplanar CBCT images. (*Courtesy of* Dr Linda Juhl and Jaynini Thakker, Loma Linda CA.)

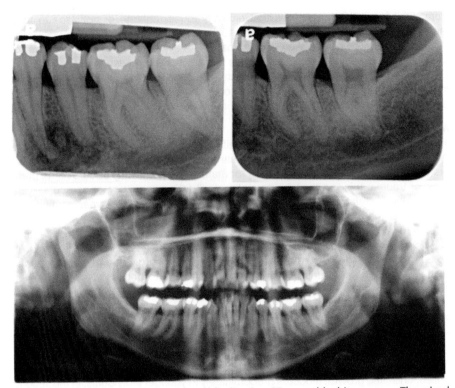

Fig. 11. A case of Fo OD was an incidental finding in a 27-year-old white woman. The mixed radiolucent-radiopaque lesion is noted in the periapical and panoramic images adjacent the apical halves of teeth #20 and #21. On histologic examination, dense woven bone was present in "moderately cellular dense fibrous connective tissue interspersed with slender trabeculae of woven bone and globular ossicles." (*Courtesy of* Dr Ryan Falke, Reno, NV.)

Radiographic features

Benign cementoblastoma presents as a radiopaque mass enlarging from the apical half of the root surface. It is attached to the root without disruption of the periodontal ligament space. Usually the outline of the original root structure is lost as a result of root resorption and development of the tumor mass. It typically has an ovoid to circumferential pattern. The periphery is radiolucent and often seems to be the disrupted outline of the periodontal ligament space. As the lesion enlarges, it expands the adjacent cortices and causes thinning and even cortical resorption (**Figs. 17** and **18**).

Management

This lesion is best managed by enucleation with extraction of the affected tooth. This treatment has the least likelihood of recurrence. There are reports of enucleating the lesion and retaining the affected tooth,[19,20] but retaining the tooth may have a poor periodontal prognosis. Hence, the decision to retain the tooth should be made on a case by case basis.

Monostotic Fibrous Dysplasia

General comments

Monostotic fibrous dysplasia is a bony hamartoma made up of an overabundance of fibrous connective tissue replacing normal bone marrow. Although the age of

A

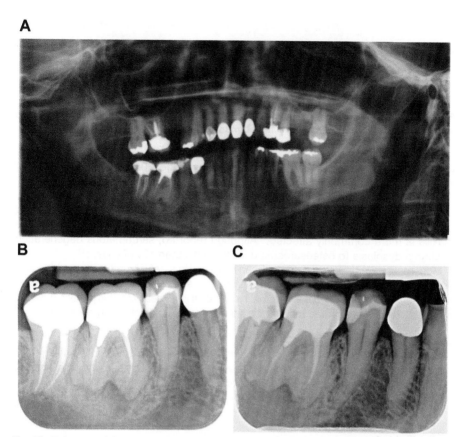

B   **C**

Fig. 12. Panoramic (*A*) and periapical images (*B, C*) of Fo OD in a 62-year-old white woman. The periapical image on the right (*C*) is taken 2 years later than the left periapical image (*B*). The mineralization is very dense making it difficult to discern the lesion from the tooth surface. The panoramic image (*A*) demonstrates that this is a unifocal lesion supporting the diagnosis of Fo OD. The stable conformation, well-demarcated inferior outlines, and the radiolucent inferior periphery further support the diagnosis of Fo OD. (*Courtesy of* Dr Ryan Falke, Reno, NV.)

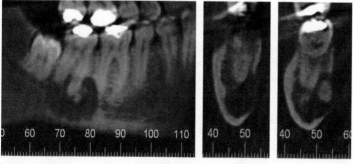

Fig. 13. Reconstructed panoramic and cross-sections of Fo OD in a 57-year-old white woman. The cross-sections demonstrate the degree of expansion and cortical changes that are manifest, as well as the tendency for the mixed radiolucent-radiopaque lesion to not to be centered at the anatomic apex of an affected tooth. (*Courtesy of* Dr Walter Schneider, Houston, TX)

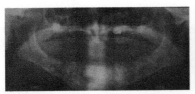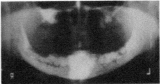

Fig. 14. Patterns of Fl OD in all 4 quadrants. Note the generalized extension of the changes well into the basal bone of the maxilla and mandible.

distribution is from 5 to 70 years, it is more common under 30 years of age. The defect is believed to arise from the abnormal differentiation of osteoblasts.

Fibrous dysplasia is known to selectively affect multiple areas of the skeletal system. Within the skull and facial area, the mandible, the maxilla, frontal, sphenoid and zygoma are the most commonly affected bones. Between the 2 jaw bones, the maxilla is more commonly affected.[8] Although reported, sarcomatous degeneration of fibrous dysplasia to osteosarcoma occurs in less than 1% of cases.[21]

More recently, a genetic cause has been identified in a gene mutation that prolongs G protein activation in osteogenesis.[22,23] This affects cell proliferation in the affected bone, which then creates the bony hamartoma. However, it is unclear why this genetic defect is only identified in the affected monostotic sites and not in the entire skeletal system.

Clinical presentation
The lesions are frequently asymptomatic and either noted as an incidental finding or as an asymptomatic facial asymmetry. If the lesions are asymptomatic, they may initially be discovered on comprehensive dental radiographic examinations. When evaluating problem-focused clinical asymmetries, the radiographic findings may be similar to those noted on comprehensive examinations.

Radiographic features
On radiographic examination, fibrous dysplasia creates bony expansion and may even thin cortical bone, but the cortical outline is maintained. The extent of the lesion in cancellous bone is typically diffuse and not readily distinguishable, with a clear delineation from the nonaffected bone. The density of the trabecular changes can range from radiolucent, to a ground glass trabecular pattern, and to a combination of ground glass with radiopaque sclerotic areas. The sclerotic areas have a greater percentage of poorly mineralized woven bone. These features are further elaborated in **Figs. 19–23**.

Management
There is no definitive treatment available for this disease process. Surgery is the most common management if lesions generate pressure symptoms, airway obstructions, or dysfunctions that arise from an enlarging tumor. Facial esthetics can also become an

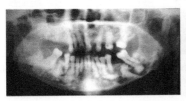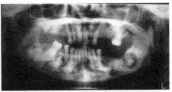

Fig. 15. Twenty-four month follow-up on a case with Fl OD. Note the increase in the extent and in the mineralized density over this time period.

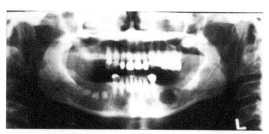

Fig. 16. Cases of FI OD are frequently associated with solitary bone cysts. This figure demonstrates the solitary bone cyst in association with one of the mineralized masses in the left mandible. Histologic confirmation or close monitoring are recommended when these solitary radiolucencies are observed.

overriding social concern necessitating cosmetic osteoplasty. Even the type and degree of surgery are complex decisions. There is little consensus on a definitive surgical approach on whether to perform excisions at an early stage or to wait until a lesion demonstrates stability in its growth. In addition, the benefits of a minimal excision osteoplasty approach versus radical resection must be considered. The latter often generates surgical dilemmas that make reconstructive surgeries more difficult.

Polyostotic Fibrous Dysplasia

McCune Albright Syndrome
General comments Multiple areas of fibrous dysplasia in association with other anomalies such as cutaneous hyperpigmentation and endocrinopathies are typically diagnostic of McCune Albright syndrome. The syndrome was originally described in 1937.[24] There is another form of polyostotic fibrous dysplasia, the Mazabraud Syndrome.[25] This polyostotic type of fibrous dysplasia also presents with multiple soft tissue myxomas, primarily intramuscular. It is far less common and is not discussed further.

McCune Albright syndrome is almost exclusive to women and presents with a similar but slightly older age range than the monostotic form. It also has a genetic cause related to the G Protein gene mutation. Hormone signaling from this mutation is related to this polyostotic manifestation.[23,26,27]

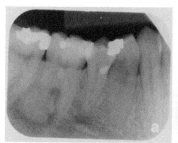
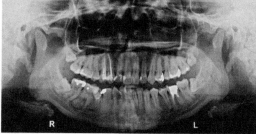

Fig. 17. Benign cementoblastoma showing classic radiographic changes. A radiopaque mass extends from the apex of the affected root in a circumferential pattern. It is fused to the root and the lesions maintain a radiolucent periphery that is often continuous with the periodontal ligament space. (*Courtesy of* Dr Murray Jacobs, Loma Linda, CA.)

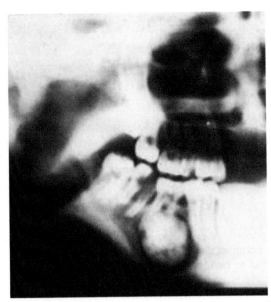

Fig. 18. Case of benign cementoblastoma with the typical changes as discussed in **Fig. 17**. Most cases are reported to affect the first molar. The radiopaque mass extends from the apex of the affected root in a circumferential pattern. It is fused to the root and the lesion maintains a radiolucent periphery.

Clinical presentation Asymmetry and esthetic concerns are most notable with the polyostotic form. When lesions affect long bones and weight-bearing areas of the skeletal system, severe deformities and dysfunction are reported.[21]

Radiographic features Multiple and coalescing fibrous dysplasia lesions are present. The severity of the extent is demonstrated by the case shown in **Fig. 24**.

Management Extension of these lesions onto adjacent anatomic structures can lead to functional and symptomatic concerns. Surgical correction for esthetic reasons, relief of symptomatology, and realignment of weight-bearing areas is often indicated.

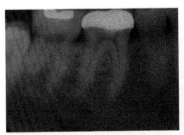
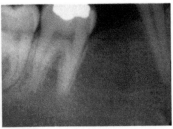

Fig. 19. Periapical radiographs illustrating the trabecular bone appearance of "ground glass" or "frosted glass." A physiologic appearing trabecular bone pattern is present on the left. The "ground glass" trabecular pattern of fibrous dysplasia in the right periapical image has the appearance of crushed or minced spicules of trabeculae with reduced or obliterated marrow spaces. This has the analogous appearance of a surface of crushed glass.

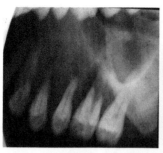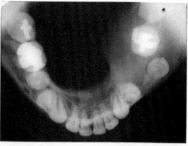

Fig. 20. Occlusal radiographs of a maxillary and a mandibular case of monostotic fibrous dysplasia. Close inspection of the trabecular pattern in both cases demonstrates the ground glass trabeculation. On the mandibular case (*right*), note the degree of lingual expansion with thin but intact cortices. It is difficult to locate the trabecular margin because of the diffuse outline of fibrous dysplasia in trabecular bone.

Craniofacial Fibrous Dysplasia

General comments

Craniofacial fibrous dysplasia is a polyostotic form of fibrous dysplasia that is not related to endocrinopathies and does not have an exclusive female gender predilection. It is seen when a seemingly localized mass of fibrous dysplasia extends to multiple contiguous bones of the craniofacial complex.[11,28] Usually cases extend from the maxilla to the zygoma or to the sphenoid bone. **Fig. 25** shows an extensive case where the fibrous dysplasia affected the maxilla, mandible, zygoma, frontal, temporal, parietal, sphenoid, ethmoid, and occipital bones.

The radiographic findings and management do not otherwise differ from the monostotic form. However, the greater degree of symptomatology and the degree of surgical correction are highly correlated to the greater extension of the polyostotic lesion.

Ossifying Fibroma

General comments

Ossifying fibroma is a true neoplasm of bone. Because of this designation it has the potential for uncontrolled and unlimited benign growth. Other names for this lesion include cementifying fibroma and cemento-ossifying fibroma. However, as discussed with the periapical, focal, and florid osseous dysplasias, a specific histologic identification of cementum is difficult to establish. The acellular amorphous mineralized structures identified in the lesion are variations of amorphous bone and similar mineralized patterns believed to be cementum have also been found in ossifying fibromas distant to the jaws. Hence, we agree with others[7,11] that the term cementum should be avoided and the term ossifying fibroma should be used.

This lesion has the highest incidence in young adults. It is more common in the mandible than the maxilla. A slight female gender predilection exists.

An aggressive variation of the ossifying fibroma occurs in the pediatric population. The juvenile ossifying fibroma is so named because of its rapid growth and large size. Two different types are classified: the trabecular and psammamatoid patterns. Differentiation between these 2 types of the juvenile variant is not discussed further.

Clinical presentation

In general, these lesions are slow growing and generally asymptomatic until esthetics, compressions on adjacent structures, or jaw function are affected. Some lesions may

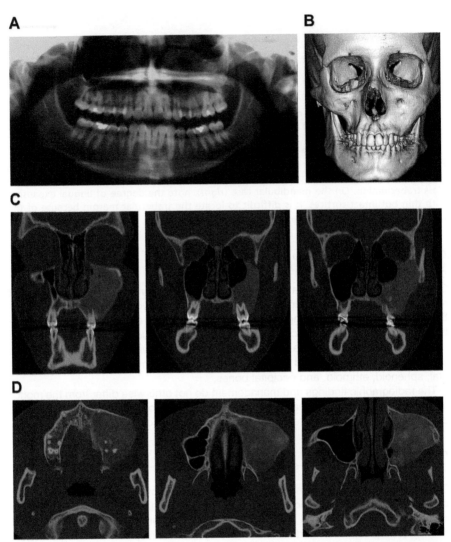

Fig. 21. Monostotic fibrous dysplasia in a 17-year-old male patient. The lesion is localized to the left maxilla causing prominent asymmetry and expansion. Note the displacement of the left orbit. The mass of the lesion demonstrates the diffuse pattern in the cancellous bone and the "ground glass" or "frosted glass" trabecular pattern. The demarcation of the lesion in the cancellous bone is diffuse. (*A*) Standard panoramic image. There is narrowing of the left maxillary sinus lumen from the expansion of the fibrous dysplasia into the sinus airspace. (*B*) 3D rendering with osseous filter demonstrating the degree of maxillary expansion and asymmetry. (*C*) Coronal CBCT multiplanar reconstructions. There is lateral expansion of the maxilla and narrowing of the maxillary sinus space. The lesion remains lateral to the nasal cavity. The superior extension of the lesion is at the inferolateral orbital rim. The medullary space has lost the trabecular pattern which is replaced by a "ground glass" appearance with a mixed radiolucent pattern and sclerotic masses within the radiolucent matrix. (*D*) Axial multiplanar reconstructions. The changes in the cancellous pattern as noted in (*C*) are also depicted here. (*Courtesy of* Dr Alan Herford, Loma Linda, CA.)

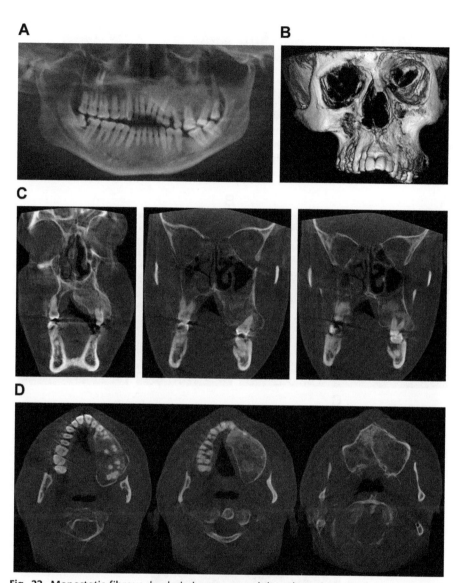

Fig. 22. Monostotic fibrous dysplasia in a young adult male patient. Similar to the case in **Fig. 21**, this lesion is also localized to the left maxilla with more prominent asymmetry and expansion in a more inferior pathway. The cancellous pattern of the lesion also demonstrates the "ground glass" pattern. The inferior extension has altered the occlusal plane with compensatory adaptive remodeling of the mandible to accommodate the altered occlusal plane. (*A*) Reconstructed panoramic image. (*B*) 3D rendering with osseous filter. (*C*) Coronal multiplanar CBCT reconstructions demonstrating similar cancellous changes as in **Fig. 21**, but to a greater extent. There is lateral expansion of the left maxilla and maxillary alveolar process, and narrowing of the maxillary sinus space. The lesion remains lateral to the nasal cavity. The caudal-cephalic extension of the lesion has elevated the left orbit and inferiorly displaced the curve of Spee. The medullary spaces manifest the "ground glass" appearance with sclerotic masses within the matrix. (*D*) Axial multiplanar CBCT reconstructions demonstrating the degree of expansion of the left alveolar and palatine processes of the maxilla. (*Courtesy of* Dr Mel Mupparapu, Philadelphia, PA; and Dr Steven Singer, New York, NY.)

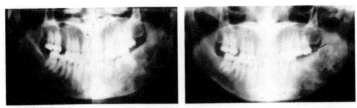

Fig. 23. Progression of monostotic fibrous dysplasia over a 5-year time interval. The 5-year follow-up image (*right*) shows how the lesion has enlarged with a more dense ground glass trabecular pattern. Enlargement is also noted by the decrease in the left side interocclusal space (*arrow*).

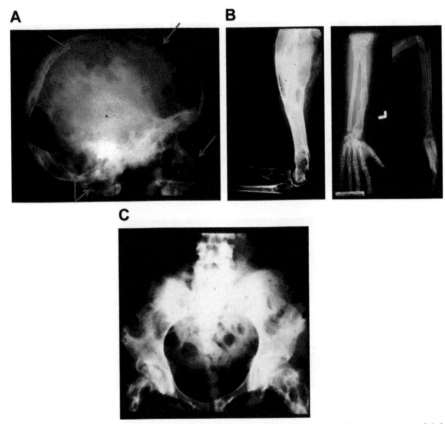

Fig. 24. McCune Albright syndrome in a 13-year-old girl. This patient demonstrates multiple lesions in several bones. Multiple sites are present in the occipital, sphenoid and ethmoid bones as noted by the arrows (*A*). The left maxilla was also affected, and this contributed to her notable facial asymmetry. The left humerus, ulna and radius (*B*) and the pelvis are similarly affected (*C*). This patient also had multiple areas of cutaneous hyperpigmentation, ie, café-au-lait spots. At this age, she also had started to develop the endocrine abnormalities associated with precocious puberty; ie, specifically in her case were early menses and enlarged breasts. (*A*) Standard lateral skull projection demonstrating the multiple skull lesions. Mixed density lesions are noted in the frontal, parietal, occipital and maxillary skull bones. (*B*) Lateral and anterioposteror projections demonstrating the multiple lesions in the humerus, ulna and radius. (*C*) Anterioposteror projection demonstrating the multiple lesions in the pelvis, and bilateral head of the humerus. (*Courtesy of* Dr Benton E. Crawford [deceased], Houston, TX.)

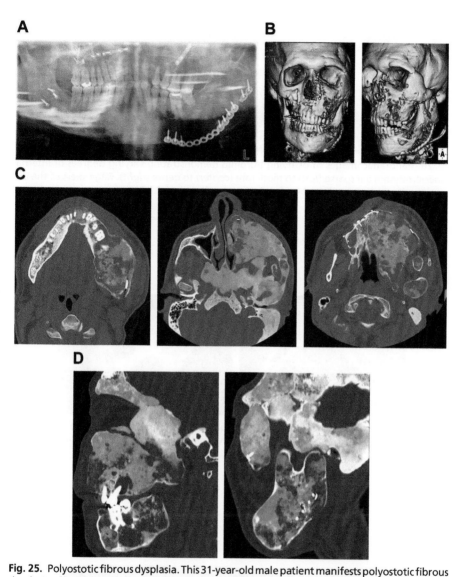

Fig. 25. Polyostotic fibrous dysplasia. This 31-year-old male patient manifests polyostotic fibrous dysplasia affecting multiple skull bones on the left side as evidenced in this series of images. The skull bones affected include the mandible, maxilla, zygoma, frontal, temporal, parietal, sphenoid, ethmoid, and occipital bones. These changes have narrowed multiple skull foraminae and obliterated the paranasal sinuses. (*A*) Standard panoramic image. Because of the degree of facial asymmetry from the lesions, the patient's left side did not fit into the panoramic focal trough. For the best fit, the patient's midline is shifted to the right, thus creating left side enlargement artifact further contributing to the appearance of the asymmetry. (*B*) 3D rendering of frontal and left lateral views with osseous filter. The enlargement of the facial bones and degree of asymmetry is evidenced from these reconstructions. (*C*) Axial multiplanar multidetector computed tomography (MDCT) reconstructions of the mandible and mid-face region. Expansion of the affected skull bones is noted with a mix of radiolucent, ground glass and sclerotic areas in the cancellous bone. (*D*) Sagittal multiplanar MDCT reconstructions further documenting the changes discussed in (*C*). Although the periapical radiolucency noted at the #14 apex has the appearance of a dentoalveolar abscess formation, it is related to the fibrous dysplasia. (*Courtesy of* Dr Andre Guerrero Fernandes, Loma Linda, CA.)

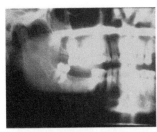
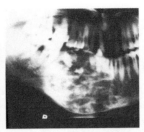
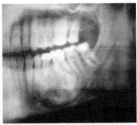

Fig. 26. Panoramic images of ossifying fibromas demonstrating varying degrees of internal mineralization from sparse (*left*) to moderate (*center*) to dense (*right*). Regardless of the degree of mineralization, all lesions demonstrate well-demarcated borders.

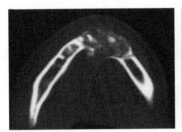
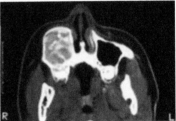

Fig. 27. MDCT axial constructions of a mandibular (*left*) and a maxillary (*right*) ossifying fibroma. Both cases have moderate amounts of internal mineralization with well-demarcated outlines.

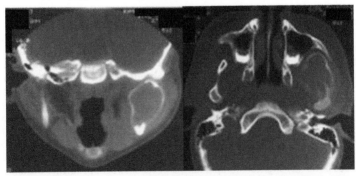

Fig. 28. Coronal (*left*) and axial (*right*) MDCT constructions of a mandibular juvenile ossifying fibroma. The lesion has well-demarcated borders with sparse amounts of internal mineralization but the aggressive growth is affecting the temporomandibular articulation.

Table 1
Summation of fibro-osseous lesions

Lesion	Age (y)	Gender	Location	Radiographic Appearance	Clinical Symptoms	Treatment
POD	30–50	F:M (14:1) Highest in black women, then Asian Lowest in whites	Anterior mandible periapical regions	Circumscribed radiolucencies at apical area of teeth transforming into mixed radiolucent-radiopaque with lucent rim Often involves multiple teeth	Vital teeth Asymptomatic	Self-limiting, monitor
Fo OD	30–70	F 90% Higher percentage in whites	Mainly posterior mandible periapical regions	1.5 cm or smaller well-defined radiolucent to densely radiopaque with thin peripheral radiolucent rim When identified, it affects 1 area of the dentition but may involve up to 3–4 teeth	Vital teeth Asymptomatic	Self-limiting, monitor

(continued on next page)

Table 1
(continued)

Lesion	Age (y)	Gender	Location	Radiographic Appearance	Clinical Symptoms	Treatment
Fl OD	40–70	F (black 90%) also high in the East Asian population	Multifocal Often bilateral and extends into basal bone of maxilla and mandible	Similar to POD and Fo OD (above) with extension to the basal bone of the maxilla and mandible	Vital teeth Often asymptomatic but episodic symptoms from adjacent periodontal or pulpal infection	Self-limiting, monitor May require surgical intervention when enlarged areas cause disfiguring asymmetry or symptoms
Benign cementoblastoma	20–40	Slight male predilection	Mandibular molar region mainly	Opaque round/ovoid mass fused to root Periphery is radiolucent	Slow growing and generally asymptomatic Facial swelling in advanced cases	Surgical extraction of tooth with attached mass Monitor for recurrence
Fibrous dysplasia (monostotic)	5–70 More common under 30	Equal	Limited to a single bone In facial area, mandible, maxilla, frontal, sphenoid and zygoma are most common Maxilla > mandible	Single expansile lesion with ground glass trabeculation and with varying foci of sclerotic opaque areas	Convex deformity with facial asymmetry Episodic symptoms from compression of paranasal sinus spaces, orbits, acoustic canal	No definitive treatment Surgical osteoplasty when disfiguring or symptomatic

	Age	Sex	Bones	Radiographic features	Clinical features	Treatment
Fibrous dysplasia- (polyostotic) McCune Albright syndrome	Slightly older than monostotic	Female Exclusive	Multiple skull and long bones Affects entire skeletal system	Multiple expansile lesions with ground glass trabeculation and with varying foci of sclerotic opaque areas	Convex deformity with facial asymmetry(s) Episodic symptoms from compression of paranasal sinus spaces, orbits, acoustic canal Deformity of long bones Pathologic fracture	No definitive treatment Surgical correction for disfiguring or symptomatic lesions Difficult to manage because of extent of lesions
Fibrous dysplasia- (polyostotic) Craniofacial	Slightly older than monostotic	Equal	Multiple cranial bones	Multiple expansile lesions with ground glass trabeculation and with varying foci of sclerotic opaque areas	Convex deformity with facial asymmetry(s) Episodic symptoms from compression of paranasal sinus spaces, orbits, acoustic canal	No definitive treatment Surgical osteoplasty when disfiguring or symptomatic; difficult to manage because of extent of lesions
Ossifying fibroma	Young adults	F > M	Mandible > maxilla	Well-defined periphery with sclerotic border Varying degrees of internal opacification Expansive and displaces adjacent dentition	Slow growing Asymptomatic Can cause secondary symptoms	Surgical enucleation with osteoplasty when disfiguring Monitor for recurrence

have a more rapid and aggressive growth pattern, but this is not common. The juvenile variant more typically shows rapid enlargement and disfigurement, and extension to neurovascular structures, paranasal airspaces, and the cranial base.

Radiographic features

Most cases have a well-defined periphery with a sclerotic border. But if a sclerotic border is not present, the well-demarcated outline remains consistent. The lesion can present with varying degrees of mineralization within its internal contents. This may be because of variations in the mineralization patterns or merely a function of time. The longer the lesion develops and matures, the greater the degree of internal mineralization that is present. **Figs. 26** and **27** demonstrate these radiographic features. **Fig. 28** demonstrates how the juvenile variant displaces and affects adjacent structures to a greater degree.

Management

Despite their size, ossifying fibromas respond well to surgical enucleation. Because of their demarcation from surrounding structures, they enucleate well with minimal recurrence. Intuitively, the larger lesions may require a more detailed imaging evaluation to assure identification of the entire outline. The juvenile variant also requires surgical removal; however, because of the growth pattern, wider resection is more common and recurrence rates are greater.

SUMMARY

Differentiating between the various fibro-osseous lesions that either are in the dentoalveolar region or extend to the facial bones have long been challenging to clinicians. Symptomatology, location, and recurrence are major discriminating factors between these entities because they often have similar histologic, and in some cases, similar radiographic features. Thus, the subtle radiographic discriminating factors play a major role in the diagnostic process when encountering these types of lesions. **Table 1** summarizes and highlights the differences that can assist the clinician in making a radiographic preliminary diagnosis.

REFERENCES

1. Waldron CA. Fibro-osseous lesions of the jaws. J Oral Surg 1970;28(1):58–64.
2. Waldron CA, Giansanti JS. Benign fibro-osseous lesions of the jaws: a clinical-radiologic-histologic review of sixty-five cases. Oral Surg Oral Med Oral Pathol 1973;35(2):190–201.
3. Waldron CA, Giansanti JS. Benign fibro-osseous lesions of the jaws: a clinical-radiologic-histologic review of sixty-five cases. II. Benign fibro-osseous lesions of periodontal ligament origin. Oral Surg Oral Med Oral Pathol 1973;35(3): 340–50.
4. Melrose RJ, Abrams AM, Mills BG. Florid osseous dysplasia. A clinical-pathologic study of thirty-four cases. Oral Surg Oral Med Oral Pathol 1976;41(1):62–82.
5. Ariji Y, Ariji E, Higuchi Y, et al. Florid cemento-osseous dysplasia. Radiographic study with special emphasis on computed tomography. Oral Surg Oral Med Oral Pathol 1994;78(3):391–6.
6. Eisenberg E, Eisenbud L. Benign fibro-osseous diseases: current concepts in historical perspective. Oral Maxillofac Surg Clin North Am 1997;7(4):551–62.
7. White SC, Pharoah MJ. Oral radiology: principles and interpretation. 7th Edition. St. Louis (MO): Elsevier; 2014.

8. Eversole LR. Clinical outline of oral pathology. 4th Edition. Shelton (CT): People's Medical Publishing House; 2011.

9. Summerlin DJ, Tomich CE. Focal cemento-osseous dysplasia: a clinicopathologic study of 221 cases. Oral Surg Oral Med Oral Pathol 1994;78(5):611–20.

10. Waldron CA. Fibro-osseous lesions of the jaws. J Oral Maxillofac Surg 1985;43(4): 249–62.

11. Neville BW, Damm DD, Allen CM, et al. Oral and maxillofacial pathology. 3rd edition. St Louis (MO): Saunders, Elsevier; 2009.

12. Young SK, Markowitz NR, Sullivan S, et al. Familial gigantiform cementoma: classification and presentation of a large pedigree. Oral Surg Oral Med Oral Pathol 1989;68(6):740–7.

13. Thakkar NS, Horner K, Sloan P. Familial occurrence of periapical cemental dysplasia. Virchows Arch A Pathol Anat Histopathol 1993;423(3):233–6.

14. Bencharit S, Schardt-Sacco D, Zuniga JR, et al. Surgical and prosthodontic rehabilitation for a patient with aggressive florid cemento-osseous dysplasia: a clinical report. J Prosthet Dent 2003;90(3):220–4.

15. Monti LM, Souza AM, Soubhia AM, et al. Cementoblastoma: a case report in deciduous tooth. Oral Maxillofac Surg 2013;17(2):145–9.

16. Lemberg K, Hagstrom J, Rihtniemi J, et al. Benign cementoblastoma in a primary lower molar, a rarity. Dentomaxillofac Radiol 2007;36(6):364–6.

17. Iannaci G, Luise R, Iezzi G, et al. Multiple cementoblastoma: a rare case report. Case Rep Dent 2013;2013:828373.

18. Ohki K, Kumamoto H, Nitta Y, et al. Benign cementoblastoma involving multiple maxillary teeth: report of a case with a review of the literature. Oral Surg Oral Med Oral Pathol Oral Radiol 2004;97(1):53–8.

19. Biggs JT, Benenati FW. Surgically treating a benign cementoblastoma while retaining the involved tooth. J Am Dent Assoc 1995;126(9):1288–90.

20. Gulses A, Bayar GR, Aydin C, et al. A case of a benign cementoblastoma treated by enucleation and apicoectomy. Gen Dent 2012;60(6):e380–2.

21. Fitzpatrick KA, Taljanovic MS, Speer DP, et al. Imaging findings of fibrous dysplasia with histopathologic and intraoperative correlation. AJR Am J Roentgenol 2004;182(6):1389–98.

22. Weinstein LS. G(s)alpha mutations in fibrous dysplasia and McCune-Albright syndrome. J Bone Miner Res 2006;21(Suppl 2):P120–4.

23. Perdigao PF, Pimenta FJ, Castro WH, et al. Investigation of the GSalpha gene in the diagnosis of fibrous dysplasia. Int J Oral Maxillofac Surg 2004;33(5):498–501.

24. Albright F, Butler AM, Hampton AO, et al. Syndrome characterized by osteitis fibrosa disseminata, areas of pigmentation and endocrine dysfunction, with precocious puberty in females. N Engl J Med 1937;216(17):727–46.

25. Iwasko N, Steinbach LS, Disler D, et al. Imaging findings in Mazabraud's syndrome: seven new cases. Skeletal Radiol 2002;31(2):81–7.

26. Lietman SA, Ding C, Levine MA. A highly sensitive polymerase chain reaction method detects activating mutations of the GNAS gene in peripheral blood cells in McCune-Albright syndrome or isolated fibrous dysplasia. J Bone Joint Surg Am 2005;87(11):2489–94.

27. Lumbroso S, Paris F, Sultan C. Activating Gsalpha mutations: analysis of 113 patients with signs of McCune-Albright syndrome–a European Collaborative Study. J Clin Endocrinol Metab 2004;89(5):2107–13.

28. MacDonald-Jankowski DS. Fibro-osseous lesions of the face and jaws. Clin Radiol 2004;59(1):11–25.

Granulomatous Diseases Affecting Jaws

Baddam Venkat Ramana Reddy, BDS, MDS[a], Kiran K. Kuruba, BDS, MDS[a],
Samatha Yalamanchili, BDS, MDS[b], Mel Mupparapu, DMD, MDS[c,*]

KEYWORDS

- Granuloma • Bacterial infection • Viral infection • Parasitic infection
- Granulomatous lesion • Trauma • Autoimmune diseases

KEY POINTS

- Identification of oral granulomatous lesions clinically and radiographically with histologic confirmation for a definitive diagnosis is the standard strategy.
- On occasion, the interventions can be undertaken by clinical and radiographic diagnosis alone to curtail the spread of the infection.
- As oral granulomatous lesions are rare, a thorough understanding of the mechanisms involved in the production of clinical symptoms is essential to identify these lesions at an early stage.

INFECTIONS

Tuberculosis

Tuberculosis (TB) is an airborne disease caused by the bacterium *Mycobacterium tuberculosis*. It spreads through air droplets. It mainly affects the respiratory tract and lungs via the nasal passage (**Table 1**).[1]

Clinical features

Primary TB is associated with episodic fever, chills, fatigability, malaise, gradual loss of weight, and a persistent cough, which may be dry or productive. Secondary TB presents with fever, cough, chest pain, and hemoptysis. Military TB shows symptoms of acute febrile illness in children. However, in adults, it is insidious with gradual development of ill health, anorexia, loss of weight, and fever.[1]

Tuberculous lymphadenitis may progress to the formation of an actual abscess or remain as granulomatous infection. They are tender because of inflammation of the overlying skin with perforation and pus discharge.[2] More than 50% of the patients with AIDS have extrapulmonary TB lesions.

[a] Department of Oral & Maxillofacial Pathology, Sibar Institute of Dental Sciences, Guntur, Andhra Pradesh, 522601, India; [b] Department of Oral Medicine & Radiology, Sibar Institute of Dental Sciences, Guntur, India; [c] Department of Oral Medicine, Robert Schattner Center, University of Pennsylvania School of Dental Medicine, #214, 240 South 40th Street, Suite 214, Philadelphia, PA 19104, USA
* Corresponding author.
E-mail address: mmd@dental.upenn.edu

Dent Clin N Am 60 (2016) 195–234
http://dx.doi.org/10.1016/j.cden.2015.08.007
0011-8532/16/$ – see front matter © 2016 Elsevier Inc. All rights reserved.

dental.theclinics.com

Table 1
Diseases and etiologic agents

Category/Disease	Etiologic Agent
Infections	
Bacterial infections	
TB	*Mycobacterium tuberculosis*
Leprosy	*Mycobacterium leprae*
Actinomycosis	*Actinomyces israelii*
Rhinoslceroma	*Klebsiella rhinoscleromatis*
Anthrax	*Bacillus anthracis*
Brucellosis	*Brucella melitensis*
Syphilis	*Treponema pallidum*
Fungal infections	
Histoplasmosis	*Histoplasma capsulatum*
Blastomycosis	*Blastomyces dermatitidis*
Phycomycosis	*Basidiobolus haptosporus*
Aspergillosis	*Aspergillus*
Cryptococcosis	*Cryptococcus neoformans*
Rhinosporidiosis	*Rhinosporidium seeberi*
Parasitic infection	
Leishmaniasis	*Leishmania* (through sandfly)
Myiasis	*Chrysomya bezziana*
Toxoplasmosis	*Toxoplasma gondii*
Traumatic cause	
Pyogenic granulomas	Trauma and local factors
Reparative granulomas	Trauma or inflammation
Foreign body cause	
Oral foreign body reaction	Inflammation
Cholesterol granulomas	Eustachian tube dysfunction
Cocaine-induced midline granulomas	Inflammation and necrosis
Gout	Excess uric acid
Neoplastic	
Langerhans cell histiocytosis (LCH)	Malignancy
Necrotizing sialometaplasia	Inflammation, trauma, reactive
Polymorphic reticulosis (lethal midline granulomas)	Epstein-Barr virus
Unknown cause	
Sarcoidosis	Unknown
Crohn diseases	Unknown
Autoimmune and vascular diseases	
Wegener granulomatosis	Autoimmune
Systemic lupus erythematosus	Autoimmune
Sjögren syndrome	Autoimmune
Developmental	
Melkersson-Rosenthal syndrome (orofacial granulomatosis)	Developmental

Oral manifestations

Direct contact with infected sputum is the most common route. There are other routes of infections, such as lymphatic spread, hematogenous spread, and extension from the involved neighboring tissues.[3] The resulting oral lesions present as ulcers, nodules, tuberculomas, and apical granulomas.[4]

Histopathologic features

Areas of infection demonstrate the formation of granulomas, circumscribed by collections of epithelioid histiocytes, lymphocytes, and multinucleated giant cells with central caseous necrosis. These granulomas are called as tubercles.[5]

Radiographic features

There are 3 patterns of nodal involvement in tuberculous lymphadenitis on CT or MRI.[6]

- Nodes are homogeneous in attenuation or signal intensity and enhance homogenously after the injection of contrast material in the early phase of the disease.
- A node with a central area of necrosis is seen as the disease progresses.
- A fibrocalcified node is usually seen in patients who have been treated for TB.

TB of the nose and paranasal sinuses in CT or MRI demonstrates nasal soft tissue nodules and thickening and involvement of the paranasal sinuses.[1]

Typically tuberculous osteomyelitis with mandibular involvement shows radiographic features that include osteopenia and poorly defined lytic lesions with minimal surrounding sclerosis.[1]

Dental considerations

The following Centers for Disease Control and Prevention recommendations apply to patients who are known or suspected to have active TB[7] and should be adopted by every dentist.

- Evaluate patients away from other patients and dental team members. When they are not being evaluated, patients should wear a surgical mask or be instructed to cover their mouth and nose when coughing or sneezing.
- Defer elective dental treatment until patients are noninfectious as confirmed by a physician.
- Refer patients requiring urgent dental treatment to a previously identified facility (such as a hospital) with TB engineering controls and a respiratory protection program.

Leprosy

Leprosy, also known as Hansen disease, is a chronic infectious disease mainly caused by *Mycobacterium leprae*. This organism requires a cold host body temperature for endurance.

Clinical features

Clinical presentations of leprosy could be in one of the 2 known forms: (1) tuberculoid leprosy and (2) lepromatous leprosy.

Tuberculoid leprosy develops in patients with high immune reactions. Lepromatous leprosy is seen in patients with reduced cell-mediated immunity.[8]

Paucibacillary leprosy Small number of well-circumscribed, hypopigmented skin lesions will be noted. Nerve involvement resulting in anesthesia of the affected skin is observed. Oral lesions are rare in this variant.

Multibacillary leprosy Numerous ill-defined hypopigmented macules or papules may be noted on the skin and becomes thickened with time. Skin enlargements can lead to distorted facial appearance, that is, leonine facies. Nerve involvement leads to loss of sweating and decreased sensations of light, touch, pain, and temperature. Sensory loss begins in the extremities and spreads to most of the body.[9]

Oral manifestations

Oral soft tissue lesions initially present as yellowish to red, sessile, firm, enlarging papules that develop ulceration and necrosis (**Fig. 1**). Deep infiltration of the soft tissue involvement leads to bone destruction.[10]

Features of facies leprosa[11]

- Atrophy of the anterior nasal spine
- Atrophy of the anterior maxillary alveolar ridge
- Endonasal inflammatory changes

Teeth show enamel hypoplasia and short tapering roots with internal resorption. Facial and trigeminal nerves can be involved with the infectious process.[10] Involvement of the tongue is not uncommon with indurated areas (**Fig. 2**). Oral erosive lesions and ulcerations can also be noted within the oral cavity (**Fig. 3**).

Histopathological features

There are well-formed granulomas with clusters of epithelioid histiocytes, lymphocytes, and Langhans-type multinucleated giant cells. There is a lepromatous pattern with sheets of lymphocytes intermixed with vacuolated histiocytes known as *lepra* cells. An abundance of organisms can be demonstrated with acid-fast stains in the lepromatous variant.[10]

Radiographic features

Facies leprosa are better visualized in lateral cephalometric radiographs because of the deficiency of the premaxillary region. Shortening of roots of the maxillary anterior teeth in a panoramic radiograph have also been reported. Gallium[67] citrate scintigraphy may be used to detect active multibacillary forms of leprosy. When gallium is used to estimate skin involvement, it is not uncommon to see a moderate to diffuse uptake of the radiopharmaceutical in the skin producing a skin outlining sign. The uptake is very important for the skin where the lepromas are commonly seen.

Dental management

Although patients with leprosy will first report to the dermatologist and rarely to the dental professional, the dental professional should be well aware of the precautions to be taken while giving any kind of treatment to these patients in a leprosy center. Appropriate treatment of dental infections will help to reduce the recurrence in leprosy reactions, as will improving the general oral hygiene of patients. Further, it is thought that oral lesions, along with nasal lesions, form an important source of bacillary dissemination in the community. Oral health status of individuals treated and healed from leprosy is poor. Better methods of oral hygiene and regular dental monitoring should be adopted in order to improve the quality of life of these patients.

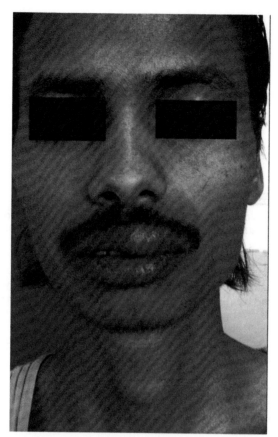

Fig. 1. A tubercular leprosy lesion (borderline) noted in the upper lip with type 1 reaction. (*From* Pallagatti S, Sheikh S, Kaur A, et al. Oral cavity and leprosy. Indian Dermatol Online J 2012;3(2):103.)

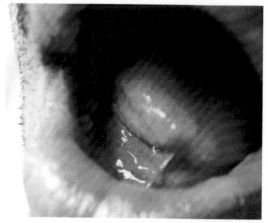

Fig. 2. Intraoral photograph of a patient with leprosy with tongue lesions. Induration of the tip and lateral border of the tongue are noted. (*From* Pallagatti S, Sheikh S, Kaur A, et al. Oral cavity and leprosy. Indian Dermatol Online J 2012;3(2):103.)

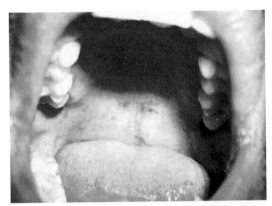

Fig. 3. Superficial erosions of the hard palate noted in a patient with leprosy. (*From* Pallagatti S, Sheikh S, Kaur A, et al. Oral cavity and leprosy. Indian Dermatol Online J 2012;3(2):103.)

Actinomycosis

Chronic granulomatous and fibrosing disease caused by *Actinomyces israelii*. It is chiefly characterized by the formation of abscesses that tend to drain by the formation of the sinus tract.[12]

> In 1938 Cope classified it into 3 types depending on the location:
>
> • Cervicofacial
>
> • Abdominal
>
> • Pulmonary forms

Pathogenesis

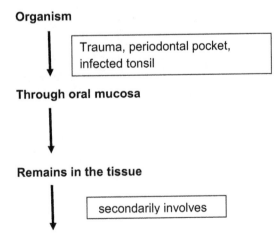

Oral manifestations

Hyperpyrexia is noted, with the presence of regional lymphadenopathy in late stages of the disease.[13] Swelling and indurations of the soft tissue may be noted. Later it may develop into abscesses that tend to discharge pus containing the typical *sulfur granules*. There are multiple sinus openings. Common sites for multiple sinus openings are mandibular or maxillary bone, which lead to *actinomycotic* osteomyelitis.[14]

Histopathologic features

Histological specimen stains with hematoxylin. There is central abscess formation noted with characteristic colonies of microorganisms within it. The colonies seem to be floating in a sea of polymorphonuclear leukocytes, associated with multinucleated giant cells and macrophages at the periphery of the lesion. The eosinophilic club-shaped ends of the *A israelii* filaments are the basis for the term *ray fungus*.[14]

Radiographic findings

Computed tomographic (CT) findings include the following:

- Cervico-facial actinomycosis is an enhancing soft tissue mass with a low-attenuating center associated with inflammatory change in the adjacent soft tissue. Invasion of the adjacent soft tissue, including the muscles, can occur.[1]
- Actinomycotic osteomyelitis of the jaws presents as an irregularly marginated lesion with increased bone marrow attenuation, osteolysis, and involvement of the skin in all patients. Periosteal reaction and intralesional gas can also be seen in patients.

T1- and T2-weighted MRI show intermediate signal intensity associated with moderate contrast enhancement. This characteristic signal intensity may be associated with the histologic feature of abundant granulation and fibrous tissue in actinomycosis. Popcornlike dystrophic calcification can also be seen occasionally.[15]

> Extensive soft tissue inflammatory and infiltrative changes in the surrounding soft tissues extending to the skin may be useful in the differentiation of actinomycosis from osteomyelitis due to other causes.[16]

Dental management

Initially, attempts are made to treat actinomycosis, including extensive disease, with aggressive antimicrobial therapy alone. Surgery is indicated to take a biopsy specimen, to drain abscesses, and to extirpate (wide excision) a fibrotic sinus tract. Follow-up should be adequate and meticulous to have a complete cure of the disease.

Klebsiella rhinoscleromatis Infection

It is a chronic, slowly progressive, localized infection caused by *Klebsiella rhinoscleromatis*. It is commonly seen in the upper respiratory tract, often originating in the nose.[17]

Clinical features

Common sites will be lacrimal glands, orbit, skin, and paranasal sinuses. It shows features, such as exudative, proliferative, and fibrotic (cicatrical).[18]

Exudative phase

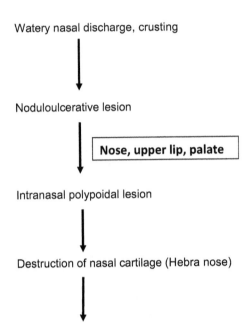

Watery nasal discharge, crusting

↓

Noduloulcerative lesion

↓   **Nose, upper lip, palate**

Intranasal polypoidal lesion

↓

Destruction of nasal cartilage (Hebra nose)

↓

Fibrosis and obstruction (Sclerotic stage)[18]

Oral manifestations
Impairment of the sensation of taste, anesthesia of the soft palate, and enlargement of the uvula and upper lip are observed.

Histopathologic features
There is a nonspecific inflammatory reaction with polymorph nuclear cells and dense plasma cell infiltration. Also noted are the Mikulicz cells: large foamy histiocytes, that is, macrophages with a size of up to 100 mm that are unable to digest phagocytosed bacteria, which persist in massively enlarged vacuoles. The sclerotic stage is characterized by granulomatous masses that result from scarring of chronically infected upper airways.[18]

Radiographic features
CT scan of the neck shows a big air pocket in the parapharyngeal spaces.[19] These findings are suggestive of a developing abscess. Gas-forming brain abscesses have been reported to result from escape of air into the cranium due to skull fracture or gas-forming organisms.[20]

Anthrax
Anthrax is caused by *Bacillus anthracis*. In cutaneous anthrax, it clinically appears as coal-like black lesions found on the skin.[21]

Clinical features
The spectrum of disease ranges from asymptomatic to severe, terminating in sepsis, septic shock, and death.[22] Oropharyngeal anthrax lesions are generally localized in the oral cavity, especially on the buccal mucosa, tongue, tonsils, or posterior pharynx

wall. The characteristic oral lesion is generally 2 to 3 cm in diameter and covered with a gray pseudomembrane surrounded by extensive edema. The main clinical features are sore throat, dysphagia, and painful regional lymphadenopathy in the involved side of the neck. The illness may progress rapidly, and edema around lymph nodes may result in extensive swelling of the neck and anterior chest wall. The overt infection leads to toxemia, acute respiratory distress, and alteration in mental state.[23]

Histopathologic features

Gram-stained smear from the lesion reveals polymorphonuclear leukocytes and gram-positive bacilli, and the culture may be positive for *B anthracis*.[24]

Radiographic features

- Disease manifests as pleural effusions, mediastinal widening, and, rarely, pneumonia. Mediastinal widening with high-attenuation mediastinal and hilar lymph nodes on CT in the absence of trauma, dissection, or bleeding diathesis is suspicious.[25]

Brucellosis

It is a multisystem disorder with a broad spectrum of nonspecific symptoms.[26] Brucellosis manifests as an acute febrile illness that may persist and progress to a chronically incapacitating disease with severe complications. Bone and joint involvement is the most frequent complication of brucellosis, occurring in up to 40% of cases.[27]

Syphilis

Syphilis is caused by *Treponema pallidum* and is characterized by episodes of active disease interrupted by periods of latency. It can be either acquired or congenital. The acquired form is contracted as a venereal disease and if untreated manifests 3 distinctive stages throughout its course: primary, secondary, and tertiary stages.[28]

Oral manifestations

The primary lesion is an elevated, ulcerated nodule that shows indurations and produces regional lymphadenopathy. The intraoral chancre can be appreciated. The secondary stage produces multiple, painless, grayish-white plaques overlying an ulcerated surface and are called mucous patches.[29] Several adjacent mucous patches fuse to form a serpentine or snail-track pattern. Commonly involved sites include the tongue, gingiva, and buccal mucosa. Occasionally papillary lesions resembling viral papillomas may arise called as condylomata lata.[30] Late congenital syphilis is diagnosed by clinical history, distinctive physical signs, and a positive serologic test. The Hutchinson triad of interstitial keratitis, Hutchinson incisors (**Figs. 4** and **5**), and eighth cranial nerve deafness are diagnostic.

Histopathologic features

The primary lesions show ulcerated surface epithelium with several vascular channels and intense chronic inflammatory infiltrate in the underlying lamina propria. The inflammatory infiltrate is chiefly composed of lymphocytes and plasma cells and demonstrates a perivascular pattern. In the secondary stages, the epithelium demonstrates hyperplasia with significant spongiosis and exocytosis. Tertiary lesions exhibit peripheral pseudoepitheliomatous hyperplasia. The foci of granulomatous inflammation with well-circumscribed collections of histiocytes and multinucleated giant cells can be observed.[31]

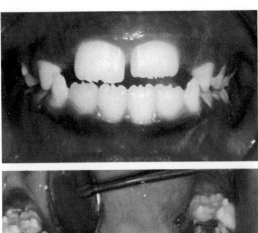

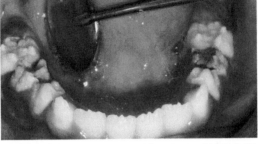

Fig. 4. Hutchinson incisors noted in a patient with suspected congenital syphilis. Note the hypoplastic mulberry molars in the mandible. (*Courtesy of* Dr R. George, Rutgers School of Dental Medicine, Newark, NJ.)

Radiographic features

- Syphilitic osteomyelitis causes osteolytic changes in the cortex and medullary space, usually with an aggressive pattern of bone destruction compared with other types of osteomyelitis that occur in jaws. Sequestra in syphilis are difficult to visualize radiographically because they are small and usually occur in cancellous bone. It should be stressed that the destructive lesions in early acquired syphilis are those of osteomyelitis and do not represent gummas.[32] MRI demonstrates marrow space involvement, periosteal process, and a degree of intracranial extension more completely than CT.[33]
- Proliferative periostitis has been well described in secondary syphilis and is most commonly seen in the tibiae, skull, clavicles, ribs, and sternum. Scintigraphy is a

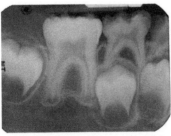
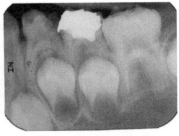

Fig. 5. Bitewing radiographs of the patient noted in **Fig. 4** demonstrating hypoplastic nature of the primary molars and permanent first molars. (*Courtesy of* Dr R. George, Rutgers School of Dental Medicine, Newark, NJ.)

sensitive means of detection in subtle cases and can be useful in the determination of the extent of disease for guiding bone biopsy.
- Syphilitic gummas in CT may present as hypodense with no contrast enhancement or mass effect or as densely enhancing masses with surrounding edema. Magnetic resonance (MR) descriptions have included lesions hypointense to isointense on T1-weighted images and hyperintense on T2-weighted images, associated with homogeneous contrast enhancement.[34]

FUNGAL INFECTIONS
Histoplasmosis

It is a granulomatous fungal infection caused by a dimorphic fungus *Histoplasma capsulatum*, first described by Samuel Darling in 1905 (see **Table 1**).[35]

Clinical features
It is acquired by the inhalation of dust containing the spores of fungus or contamination occurring from excreta of birds, such as pigeons, starlings, and black birds. It is clinically classified into the following:

- Acute primary pulmonary histoplasmosis
- Chronic pulmonary histoplasmosis
- Disseminated histoplasmosis[35]

It is characterized by chronic low-grade fever, productive cough, splenomegaly, hepatomegaly, and lymphadenopathy. The infection may be mild and manifests only as local lesions, such as subcutaneous nodules or supportive arthritis.[36] Oral lesions appear as nodular, ulcerative, or vegetative lesions on the buccal mucosa, gingiva, tongue, palate, or lips. Ulcerated areas are covered by a gray membrane that is indurated with raised and rolled-out borders resembling carcinoma. It is solitary and very painful.[37]

Histopathologic features
The classic feature of histoplasmosis is granuloma formation, a collection of macrophages organized into granulomas. Granulomatous inflammation is associated with multinucleated giant cells. Special stains, such as periodic acid-Schiff and Grocott–Gomori methenamine silver methods, can be used. They demonstrate characteristic 2- to 4-µm oval, narrow-based budding yeasts of *H capsulatum*. Yeasts are found within the macrophages and can also be seen free in the tissues.[38]

Radiographic features
In chronic pulmonary histoplasmosis, chest radiographs often reveal emphysematous lungs with apical bullae surrounded by segmental airspace disease. Progressive thickening of cavity walls and retraction of adjacent lung tissue occur over time, but lymphadenopathy is typically absent. In disseminated histoplasmosis, chest radiographs may be normal but usually display small, diffuse, nodular opacities.[39]

Treatment of histoplasmosis depends on the severity of the clinical syndrome. Mild cases may require only symptomatic measures, but antifungal therapy is indicated in all cases of chronic or disseminated disease and in severe or prolonged acute pulmonary infection.

Blastomycosis

It is also called as Gilchrist disease. It is caused by *Blastomyces dermatitidis*, which is a dimorphic fungus. It is endemic in South, South Central, and the Great Lakes regions of the United States as well as parts of Canada.[40]

Clinical features

The source of infection in humans is unknown. Most commonly affected individuals are those who work in the outdoors for longer time periods. It occurs in the middle-aged population, and men are more commonly affected than women. It manifests on the skin as small red papules that gradually increase in size and form tiny miliary abscess or pustules that tend to ulcerate and discharge pus. It presents as crateriform lesions with induration and elevated borders. It is associated with fever, sudden weight loss, and productive cough.[41] Oral manifestations are either primary or secondary to lesions present on the body. It is characterized by tiny ulcers. These lesions may bear resemblance to epidermoid carcinoma.[42]

Histopathologic features

It is characterized by acute inflammatory cell infiltrate followed by histiocytic response and granuloma formation. Inflamed connective tissue shows multinucleated giant cells, and microabscesses are found frequently.[42] The granulomas are noted with central necrotic neutrophils surrounded by epithelioid histiocytes. The yeasts are present within the purulent centers of the granulomas and within the histiocytes measuring between 5 µm and 15 µm in diameter. They are round and have a double refractive capsule. Nonulcerated lesions present pseudoepitheliomatous hyperplasia.[41]

Radiological features

There are reported cases of radiolucent bone lesions in the jaws in blastomycosis. Chest radiographs show concomitant pulmonary involvement in all cases. The major radiologic features of pulmonary involvement fall into the following categories: airspace consolidation, masses, intermediate sized nodules, interstitial disease, miliary disease, and cavitary lesions. Unlike histoplasmosis, blastomycotic infections rarely have parenchymal or lymph node calcifications.[43]

Treatment

Ketoconazole, fluconazole, or itraconazole is used for the management of mild to moderate disease and amphotericin B for severe disease.

Phycomycosis

It is also called mucormycosis and zygomycosis. It was first described by Paultauf in 1885.[1] It is caused by numerous Phycomycetes organisms of the Eumycetes class, such as *Rhizopus*, *Mucor*, *Absidia*, and, rarely, *Saksenaea* and *Cunninghamella*.[44]

Clinical features

- There are 5 forms of the disease:
  o Rhinocerebral
  o Pulmonary
  o Gastrointestinal (GI) tract
  o Cutaneous
  o Disseminated[45]
- It occurs in 2 main forms:
  o Superficial
  o Visceral[46]
- It is an opportunistic infection manifesting in those with malignant lymphomas, patients having renal failure, organ transplant, AIDS, and cirrhosis. It is more common in patients with uncontrolled diabetes mellitus who are ketoacidotic.

Ketoacidosis inhibits the binding of iron to transferrin and raises the levels of iron, which in turn enhances the growth of these fungi.[47]

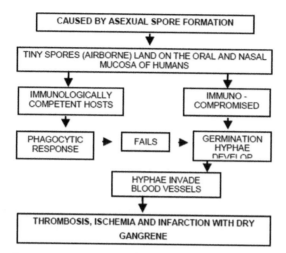

Pathophysiology of mucormycosis. (*Adapted from* Hingad N, Kumar G, Deshmukh R. Oral mucormycosis causing necrotizing lesion in diabetic patient: a case report. Int J Oral Maxillofac Pathol 2012;3(3):8–12.)

It is characterized by nasal obstruction, bloody nasal discharge, facial pain, facial swelling, and visual disturbances with proptosis. As the disease progresses into the cranial vault, it results in blindness, lethargy, and seizures followed by death. The maxillary sinus is frequently involved and presents as an intraoral swelling of the maxillary alveolar process and palate. Eventually, ulceration may develop. It is typically black in color and is necrotic.[47]

Histopathologic features
On microscopic examination, extensive tissue necrosis with numerous branching and nonseptate hyphae, which tend to branch at 90°, are seen at the periphery. Fungi have a preference for invasion of small blood vessels, which disrupt normal blood flow to the tissues resulting in necrosis.[45] The inflammatory infiltrate is primarily made of neutrophils and is predominant in the viable tissue.

Radiographic features
Radiographically, rhinocerebral mucormycosis demonstrates nodular thickening of the sinus, sinus opacification without fluid level, and spotty destruction of paranasal sinuses.[48] CT scan with contrast/MRI scan may demonstrate erosion or destruction of bone and may help to delineate the extent of the disease.

Dental management
Surgical management should be initiated early in the course of treatment. This management should involve debridement of all infected tissues. In some cases, radical resection may be required, which can include partial or total maxillectomy, mandibulectomy, and orbital exoneration. The use of amphotericin B in patients with mucormycosis has been a widely published and accepted treatment, with a survival rate of up to 72%.

Aspergillosis

It is fungal disease caused by *Aspergillus*, a ubiquitous fungus that belongs to Asco-mycetes molds. It is introduced by inhalation and inhabits the human upper respiratory tract.[49]

Clinical features

The classification has been put forth by Rowe-Jones and Moore-Gillon[50] in 1994, which includes 3 main types:

1. Noninvasive
2. Invasive
3. Destructive noninvasive types, which are further classified into the following:
   a. Aspergilloma
   b. Fungus ball
   c. Mycetoma (usually affecting one sinus) or aspergillus sinusitis (involving more than one sinus)[50]

More extensive invasive infection is evident in immune compromised conditions, such as AIDS or in those with organ transplantation.[51] A low-grade infection estab-lished in the maxillary sinus results in a mass of fungal hyphae called aspergilloma. It may undergo dystrophic calcification and results in a radiopaque body within the si-nus called an antrolith. It may also occur after tooth extraction or endodontic treat-ment, particularly in the maxillary posterior segments. Symptoms of localized pain and tenderness along with nasal discharge can be evident. It could also result in pain-ful gingival ulcerations, as the main portal of entry to the oral cavity is the marginal gingiva or the gingival sulcus. Long-standing diseases could result in necrosis and clinically present as a yellow or black ulcer.[52]

Histopathologic features

Histopathologic features of aspergillosis shows septate hyphae of 3 to 4 μm in diam-eter that tend to branch at acute angles (**Fig. 6**). They tend to invade small blood ves-sels, occlusion of which results in necrosis. In immunocompromised patients, granulomatous inflammatory response can be expected.[53]

Radiographic features

Each form of paranasal aspergillosis has a specific radiologic profile. The presence of radiodense foci in association with homogenous opacity of the sinus is highly

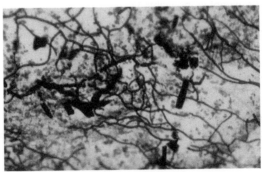

Fig. 6. Stain shows branching septate hyphae with acute angle (Grocott-Gomori methena-mine silver stain, original magnification ×20). (*Courtesy of* Dr C. Padmavathi Devi, Professor & Head, Department of Pathology, Guntur Medical College & Hospital, Guntur, India.)

suggestive of a noninvasive mycetoma. Opacity of the sinus with or without destruction may be demonstrated in the invasive form. MRI was found to be even more sensitive than CT in diagnosing fungal sinusitis (**Figs. 7** and **8**). Fungal sinusitis has a characteristic low T2 hyperintensity.[54]

Cryptococcosis

Cryptococcosis is a fungal disease caused by *Cryptococcus neoformans*, which was discovered in 1894 as an encapsulated yeastlike fungus.[55] It can be destructive to immune-compromised individuals, such as those with AIDS, malignancy, or receiving systemic corticosteroid therapy or cancer therapy.[56]

Clinical features
Primary cryptococcal infection of lungs results in mild flulike illness with productive cough, chest pain, fever, and malaise. The disseminated form involves the meninges, skin, bone, and prostate gland.[57] Cutaneous lesions appear as erythematous papules or pustules, which ulcerate and discharge puslike material. Oral lesions are characterized by craterlike nonhealing ulcers or as friable papillary erythematous plaques that are tender on palpation.[58]

Histopathologic features
Histopathologic features are suggestive of a granulomatous inflammatory response, which is recognized as a compact aggregate of macrophages with epithelioid features and multinucleated giant cells, of both foreign-body reaction and Langerhans type, with yeasts appearing as round to ovoid structures of 4 to 6 μm in diameter and surrounded by a clear halo.[59]

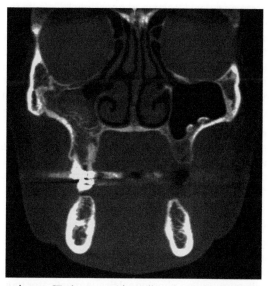

Fig. 7. Coronal cone beam CT view at midmaxillary level demonstrating radiopaque foci within the soft tissue density in the right maxillary sinus without any fluid levels, a characteristic feature of fungal sinusitis. (*Courtesy of* Dr Mansur Ahmad, University of Minnesota School of Dentistry, Minneapolis, MN.)

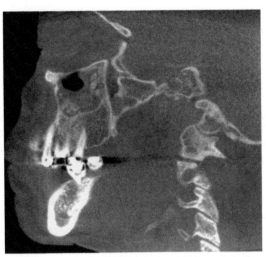

Fig. 8. Sagittal cone beam CT view showing the right maxillary sinus and its contents. Note the soft tissue opacity within the sinus interspersed with calcific foci, and absence of air-fluid interface suggests maxillary sinusitis of fungal origin. (*Courtesy of* Dr Mansur Ahmad, University of Minnesota School of Dentistry, Minneapolis, MN.)

Rhinosporidiosis

It is a chronic granulomatous infection caused by *Rhinosporidium seeberi*.[60]

Clinical features

It commonly manifests as a nasal lesion and occasionally affects the skin. Extranasal sites, such as the eye, ear, trachea, and parotid duct, may also be involved.[1] Nasal lesions are painless, friable, polypoidal growths, which may hang anteriorly into the nares or posteriorly into the pharynx.[61] Cutaneous lesions manifest in the form of verrucous plaques, polypoidal growths, subcutaneous nodules, furunculoid lesions, and ecthymatoid lesions.[62] Rhinosporidiosis involving the parotid duct manifests itself as a facial swelling. Oronasopharyngeal lesions appear as soft, red, polypoid growths.[63]

Histopathologic features

Histopathologic features are suggestive of sporangia containing large numbers of round or ovoid endospores, measuring approximately 5 to 7 μm in diameter (**Fig. 9**). The surrounding connective tissue shows vascular granulation tissue and mixed inflammatory cells.[64]

Radiographic features

The role of imaging in rhinosporidiosis is to evaluate the number of lesions, the location and extent of disease, surrounding bone involvement, nasolacrimal duct involvement, and any associated complications. CT shows moderate to intense enhancement in the lesion compared with surrounding pharyngeal tissue/masticator muscles with Hounsfield units ranging from 70 to 160. Contrast MRI demarcates the extent; it appears as an intensely enhancing lesion in the respective area, which may be due to the rich vascularity of this lesion.[65]

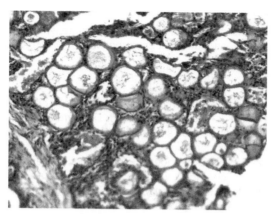

Fig. 9. Stain shows multiple granulomas containing sporangias with lymphocytes (hematoxylin-eosin, original magnification ×10). (*Courtesy of* Dr C. Padmavathi Devi, Professor and Head, Department of Pathology, Guntur Medical College & Hospital, Guntur, India.)

Dental management

The mainstay of treatment is surgical excision. Limited excision with cauterization at the base of the lesion is preferred, as radical surgery may lead to perforation, hemorrhage, increased recurrence, and dissemination. However, those with oropharyngeal extension may require a more extensive approach. Dapsone is a promising drug that is used as an adjunct to surgery as it arrests the maturation of sporangia and promotes fibrosis.

PARASITIC INFECTIONS
Leishmaniasis

Leishmaniasis is caused by *Leishmania donovani* (see **Table 1**). It is a parasitic infection affecting the organs.[66] Leishmaniasis is endemic. It is commonly seen in Lahj, Abyan, and Hagga governorates in Yemen.[67]

Clinical features

The incubation period is usually from 2 to 6 months.[68] The mode of transmission is through blood, transfusion, and sexual contact.[69] Patients present with a history of fever with splenomegaly, hepatomegaly, and lymphadenopathy.[70] Anemia with epistaxis and bleeding is common.[71]

Histopathologic features

Parasitic macrophages with amastigotes multiply in the spleen, liver, and bone marrow.[72] Marked proliferation of the reticuloendothelial proliferation is loaded with *Leishmania donovani* bodies and lymphocytic infiltration.[73]

Management

The treatment of choice in all clinical forms of leishmaniasis is based on the administration of pentavalent antimonial drugs, such as meglumine antimonate and sodium stibogluconate. The former drug is more widely used, preferentially via the intramuscular route, with intravenous dosing as secondary alternative.[74]

Myiasis

It is parasitic infestation of the body of a living mammal by fly larvae (maggots).[75] Myiasis is more prevalent in regions where the climate is more humid and warm.[76] The most common predisposing factors are diabetes and peripheral vascular diseases.[77]

Clinical features

Myiasis is initially asymptomatic. When the lesion progress, it may show acute pain with irritation of the mucosa. The most common location is the anterior maxilla.[78]

DIAGNOSIS

Ultrasound can be very useful to confirm a case of furuncular myiasis and also for the complete removal of the larvae. On ultrasound, *Dermatobia hominis* presents as a well-defined, highly echogenic area surrounded by a hypoechoic area. Other features include the presence of segmentations on longitudinal sections and distal shadowing. The strong posterior acoustic shadowing may reflect the external coating of the larva.[79] Color Doppler sonography, which is able to visualize the continuous movement of internal fluids of the larva, has proven to be useful for the detection of *D hominis* and *Cordylobia anthropophaga* larvae when ultrasound is not able to detect the parasite.[79] MR and CT are able to identify a subcutaneous segmented nodule; however, its morphology does not aid in the diagnosis.

Dental Management

- Surgical debridement of the wound and extraction of larvae are most commonly done under local anesthetic or general anesthesia. The occlusion or suffocation approach forces aerobic larvae to surface in search of air where they can be removed with the aid of forceps or tweezers (**Figs. 10** and **11**).
- Some of the agents that have been used to suffocate are petroleum jelly, heavy oil, beeswax, raw meat, mineral oil, nail polish, adhesive tape, butter, chewing gum, turpentine oil, whitehead varnish, native tobacco leaf, chloroform, and ether.
- Topical and oral ivermectin have been used against maggots in humans.[80] It is assumed that ivermectin blocks nerve impulses to the nerve endings through the release of gamma aminobutyric acid, linking to the receptors and causing palsy and death of maggots.

Toxoplasmosis

It is a protozoan parasitic infection caused by *Toxoplasma gondii*. *Toxoplasma gondii* will be presented with the cell.[81] Spreading of toxoplasmosis will take up a complex

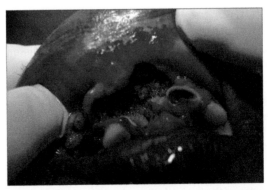

Fig. 10. Maggots noted within the oral lesion in a patient with special needs. (*From* Sankari LS, Ramakrishnan K. Oral myiasis caused by Chrysomya bezziana. J Oral Maxillofac Pathol 2010;14(1):17.)

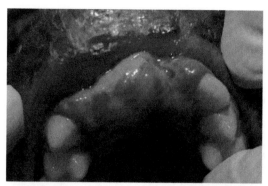

Fig. 11. Intraoral lesion of myiasis healing after surgical debridement and irrigation. (*From* Sankari LS, Ramakrishnan K. Oral myiasis caused by Chrysomya bezziana. J Oral Maxillofac Pathol 2010;14(1):17.)

life cycle. The primary host will be epithelial cells of the digestive tract of cats and secondary will be the mammals and birds.[82]

Clinical features

Patients with *Toxoplasmosis gondii* do not show any symptoms.[3] Sometimes patients may present with a history of low-grade fever, cervical lymphadenopathy, fatigue of muscles, and joint pains.[83] *Toxoplasmosis gondii* can cause sever myocarditis, pneumonitis, and encephalitis as a latent infection.[84]

Histopathologic features

Histopathologic features show reactive germinal centers, which exhibit an accumulation of eosinophilic macrophages.[81] These macrophages are seen in the subcapsular and sinusoidal region of the lymph node.[85]

TRAUMATIC CAUSE
Pyogenic Granulomas

It is an inflammatory hyperplasia of the soft tissue growth intraorally (**Figs. 12** and **13**; see **Table 1**).[86] Pyogenic granulomas can occur on the skin but very rarely in the GI tract.[87] Hullihen[88] first reported the finding in 1844, and Hartzell[89] coined the term *pyogenic granulomas*.

Clinical features

Seventy percent to 80% of the cases of pyogenic granulomas are seen in the gingival region.[90] Other sites, such as the lip, buccal mucosa, and tongue, have also been reported.[91] Women are more commonly affected than men. Pyogenic granulomas clinically present as smooth, lobulated, pedunculated lesions.[92] The size of the lesion can vary from a few millimeters to a few centimeters.[93] The surface appears as an ulceration with a yellow fibrous membrane covered with an ulcerated area.[94]

Histopathologic features

It presents as numerous blood vessels with endothelial cell proliferation, which may resemble a granuloma.[93] These blood vessels appear as clusters that are separated with thin fibrous connective tissue septa, leading to an overall appearance of lobular hemangioma (**Fig. 14**).[94] Connective tissue stroma shows fibroblasts and typically appears plump with extravasated red blood cells.[94] Long-standing pyogenic granulomas may show the features of peripheral ossifying fibromas.[95]

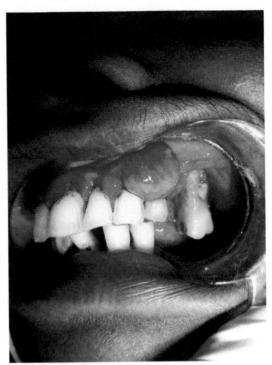

Fig. 12. A patient with a large pyogenic granuloma in relation to maxillary left canine and first premolar region. The lesion seems to be very vascular. The patient has generalized advanced periodontitis. (*Courtesy of* Department of Oral Pathology, Sibar Institute of Dental Sciences, Guntur, India.)

Treatment

- Conservative surgical excision and removal of causative irritants are used.[95]
- Nd:YAG, carbon dioxide, and flashlamp-pulsed dye lasers have also been used for the treatment of pyogenic granulomas.

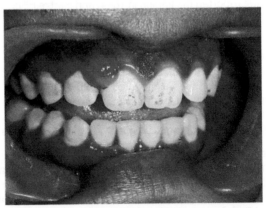

Fig. 13. A patient with moderate-sized pyogenic granuloma in relation to the papilla between maxillary right central and lateral incisors. (*Courtesy of* Department of Oral Pathology, Sibar Institute of Dental Sciences, Guntur, India.)

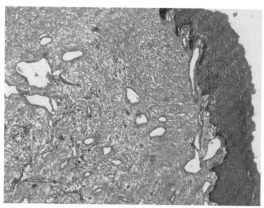

Fig. 14. Parakeratinized stratified squamous epithelium, fibrocellular connective tissue, numerous dilated blood vessels, and endothelial cell proliferation (hematoxylin-eosin, original magnification ×4). (*Courtesy of* Dr C. Padmavathi Devi, Professor and Head, Department of Pathology, Guntur Medical College & Hospital, Guntur, India.)

- Cryotherapy with liquid nitrogen or nitrous oxide is another treatment modality.
- Sclerotherapy with sodium tetra decyl sulfate, monoethanolamine oleate, and polidocanol has been described as a conservative method with effective results.

FOREIGN BODY CAUSE
Oral Foreign Body Reaction

Foreign body reaction is a circumstance in which the substances that aggravate the inflammatory cells lead to either an acute or chronic reaction, characterized by phagocytes, and cannot be digested by the neutrophils (see **Table 1**). This reaction may lead to granulomatous inflammation with the collection of epithelioid cells and multinucleated giant cells.[96]

Clinical features

It is asymptomatic, but occasionally patients may give a history of foreign bodies that have entered into the soft tissue because of laceration or trauma.[97] There are some evidence literature shown that food substances, like fish bones and teeth, and some filling components, such as amalgam and composite material, cause granulomas.[98]

Histopathologic Features

Histopathologic features of foreign body reactions seem similar to other granulomatous inflammation, with epithelioid histiocytes surrounded by lymphocytes and multinucleated giant cells.[99]

Cholesterol Granulomas

They are slow-growing extradural lesions that cause an inflammatory granulation tissue response in the presence of cholesterol crystals.[100] First reported by Manasse in 1894, cholesterol granulomas are associated with cerebellopontine angle syndrome.[101] It is a foreign body reaction, mainly associated with cholesterol crystals, and it leads to granulomas.[102] It can occur anywhere in the body, including the mastoid process, temporal bone, kidney, lung, testis, and brain. It is rarely seen in paranasal sinuses.[103] Only few cases are associated with jawbones.

Pathogenesis
The pathogenesis is still unknown. Yamazaki suggested that perlecan, which is predominantly seen in the cyst wall of immature granulomas, may cause cholesterol granulomas.[104]

Clinical features
It is more commonly seen in men compared with women. The maxillary sinus is the most common site, followed by the mandible, as reported by Hirschberg and colleagues.[105] Kaffe and colleagues[106] reported cholesterol granulomas associated with maxillary odontoma. It is the first reported case of cholesterol granulomas within a mandibular odontogenic cyst.

Histopathologic features
There are nonkeratinized epithelial cells surrounded by a thin fibrous capsule without inflammatory cells. There is granulomatous tissue with heavy lymphocytic infiltration between cholesterol clefts within a fibrous capsule. There is dense diffuse chronic inflammatory cell infiltration made up chiefly by lymphocytes with multinucleated giant cells.[106]

Radiographic features
Cholesterol granuloma of the maxillary sinus in a radiograph manifests as an opacification with cystic arrangement or soft tissue density, usually well defined by a sclerotic cortical bone, although bone expansion and erosion can also be observed.[107]

Treatment
The treatment of choice for maxillary sinus cholesterol granuloma is surgical excision, usually through a Caldwell-Luc approach; but the transnasal endoscopic technique has also been reported to be useful. Generally, patients with symptoms are managed surgically, whereas nonsurgical management is advocated for asymptomatic patients. The prognosis is good, and recurrences are rare with effective treatment.

Cocaine-Induced Granulomas

Cocaine is a crystalline alkaloid derived from the coca leaves of the coca plant.[108] Cocaine can be converted into cocaine chlorhydrate with catalyst agents like ether, sulfuric acid, and gasoline. Cocaine mainly causes vasoconstriction, which leads to necrosis in the paranasal mucosa and destruction of the nasal septa, paranasal sinus walls, and palate.[109] Clinically it may mimic leishmaniasis, lymphoma, blastomycosis, and Wegener granulomatosis.[110]

Clinical features
Acute administration may cause feelings of increased energy and motor activity and decreases need for food and sleep. Clinically, cocaine-induced lesions appear similar to lymphoma, infection, and granulomatosis polyangitis.[109] Dermatologic manifestations include frank extensive necrosis and crusting eschars. There is literature available on Stevens-Johnson syndrome associated with cocaine abusers[111] as well as musculoskeletal manifestations, such as arthralgia and myalgia.[112]

Histopathologic features
There are necrotic areas admixed with chronic inflammatory cell infiltration. There is squamous metaplasia in minor salivary glands. Along with chronic inflammatory cell infiltration, there are few giant cells seen.[112]

Radiographic features

Radiographs reveal a relative radiolucency in the palatal aspect. A CT scan of the head might reveal an absence of the nasal septum with destruction of the medial wall of the maxillary sinus.[113] Surgical removal followed by the use of obturators and psychological consultation remains the mainstay of treating such lesions.

Gout

It is a systemic disease characterized by chronic hyperuricemia, which leads to the deposition of monosodium urate crystals.[114] Urate crystal deposition may initiate inflammatory changes and causes inflammatory arthropathy. Urate crystal deposition is episodic and leads to renal calculi and urate nephropathy.[115]

Pathogenesis[116]

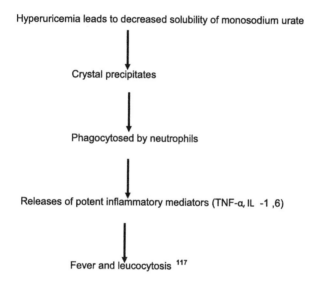

Hyperuricemia leads to decreased solubility of monosodium urate

↓

Crystal precipitates

↓

Phagocytosed by neutrophils

↓

Releases of potent inflammatory mediators (TNF-α, IL -1 ,6)

↓

Fever and leucocytosis [117]

Clinical features

Clinically gout will show 4 stages:

1. Asymptomatic hyperuricemia
2. Intermittent acute gout
3. Intercritical gout
4. Advanced or chronic tophaceous gout

   Although initially asymptomatic, acute gout is characterized by joint pain and inflammation that is typically monoarticular.[2] As the disease progresses, it may become polyarticular, and it will be associated with pain. In advanced cases, it leads to pain and swelling in the joints.[117]

Histopathologic features

Cutaneous gout shows a granulomatous reaction. Small to large granulomas are separated with fibrous septa and degenerative pseudonecrotic changes.[118]

Radiographic features

Patients with temporomandibular joint involvement may present with degenerative articular changes of the condyle and temporal bone. Punched-out radiolucency may be seen on the condylar cartilage. CT usually demonstrates a calcified mass involving the joint space with degenerative changes of the surrounding bones (articular space narrowing, osteophytosis).[119]

MR features have rarely been described, except in tumoral forms, which demonstrate low-signal-intensity periarticular formation on T2-weighted images.

Treatment

Treatment of gout is based on the prevention of crystal formation, dissolution of crystals, and decrease of biological consequences of crystal-cell interactions. Administration of uricosuric agents like colchicine and allopurinol to increase elimination of uric acid is helpful.[6]

NEOPLASTIC
Histiocytosis X

Histiocytosis X, currently described as Langerhans cell histiocytosis (LCH), was first identified in 1893 by Hand (see **Table 1**).[120] It is a rare disorder in which the pathologic cells derived from bone marrow infiltrate and destroy the tissue.[121] It can present clinically as a single-system disorder, which mainly affects the bone (single or multifocal), or as a multisystem disorder.[121] Eosinophilic granulomas make up the most common and indolent form of LCH affecting a single system (the bone).[121]

Clinical features

It can affect at any age, but more than 50% of the patients are diagnosed before 6 years of age.[122] Bones of the skull are most commonly affected. It can also affect the long bones, pelvis, and the vertebrae.[122] Hand-Schüller-Christian disease is a multisystem form of LCH that occurs in children between 1 and 5 years of age. These patients show a classic triad of symptoms: exophthalmos, diabetes insipidus, and osteolytic skull lesions. In some patients, the brain, viscera, and skin might also be affected.[123]

Letterer-Siwe disease is probably the most dangerous form of LCH, which affects children predominantly younger than 3 years.[124] It is associated with fever, rashes, and pancytopenia, along with enlargement of the liver, spleen, and lymph nodes.[124] It is a rapidly progressive disorder and has a high mortality rate. Pulmonary and hepatic dysfunction are common findings in these patients.[125]

Histopathology

LCH cells exhibit a homogeneously eosinophilic cytoplasm and lobulated nucleus.[120] These aggregates of LCH cells are admixed with a variable number of lymphocytes, macrophages, and eosinophils; occasionally a few multinucleated giant cells can also be seen.[126] A confirmatory diagnosis with hematoxylin-eosin is not always possible, and demonstration of CD1a immunohistochemically or Birbeck granules electron microscopically usually gives a definitive diagnosis.[127]

Radiographic findings

The different types of lesions produced by LCH in the maxilla and mandible are described according to their radiographic characteristics.[128]

1. Solitary intrabony lesions appear as circular or elliptical, solitary or unifocal lesions principally in the body and ramus of the mandible. They are incidental radiographic findings.
2. Multiple alveolar lesions, in most cases, appear well defined. In 37.7% of cases, they may have poorly defined or invasive margins (**Figs. 15** and **16**).

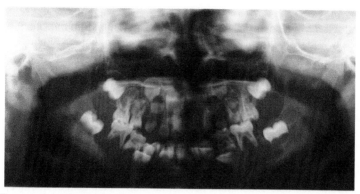

Fig. 15. Panoramic radiograph of a 3-year-old man patient showing multiple destructive mandibular lesions essentially giving the appearance of floating teeth. The patient was diagnosed with histiocytosis X and was treated with surgery and chemotherapy. (*Courtesy of* Dr Mansur Ahmad, University of Minnesota School of Dentistry, Minneapolis, MN.)

3. Scooped-out alveolar lesions result from bony destruction beginning below the alveolar crest (either at furcation level or one-half of the tooth root).
4. There are alveolar lesions with bone sclerosis.
5. There are alveolar lesions with bone neoformation.
6. There is a floating teeth appearance.[129]

Management

Antibiotic therapy, chemotherapy, radiotherapy, surgery, adrenocorticotropic hormone, and corticoids (both systemic and intralesional) have been advocated in the management of these lesions.

Necrotizing Sialometaplasia

Necrotizing sialometaplasia is a benign, self-limiting disease affecting mainly the minor salivary glands, which was first reported by Abrams and colleagues.[130]

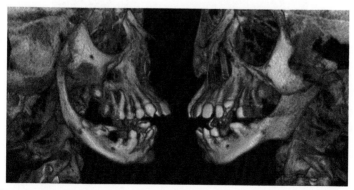

Fig. 16. Cone beam CT reconstruction of the same patient as in **Fig. 15** 10 years after initial diagnosis of histiocytosis X. Note the healed lesions, although there are multiple jaw deformities and malocclusion. (*Courtesy of* Dr Mansur Ahmad, University of Minnesota School of Dentistry, Minneapolis, MN.)

Clinical features

The site affected most commonly is the hard palate. It mimics a malignant neoplasm both clinically and histologically and, hence, is very important.[130] Although the exact cause is not known, ischemia to the minor salivary glands, precipitated by a history of trauma is the most acceptable explanation for this entity.[131] Reduced blood supply to the lobules ultimately leads to necrosis, which is the characteristic feature of necrotizing sialometaplasia.[132]

Although trauma is considered to be the cause, smoking, alcohol consumption, radiation, and upper respiratory tract infection are also considered to be factors precipitating ischemia to the minor salivary glands.[133]

Histopathology

It shows lobular necrosis associated with squamous metaplasia of ductal epithelium (**Fig. 17**).[131] The most striking feature is that the normal salivary lobular architecture is maintained.[132]

Radiographic features

Usually no radiographic manifestations are seen. In rare instances, CT findings show a craterlike defect in the palatal region.[134]

Management

These lesions are usually self-healing (4–10 weeks) and do not require any specific treatment. The healing time is primarily related to the size rather than the nature of the lesions. Analgesics can be given for pain management. These lesions should always include an incisional biopsy and close follow-up until they entirely disappear and they have minimal chances of recurrence.[135]

Polymorphic Reticulosis (Lethal Midline Granulomas)

It is a midfacial necrotizing disease that is characterized by the presence of destructive lesions in the mucosa of the upper aerodigestive tract.[136]

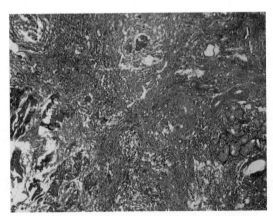

Fig. 17. Minor salivary gland acini (*asterisk*) with squamous metaplasia (*plus*) and lymphocytic infiltration (hematoxylin-eosin, original magnification ×4). (*Courtesy of* Dr C. Padmavathi Devi, Professor and Head, Department of Pathology, Guntur Medical College & Hospital, Guntur, India.)

Clinical features

The nasal septum, hard palate, lateral nasal walls, paranasal sinuses, skin of the face, orbit, and nasopharynx are the most commonly affected sites.[136] Nasal stuffiness with discharge, rhinorrhea, epistaxis, and nasal obstruction along with pain are some of the characteristic complaints of patients.[137] The most common age is in the fourth decade, and the man to woman ratio is 8:1 to 2:1. Epstein-Barr virus is considered to be associated with these lesions.[138]

Histopathology

There is dense cellular infiltrate, primarily consisting of atypical lymphoid and reticulum cells.[139] Areas of necrosis with leukocytic reactions are a common finding in the infiltrated tissue.[140]

Radiographic features

CT scans reveal radiopacity of a degree consistent with the soft tissue encroaching into the nasal cavity, maxillary sinuses, ethmoidal, frontal and sphenoidal sinuses, and the nasopharynx.[141]

Management

Treatment varies from the use of radiation therapy to corticosteroid and chemotherapy.

UNKNOWN CAUSE
Sarcoidosis

It is a skin manifestation with hilar lymphadenopathy and pulmonary infection (see **Table 1**). The World Congress in KYOTO 1991 defined it as a "multisystem disorder of unknown cause. It may affect young and middle aged adults and frequently presents with bilateral hilar lymphadenopathy, pulmonary infiltration; ocular and skin lesion."[142] In a joint statement of the American Thoracic Society, The European Respiratory Society, and the World Association of Sarcoidosis in 1991 "Sarcoidosis is a multisystem disorder of unknown cause the diagnosis established when clinicopathologic evidence of non caseating epithelioid cell granulomas. Granulomas of known cause and local sarcoid reactions must be excluded."[143]

Clinical features

There is formation of noncaseating epithelioid granulomas. It has cutaneous involvement as well as lung, lymph node, and eye involvement. Clinically, it appears as papules, nodules, plagues, subcutaneous tumors, and lupus pernio.[144,145] The working diagnosis of patients with sarcoidosis without histopathology is involvement of erythema nodosum or fibril arthropathy, bilateral hilar lymph node enlargement, and low tuberculin sensitivity.[144] Radiographs may show evidence of osteopenia (**Fig. 18**).

Histopathologic features

There are granulomatous inflammation features. Clusters of epithelioid histiocytes surround the rim of lymphocytes. Langerhans giant cells are seen with lamilated basophilic calcifications known as Schaumann bodies or asteroid bodies. In the lymph node, small yellow structures called Hamazaki–Wesenberg bodies can be seen in subcapsular sinuses.[14]

Crohn Disease

It is a chronic inflammatory bowel disease with an unknown cause. It is characterized by exacerbations and spontaneous or drug-induced remission.[146] Crohn disease was

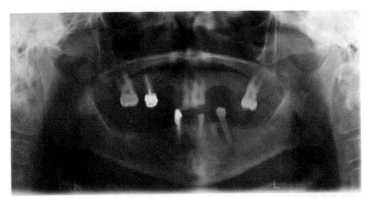

Fig. 18. A panoramic radiograph of a patient with sarcoidosis. Note the generalized reduction in trabeculae and thinning of the cortices suggestive of significant osteopenia.

first described by Crohn and colleagues[147] in 1932.[147] It is a transmural disease that can affect the entire GI tract and oral cavity. It can be multifactorial, and there are alterations in the immune system.[148]

Clinical features
It is usually associated with anemia, ocular problems, renal dysfunction, and mucocutaneous lesions.[149] Crohn disease is associated with skin disorders.[150] The clinical types that are associated with mucocutaneous Crohn disease are granulomatous, oral and perianal, caused by direct involvement of GI diseases; reactive conditions associated with erythema nodosum and Sweet syndrome; and nutritional deficiency, such as acrodermatitis entropathica.[151] Some cases of Crohn disease are associated with *Staphylococcus aureus*.

Histopathologic features
Histopathologic features are similar to other granulomatous lesions. Subepithelially non-necrotizing granulomatous inflammation is noted within the submucosal connective tissues. These granulomas vary from patient to patient. Chronic inflammatory cell infiltration is made up of predominantly plasma cells and lymphocytes and occasionally polymorphonuclear leukocytes. Focal areas show areas of degeneration and necrosis.[152]

AUTOIMMUNE AND VASCULAR DISEASES
Wegener Granulomatosis

It is an idiopathic systemic inflammatory disease. It is characterized by granulomatous inflammation (see **Table 1**).[153] It is usually associated with the upper and lower respiratory tract.[154] Renal involvement most commonly causes segmental necrotizing glomerulonephritis, a proliferative glomerulonephritis.[155]

Clinical features
It can affect a wide spectrum of systems.[156] It commonly involves the upper respiratory tract, lungs, and kidneys. Less commonly it involves the skin, heart, salivary gland, eye and orbit, breast, gastro intestinal tract (GIT), spleen, and thyroid gland.[157] Initial symptoms include prodromal symptoms and persistent rhinorrhea or epiphora.[158] It can be associated with other systems, such as the respiratory tract, pulmonary airways, ocular, renal, cutaneous, and vascular and neural systems.

Oral manifestations features

Six percent to 13% of cases are associated with oral manifestations.[159] Oral manifestations will be the primary features of Wegener granulomatosis.

The common site for Wegener granulomatosis are as follows[160,161]:

- Oral mucosa
- Lip
- Gingival
- Alveolar mucosa
- Plate

Histopathologic features

It shows features of granulomatous inflammation. Characteristic features include a necrotic area with a serpiginous border surrounded by multinucleated giant cells. The lesion may be admixed with acute and chronic inflammatory cell infiltration.[162]

Radiographic findings

Radiographic examination shows alveolar bone loss, often associated with the gingival lesions. Chest radiographs may show lesions in the lungs suggestive of pulmonary involvement of Wegener granulomatosis.

Dental management

Symptomatic treatment starts from oral prophylaxis[1] Excision can be done for hyperplastic gingiva.[163] The mainstay of treatment is to administer corticosteroids and cytotoxic drugs, such as cyclophosphamide.[163] Methotrexate and azathioprine have been effectively used for remission-maintenance treatment.[164]

Systemic Lupus Erythematosus

It is a multisystem autoimmune disorder that affects organs and oral tissues.[165] It is mainly observed in UK residents of Afro-Caribbean descent and the nonwhite population.[166]

Types

1. Systemic lupus erythematosus
2. Chronic cutaneous lupus erythematosus
3. Subacute cutaneous lupus erythematosus

Clinical features

Most common manifestations in systemic lupus erythematosus are arthritis, pleuritis, photosensitivity, pericarditis, and hematological disorders.[167] Women are commonly affected more commonly than men with a 9:1 ratio with the age group of 15 and 40 years.[168] Patients will give history of fever, weight loss, arthritis, and fatigue with prodromal symptoms. The characteristic feature of systemic lupus erythematosus is a butterfly rash seen over the malar region of the nose.[169] Other organ involvement, such as the kidney and heart, may be observed in these cases. Literature shows that in a small group of patients with systemic lupus erythematous, cardiac values can be thickened.[170]

Oral manifestations
The most common sites include the palate, buccal mucosa, and gingiva. Lupus cheilitis is seen on the lip manifestations as ulceration, pain, hyperkeratosis, and erythema. Other oral manifestations include xerostomia, stomatodynia, candidiasis, and dyspepsia.[171]

Histopathologic features
Hyperkeratosis with follicular plugging is noted. Connective tissue stroma shows patchy to dense aggregates of chronic inflammatory cell infiltration. There is hyperkeratosis with atrophy and basal cell degeneration of the basal cells.[172]

Dental management
Appropriate dental management of these patients requires an understanding of the cause, clinical manifestations, current treatment recommendations, and psychological aspects of the disease.

- Hydroxychloroquine is commonly used for discoid lesions on the skin and mucosa. Topical steroids or intralesional steroids are recommended for discoid and ulcerative lesions.[173]
- Dentists must enforce preventive dental care and monitor patients with systemic lupus erythematosus closely for head and neck infections because they are predisposed to severe infections, bleeding, and adrenal suppression. The risk of infection can be managed by recommending prophylactic antibiotics. The risk of bleeding can be prevented by preoperative platelet transfusion. Bleeding control should be done by local measures, such as pressure and application of hemostatic agents.[173]

Recent studies regarding the adrenal suppression show replacement or doubling of the dosage for patients using steroids is unnecessary for oral surgical procedures.[165]

Sjögren Syndrome

It is a slowly progressive, inflammatory autoimmune disease affecting mainly exocrine glands.[174] It mainly consists of SSA(Ro) and SSB(La) autoantibodies.[175]

Sjögren syndrome is broadly divided into 2 forms:

- Primary Sjögren syndrome: mainly xerostomia and xerophthalmia
- Secondary Sjögren syndrome–associated autoimmune rheumatoid diseases

---

Clinical features
It is mainly associated with autoimmune exocrinopathy to extraglandular disease. Sjögren syndrome mainly affects the lungs, kidneys, blood vessels, and muscles.[176] It may also involve glandular, ocular, oral, ontological, and laryngeal tissues as well as the thyroid and sinus.

Ocular manifestations There are decreases in the lacrimal flow, conjunctiva damage, dryness of the eyes, and photosensitivity.[177]

Oral manifestations The oral manifestations include dryness of the mucosa, burning sensations, difficulty swallowing, and decrease in taste sensation.[178] Patients may present with hearing loss secondary to immune complexes in the stria vascularis.[179] Ten percent to 15% of the patients with Sjögren syndrome will have altered thyroid functions, which may lead to Hashimoto thyroiditis.[174]

Histopathologic features
Inflammatory cell infiltration is predominantly made up of lymphocytes. Lymphocytes are replaced with acinar structure. The histopathologic characteristic feature is that it maintains the acinar architecture.[180] Focal areas show proliferation of both ductal and myoepithelial cells.[181]

Radiographic features
Sialography has been one of the mainstay investigation tools because it establishes disease and it produces a characteristic radiographic appearance referred to as sialectasis (focal collections of contrast medium seen uniformly scattered throughout the gland). When they are small, these lesions are described as punctuate; when larger, they are referred to as globular or cavitary, suggesting a greater amount of glandular damage.[182]

In ultrasound examination, the affected glands become less well defined, appear slightly darker (hypoechoic) than a normal gland, and lose their uniform (homogenous) structure to show numerous, dark circular areas. The number and size of these dark areas seem to match the severity of the condition. Typically, the foci vary in size but are usually round or ovoid, about 2 to 5 mm in diameter, and nonvascular.[182]

MRI and MR sialography offer good accuracy in visualizing glandular structural changes.[2] Areas of high signal intensity on T1-weighted MRI that may indicate increased amounts of fat tissue are evident in the glands of patients with Sjögren syndrome.[183]

Salivary scintigraphy is a valid investigative procedure used to assess salivary gland function. After intravenous 99mTc-sodium pertechnetate administration, sequential images of the head, on anterior projection, are acquired during a variable time interval, usually between 20 and 40 minutes. Abnormal salivary scintigraphy findings include delayed uptake, reduced concentration, and/or delayed uptake of the tracer by the glandular tissue.[184]

Dental management
The primary dental concern of patients with Sjögren syndrome is managing their xerostomia. Symptomatic treatment includes stimulation of salivary flow by sugar-free, highly flavored lozenges. Systemic salivary stimulation can be done by using parasympathomimetic secretagogues like cevimeline and pilocarpine.[185] These secretagogues must be sugar free because of the risk of rampant dental caries. In contrast, dry food, heavy smoking, and drugs with anticholinergic side effects, which further decrease the salivary flow, should be avoided. Adequate oral hygiene after meals is a prerequisite for prevention of dental disease.[184]

Therapeutic strategies like hormone modulation, general and targeted antiinflammatory approaches, blunting of the B-cell response, and treatment of potential viral causes have also been advocated in the management of Sjögren syndrome.[184]

DEVELOPMENTAL
Melkersson-Rosenthal Syndrome

It is a complex neurocutaneous disorder. It is characterized by orofacial edema and craniofacial nerve dysfunction (see **Table 1**).[185] It was first described by Melkersson in 1928 and later described by Rosenthal in 1930 as a facial palsy with swelling of the lip and fissured tongue.[186]

Etiologic factors
• Allergies
• Syphilis
• Bacterial mouth infection
• Basal arachnoiditis
• Benign lymphogranulomatosis
• Hereditary
• Herpes virus[187]

Clinical features
There is swelling of one or both of the lips (upper and lower).[188] There are unilateral or bilateral and nonpitting edema, leading to nontender enlargement with a reddish-brown appearance. The lips may appear as swollen.[187] The eyelids, nose, chin, and forehead may appear as swollen.[187] Swelling may be soft to firm, and some of the swelling may be elastic.[188] Secretion alterations in salivary and lacrimal glands may occur.[188]

Histopathologic features
Histologically, it appears as a granulomatous lesion, such as a TB and sarcoidosis.[189] Granulomas are nonspecific with chronic inflammatory cell infiltration, such as lymphocytes and histiocytes with multinucleated giant cells.[189] These granulomas may be seen in the lamina propria.[189]

REFERENCES

1. Phelan JA, Jimenez V, Tompkins DC. Tuberculosis. Dent Clin North Am 1996;40: 327–41.
2. Sachs SA, Elsenbud L. Tuberculous osteomyelitis of the mandible. Oral Surg Oral Med Oral Pathol 1977;44:425–9.
3. Kumar PM, Kumas SM, Sarkar S, et al. Oral manifestations in patients with primary tuberculosis. Int J Bio Med Res 2012;3(2):1565–7.
4. Jain P, Jain I. Oral manifestations of Tuberculosis: Step toward early diagnosis. J Clin Diagn Res 2014;8(12):ZE 18–21.
5. Curto A. Oral tubercoulous lesions. Br Dent J 2015;218(12):662.
6. Moon KY, Han MH, Chang KH, et al. CT and MR imaging of head and neck tuberculosis. Radiographics 1997;17(2):391–402.
7. Siegel JD, Rhinehart E, Jackson M, et al, the Healthcare Infection Control Practices Advisory Committee. 2007 Guideline for isolation precautions: preventing transmission of infectious agents in healthcare settings. Available at: http://www.cdc.gov/ncidod/dhqp/pdf/isolation2007.pdf. Accessed July 10, 2015.

8. Girdhar BK, Desikan KV. A clinical study of the mouth in untreated lepromatous patients. Lepr Rev 1979;50:25–35.
9. Prabhu SR, Daftary DK. Clinical evaluation of oro-facial lesions of leprosy. Odontostomatol Trop 1981;4:83–95.
10. Scheepers A, Lemmer J, Lownie JF. Oral manifestations of leprosy. Lepr Rev 1993;64:37–43.
11. Pereira RM, Silva TS, Silva LS, et al. Orofacial and dental condition in leprosy. Braz J Oral Sci 2013;12(4):330–4.
12. Volante M, Contucci AM, Fantoni M, et al. Cervicofacial actinomycosis: still a difficult differential diagnosis. Acta Otorhinolaryngol Ital 2005;25:116–9.
13. Habibi A, Salehininjad J, Saghafi S, et al. Actinomycosis of the tongue. Arch Iran Med 2008;11(5):566–8.
14. Oosteman O, Smego RA. Cervicofacial actinomycosis: diagnosis and management. Curr Infect Dis Rep 2005;7:170–4.
15. Park JK, Lee HK, Ha HK, et al. Cervicofacial actinomycosis: CT and MR imaging findings in seven patients. AJNR Am J Neuroradiol 2003;24:331–5.
16. Sasaki Y, Kaneda T, Uyeda JW, et al. Actinomycosis in the mandible: CT and MR findings. AJNR Am J Neuroradiol 2014;35(2):390–4.
17. Catano JC, Gallego S. Rhinoscleroma. Am J Trop Med Hyg 2015;92(1):3.
18. Fevre C, Almeida AS, Taront S, et al. A novel murine model of rhinoscleroma identifies Mikulicz cells, the disease signature, as IL-10 dependent derivatives of inflammatory monocytes. EMBO Mol Med 2013;5(4):516–30.
19. Ibrahim FM, Mohamad I. Klebsiella pneumonia as a rare cause of parapharyngeal abscess. Pak J Med Sci 2011;27(1):214–5.
20. Cho KT, Park BJ. Gas-forming brain abscess caused by Klebsiella pneumoniae. J Korean Neurosurg Soc 2008;44:382–4.
21. Lnglesby V, Henderson D, Bartlett J, et al. Anthrax as a biological weapon: medical and public health management. Working Group on Civilian Biodefense. JAMA 1999;281:1735–45.
22. Bartlett J, Inglesby T, Borio L. Management of anthrax. Clin Infect Dis 2002;35:851–7.
23. Brossier F, Weber-Levy M, Mock M, et al. Role of toxin functional domains in anthrax pathogenesis. Infect Immun 2000;68:1781–6.
24. World Health Organisation. Anthrax in humans and animals. 4th edition. Geneva, Switzerland: WHO Publications; 2008. p. 43–52.
25. Wood BJ, DeFranco B, Ripple M, et al. Inhalational anthrax: radiologic and pathologic findings in two cases. AJR Am J Roentgenol 2003;181(4):1071–8.
26. Sauret JM, Vilissova N. Human Brucellosis. J Am Board Fam Pract 2002;15:401–6.
27. World Health Organisation. Brucellosis in humans and animals. Geneva, Switzerland: WHO Publications; 2006. p. 1–10.
28. Fiumara NJ. Venereal diseases of the oral cavity. J Oral Med 1976;31:36–40.
29. Fiumara NJ, Lessel S. Manifestations of late congenital syphilis: an analysis of 271 patients. Arch Dermatol 1970;102:78–83.
30. Meyer I, Seklar G. The oral manifestations of acquired syphilis. A study of eighty-one cases. Oral Surg Oral Med Oral Pathol 1967;23:45–61.
31. Singh AE, Romanowski B. Syphilis review with emphasis on clinical and epidemiologic and some biologic features. Clin Microbiol Rev 1999;12:187–209.
32. Ehrlich R, Kricun ME. Radiographic findings in early acquired syphilis: case report and critical review. AJR Am J Roentgenol 1976;127:789–92.

33. Huang I, Leach JL, Fichtenbaum CJ, et al. Osteomyelitis of the skull in early-acquired syphilis: evaluation by MR imaging and CT. AJNR Am J Neuroradiol 2007;28:307–8.
34. Brightbill TC, Ihmeidan IH, Post MJD, et al. Neurosyphilis in HIV-positive and HIV-negative patients: neuroimaging findings. AJNR Am J Neuroradiol 1995; 16:703–11.
35. Patil K, Mahima VG, Prathiba Rani RM. Oral histoplasmosis. J Indian Soc Periodontol 2009;13(3):157–9.
36. Cano M, Hajjeh A. The epidemiology of histoplasmosis: a review. Semin Respir Infect 2001;16:109–18.
37. Samaranayake LP. Oral mycoses in HIV infection. Oral Surg Oral Med Oral Pathol 1992;73:171–80.
38. Kauffman CA. Histoplasmosis: a clinical and laboratory update. Clin Microbiol Rev 2007;20(1):115–32.
39. O'Sullivan MV, Whitby M, Chahoud C, et al. Histoplasmosis in Australia: a report of a case with a review of the literature. Aust Dent J 2004;49(2):94–7.
40. Sarosi G, Davies S. Blastomycosis. Am Rev Respir Dis 1979;120:901.
41. Davies SF, Sarosi GA. Epidemiological and clinical features of pulmonary blastomycosis. Semin Respir Infect 1997;12:206–18.
42. Vanek J, Schwarz J, Hakim S. North American blastomycosis. A study of ten cases. Am J Clin Pathol 1970;54:384.
43. Bell WA, Gamble J, Garrington GE. North American blastomycosis with oral lesion. Oral Surg Oral Med Oral Pathol 1969;18(6):914–23.
44. Paulltauf A. Mycosis mucorina. Virchows Arch 1885;102:543–9.
45. Branscomb R. An overview of mucormycosis. Lab Med 2002;33(6):453–5.
46. Economopoulous P, Laskaris G, Ferekidis E. Rhinocerebral mucormycosis with severe oral lesion. A case report. J Oral Maxillofac Surg 1995;53:215–7.
47. De Biscop J, Mondie JM, Venries de la GB. Mucormycosis in a apparently normal host. Case report and literature review. J Craniomaxillofac Surg 1991; 19:275–8.
48. Doni BR, Peerapur BV, Thotappa LH, et al. Sequence of oral manifestations in rhino-maxillary mucormycosis. Indian J Dent Res 2011;22(2):331–5.
49. Warder FR, Chikes PG, Hudson WR. Aspergillosis of the paranasal sinuses. Arch Otolaryngol 1975;101:683–5.
50. Rowe-Jones JM, Moore-Gillon V. Destructive noninvasive paranasal sinus aspergillosis: component of a spectrum of disease. J Otolaryngol 1994;23:92–6.
51. Denning DW. Invasive aspergillosis. Clin Infect Dis 1998;26:781–803.
52. Falworth MS, Herold J. Aspergillosis of the para nasal sinuses. A case report and radiographic review. Oral Surg Oral Med Oral Pathol Oral Radiol Endod 1996;81:255–60.
53. Clancy CJ, Nguyen MH. Invasive sinus aspergillosis in apparently immune competent host. J Infect 1998;37:229–40.
54. Taneja T, Saxena S, Aggarwal P, et al. Fungal infections involving maxillary sinus – a difficult diagnostic task. J Clin Exp Dent 2011;3(2):e172–6.
55. Gazzoni FA, Elsemann RB, Conde A, et al. Updating: cryptococcosis diagnostic aspects. J AIDS Clin Res 2014;5(12):391.
56. Gazzoni FA, Oliveria FM, Salles EF, et al. Unusual morphologies of Cryptococcus spp. in tissue specimens. Report of 10 cases. Rev Inst Med Trop Sao Paulo 2010;52(3):145–9.
57. Levitz SM. The ecology of Cryptococcus neoformans and the epidemiology of cryptococcosis. Rev Infect Dis 1991;13:1163–9.

58. Scully C, Peas De Almeida O. Oro facial manifestations of the systemic myco-ses. J Oral Pathol Med 1992;21:289–94.
59. Shibuya K, Coulson WF, Wollman JS, et al. Histopathology of cryptococcosis and other fungal infections in patients with acquired immunodeficiency syn-drome. Int J Infect Dis 2001;5:78–85.
60. Panda S, Lenka S, Padhiary SK, et al. Rhinosporidiosis in the parotid duct: a rare case report. J Investig Clin Dent 2013;4:271–4.
61. Vijaikumar M, Thappa DM, Karthikeyan K, et al. Verrucous lesion of the palm. Postgrad Med J 2002;78(302):305–6.
62. Kumari R, Laxmisha C, Thappa DM. Disseminated cutaneous rhinosporidiosis. Dermatol Online J 2005;11:19.
63. Topazian RG. Rhinosporidiosis of parotid duct. Br J Oral Surg 1966;4(1):12–5.
64. Rameshkumar A, Gnanaselvi UP, Dineshkumar T, et al. Rhinosporidiosis pre-senting as a facial swelling: a case report. J Int Oral Health 2015;7(2): 58–60.
65. Rath R, Baig SA, Debata T. Rhinosporidiosis presenting as an oropharyngeal mass: a clinical predicament? J Nat Sci Biol Med 2015;6:241–5.
66. Deneshbod K. Visceral leishmaniasis (kala-azar) in Iran: a pathologic and elec-tron microscopic study. Am J Clin Pathol 1972;57(2):156–66.
67. World Health Organization. Global health situation in selected infection and parasitic diseases due to identification organism. Wkly Epidemiol Rec 1993; 68:641–3.
68. Thakur CP, Kumar M, Pathak PK. Kala-azar hits again. J Trop Med Hyg 1981;84: 271–6.
69. Compose JD. Clinical and epidemiological features of kala azar in children. J Pediatr 1995;71:238–40.
70. Singh K, Singh R, Parija SC, et al. Clinical and laboratory study of kala–azar in children in Nepal. J Trop Pediatr 1999;45:95–7.
71. Mehata BC. Approach to a patient with anemia. Indian J Med Sci 2004;58:26–9.
72. Silveira TG, Arraes SM, Bertolini DA. The laboratory diagnosis and epidemiology of cutaneous leishmaniasis in parana state, South Brazil. Rev Soc Bras Med Trop 1999;32(4):413–23.
73. Singh S, Siva kumar R. Recent advances in the diagnosis of leishmaniasis. J Postgrad Med 2003;49(1):55–60.
74. García-de Marcos JA, Dean-Ferrer A, Alamillos-Granados F, et al. Localized leishmaniasis of the oral mucosa. A report of three cases. Med Oral Patol Oral Cir Bucal 2007;12:E281–6.
75. Shinohara EH, Martin HZ, Oliveira Neto HG, et al. Oral myiasis treated with iver-mectin; a case report. Braz Dent J 2005;15:79–81.
76. Hira PR, Assad PM, Okasha G, et al. Myiasis in Kuwait: nosocomial infections caused by Lucilia sericate and Megaselia scalaris. Am J Trop Med Hyg 2004; 70:386–9.
77. Joo CY, Kim JB. Nosocomial submandibular infection with dipterous fly larvae. Korean J Parasitol 2001;39:255–60.
78. Caca I, Unlu K, Calcmak SS, et al. Orbital myiasis: case report. Jpn J Opthalmol 2003;47:412–4.
79. Francesconi F, Lupi O. Myasis. Clin Microbiol Rev 2012;25:79–105.
80. Verma N, Marya J. Oral myiasis in maxillofacial trauma - treated with ivermectin. Int J Den Clin 2011;3(2):97–8.
81. Skariah S, McIntyre MK, Mordue DG. Toxoplasma gondii: determinants of tachy-zoite to bradyzoite conversion. Parasitol Res 2010;107(2):253–60.

82. Elmore SA, Jones JL, Conrad PA, et al. *Toxoplasma gondii*: epidemiology, feline clinical aspects, and prevention. Trends Parasitol 2010;26(4):190–6.

83. Boyer KM, Hilfels E, Roizen Z, et al. Toxoplasmosis study group. Risk factor for Toxoplasma gondii infection in mother of infants with congenital toxoplasmosis implications for prenatal management and screening. Am J Obstet Gynecol 2005;192(2):564–71.

84. Jones J, Lepez A, Wilson M. Congenital toxoplasmosis. Am Fam Physician 2003;67(10):2131–8.

85. Moran WJ, Tom DW, King D. Toxoplasmosis lymphadenitis occurring in a parotid gland. Otolaryngol Head Neck Surg 1986;94:237–40.

86. Bhaskar SN, Lacoway JR. Pyogenic granulomas – clinical features, incidence, histology, and result of treatment: report of 242 cases. J Oral Surg 1966;24: 391–8.

87. Yao T, Nagai E, Utsunomiya T, et al. An intestinal counterpart of pyogenic granulomas of the skin. A newly proposed entity. Am J Surg Pathol 1995;19: 1054–60.

88. Hullihen SP. A case of aneurism by anastomosis of the superior maxilla. Am J Dent Sci 1844;4:160–2.

89. Hartzell MB. A further contribution to the study of benign cystic epithelioma. J Med Res 1908;18(1):159–64.

90. Kerr DA. Granuloma pyogenicum. Oral Surg Oral Med Oral Pathol 1951;4: 158–76.

91. Eversol LR. Clinical out line of oral pathology: diagnosis and treatment. 3rd edition. Hamilton, Ontario: BC Decker Hamilton; 2002. p. 113–4.

92. Regezi JA, Sciubba JJ, Jordon RC. Oral pathology: clinico pathologic considerations. 4th edition. Philadelphia: WB Saunders; 2003. p. 115–6.

93. Neville BW, Damm DD, Allen CM, et al. Oral & maxillofacial pathology. 2nd edition. Philadelphia: WB Saunders; 2002. p. 437–95.

94. Bouquot JE, Nikai H. Lesions of the oral cavity. In: Gnapp DR, editor. Diagnostic surgical pathology of head and neck. 3rd edition. Philadelphia: WB Saunders; 2001. p. 141–233.

95. Samata Y, Reddy TH, Jyothirrmai, et al. Management of oral pyogenic granuloma with sodium tetra decyl sulphate- a case series. N Y State Dent J 2013; 79:55–7.

96. Mariano M. The experimental granulomas. A hypothesis to explain the persistence of the lesion. Rev Inst Med Trop Sao Paulo 1995;37(2):161–76.

97. Oikarinen KS, Nieminen TM, Mäkäräinen H, et al. Visibility of foreign bodies in soft tissue in plain radiographs, computed tomography, magnetic resonance imaging, and ultrasound. An in vitro study. Int J Oral Maxillofac Surg 1993;22(2): 119–24.

98. Girdler NM. Unusual delayed sequel to facial trauma. Oral Surg Oral Med Oral Pathol 1993;75(2):264.

99. Manjunath BS, Kumar GS, Raghunathan V. Histochemical and polarization microscopic study of two cases of vegetable/pulse granulomas. Indian J Dent Res 2008;19(1):74–7.

100. Friedman I. Epidermoid cholesteatoma and cholesterol granulomas: experimental and human. Ann Otol Rhinol Laryngol 1959;68:57–60.

101. Gacek RR. Diagnosis and management of primary tumors of the petrous apex. Ann Otol Rhinol Laryngol Suppl 1975;18:1–20.

102. Graham J, Michael L. Cholesterol granulomas of the maxillary antrum. Clin Otolaryngol 1978;3:155–60.

103. Chao TK. Cholesterol granulomas of the maxillary sinus. Eur Arch Otorhinolaryngol 2006;263:592–7.
104. Yamazaki CJ, Hao N, Takagi R, et al. Basement membrane type heparin sulfate proteoglycan (perlecan) and low density lipoprotein (LDL) are co–localized in granulation tissues; a possible pathogenesis of cholesterol granulomas in jaw cysts. J Oral Pathol Med 2004;33:177–84.
105. Hirschberg A, Dayan D, Buchner A, et al. Cholesterol granulomas of the jaws. Int J Oral Maxillofac Surg 1988;17:230–1.
106. Kaffe I, Littner MM, Buchner A, et al. Cholesterol granulomas embedded in an odontoma of the maxilla. J Oral Maxillofac Surg 1984;42:319–22.
107. Almada CB, Fonseca DR, Vanzillotta RR, et al. Cholesterol granuloma of the maxillary sinus. Braz Dent J 2008;19(2):171–4.
108. Di Paolo T, Rouillard C, Morissette M, et al. Endocrine and neurochemical action of cocaine. Can J Physiol Pharmacol 1989;67:1177–8.
109. Seyer AB, Grist W, Muller S. Aggressive destructive mid facial lesions from cocaine abuse. Oral Surg Oral Med Oral Pathol Oral Radiol Endod 2002;44:465–70.
110. Armstrong M Jr, Shikani AH. Nasal septal necrosis mimicking Wegener's granulomatosis in a cocaine abuser. Ear Nose Throat J 1996;75(9):623–6.
111. Ching JA, Smith DJ Jr. Levamisole-induced necrosis of skin, soft tissue, and bone: case report and review of literature. J Burn Care Res 2012;33:1–5.
112. Khan TA, Cuchacovich R, Espinoza LR, et al. Vasculopathy, hematological, and immune abnormalities associated with levamisole-contaminated cocaine use. Semin Arthritis Rheum 2011;41:445–54. Comprehensive report with complete literature review of clinical and laboratory manifestations associated with levamisole-contaminated cocaine use.
113. Padilla-Rosas M, Jimenez-Santos CI, García-González CL. Palatine perforation induced by cocaine. Med Oral Patol Oral Cir Bucal 2006;11:E239–42.
114. Choi HK, Curhan G. Gout: epidemiology and life style choices. Curr Opin Rheumatol 2005;17:341–5.
115. Yu TF. Diversity of clinical features in gouty arthritis. Semin Arthritis Rheum 1984;13:360–8.
116. Terkeltaub RA. Gout: epidemiology, pathology and pathogenesis. In: Klippel JH, Crofford L, Stone JH, et al, editors. Primer on the rheumatic diseases. 12th edition. Atlanta (GA): Arthritis Foundation; 2001. p. 307–12.
117. Pascual E. Persistence of monosodium urate crystals and low grade inflammation in the synovial fluid of treated gout. Arthritis Rheum 1991;34:141–5.
118. Snider AA, Barsky S. Gouty panniculitis: a case report and review of the literature. Cutis 2005;76:54–6.
119. Bhattacharyya I, Chehal H, Gremillion H, et al. Gout of the temporomandibular joint: a review of the literature. J Am Dent Assoc 2010;141(8):979–85.
120. Henter JI, Tondini C, Pritchard J. Histiocyte disorders. Crit Rev Oncol Hematol 2004;50:157–74.
121. Murray M, Dean J, Slater L. Multifocal oral Langerhans cell histiocytosis. J Oral Maxillofac Surg 2011;69:2585–91.
122. Al-Ammar AY, Tewfik TL, Bond M, et al. Langerhans' cell histiocytosis: paediatric head and neck study. J Otolaryngol 1999;28:266–72.
123. Bluestone CD, Stool SE, Kenna MA. Pediatric otolaryngology. 3rd edition. Philadelphia: WB Saunders; 1996. p. 710–1.
124. Nicollas R, Rome A, Belaïch H, et al. Head and neck manifestation and prognosis of Langerhans' cell histiocytosis in children. Int J Pediatr Otorhinolaryngol 2010;74:669–73.

125. Greinix HT, Storb R, Sanders JE, et al. Marrow transplantation for treatment of multisystem progressive Langerhans' cell histiocytosis. Bone Marrow Transplant 1992;10:39–44.

126. Nanduri VR, Pritchard J, Levitt G, et al. Long term morbidity and health related quality of life after multi-system Langerhans cell histiocytosis. Eur J Cancer 2006;42:2563–9.

127. Favara BE, Feller AC, Pauli M, et al. Contemporary classification of histiocytic disorders. The WHO Committee on Histiocytic/Reticulum Cell Proliferations. Reclassification Working Group of the Histiocyte Society. Med Pediatr Oncol 1997; 29:157–66.

128. Histiocytosis syndromes in children. Writing Group of the Histiocyte Society. Lancet 1987;1:208–9.

129. Madrigal-Martínez-Pereda C, Guerrero-Rodríguez V, Guisado-Moya B, et al. Langerhans cell histiocytosis: literature review and descriptive analysis of oral manifestations. Med Oral Patol Oral Cir Bucal 2009;14(5):E222–8.

130. Abrams AM, Melrose RJ, Howell FV. Necrotizing sialometaplasia. A disease simulating malignancy. Cancer 1973;32:130–5.

131. Tanna N, Brown J, Beneng K, et al. Necrotising sialometaplasia – an unusual cause. Oral Surg 2014;7:232–5.

132. Alves MG, Kitakawa D, Carvalho YR, et al. Necrotizing sialometaplasia as a cause of a nonulcerated nodule in the hard palate: a case report. J Med Case Rep 2011;5:406.

133. Garcia NG, Oliveira DT, Faustino SE, et al. Necrotizing sialometaplasia of palate: a case report. Case Rep Pathol 2012;12:1–3.

134. Bascones-Martínez A. Case report of necrotizing sialometaplasia. Med Oral Patol Oral Cir Bucal 2011;16(6):e700–3.

135. Suomalainen A. CT findings of necrotizing sialometaplasia. Dentomaxillofac Radiol 2012;41:529–32.

136. Mendenhall WM, Olivier KR, Lynch JW, et al. Lethal midline granuloma-nasal natural killer/T cell lymphoma. Am J Clin Oncol 2006;29:202–6.

137. Mills CP. Midline Granuloma. Proc R Soc Med 1964;57(4):297–9.

138. Mallya V, Singh A, Pahwa M. Lethal midline granuloma. Indian Dermatol Online J 2013;4:37–9.

139. Aozasa K. Biopsy findings in malignant histiocytosis presenting as lethal midline granuloma. Clin Pathol 1982;35(6):599–605.

140. Tauro L, Aithala S, Menezes L, et al. Lethal midline granuloma-epithelioid angiosarcoma face. Indian J Surg 2003;65:438–40.

141. Tlholoe M, Kotu M, Khammissa RA, et al. Extranodal natural killer/T-cell lymphoma, nasal type: 'midline lethal granuloma.' A case report. Head Face Med 2013;9:4.

142. Yamamoto M, Sharma OP, Hosoda Y. Special report: the 1991 descriptive definition of sarcoidosis. Sarcoidosis 1992;9(Suppl 1):33–4.

143. Statement on sarcoidosis. Joint Statement of the American Thoracic Society (ATS), the European Respiratory Society (ERS) and the World Association of Sarcoidosis and Other Granulomatous Disorders (WASOG) adopted by the ATS Board of Directors and by the ERS Executive Committee, 1999. Am J Respir Crit Care Med 1999;160:736–55.

144. Bashour FA, Mc Connell T, Skinner W, et al. Myocardial sarcoidosis. Dis Chest 1968;53:413–20.

145. Tazman EC. Sarcoidosis : clinical manifestations, epidemiology, therapy, and pathophysiology. Curr Opin Rheumatol 1991;3:155–9.

146. Hanauer SB, Sandborn W, Practice Parameters Committee of the American College of Gastroenterology. Management of Crohn's diseases in adults. Am J Gastroenterol 2001;96:635–43.
147. Crohn's BB, Ginzbur L, Oppenheimmer GD. Regional ileitis. JAMA 1932;99: 1323–9.
148. Basu MK, Asquith P, Thompson RA, et al. Oral manifestation of Crohn's diseases. Gut 1975;16:249–54.
149. Palamarus I, El-Jabbour J, Pietropaolo N, et al. Metastatic Crohn's diseases: a review. J Eur Acad Dermatol Venereol 2008;22:1033–43.
150. Lebwohl M, Fleischmajer R, Janowitz H, et al. Metastatic Crohn's disease. J Am Acad Dermatol 1984;10:33–8.
151. Greenstein AJ, Janowitz HD, Sachar DB. The extra-intestinal complications of Crohn's diseases and ulcerative colitis: a study of 700 patients. Medicine 1976;55:401–12.
152. Dunlap CL, Friesen CA, Shultz R. Chronic stomatitis: an early sign of Crohn's disease. J Am Dent Assoc 1997;128:347–8.
153. Jennette JC. Nomenclature by granulomatous inflammation of vasculitis: lesions learned from granulomatosis with polyangiitis (Wegener's granulomatosis). Clin Exp Immunol 2011;164(Suppl 1):7–10.
154. Yi ES, Colby TV. Wegener's granulomatosis. Semin Diagn Pathol 2001;18:34–46.
155. Stevic R, Jovanovic D, Obradovic LN, et al. Wegener's granulomatosis clinic – radiological findings at initial presentation. Coll Antropol 2012;36:505–11.
156. Khan AM, Elahi F, Hashmi SR, et al. Wegener's granulomatosis: a rare, chronic and multisystem diseases. Surgeon 2006;4:45–52.
157. Berge S, Niederhagen B, Von Lindern JJ, et al. Salivary gland involvement as an initial presentation of Wegener's disease. A case report. Int J Oral Maxillofac Surg 2000;29:450–2.
158. Graves N. Wegener's granulomatosis. Proc (Bayl Univ Med Cent) 2006;19:342–4.
159. Ponniah I, Shaheem A, Shankjar KA, et al. Wegener's granulomatosis; the current understanding. Oral Sug Oral Med Oral Pathol Oral Radiol Endod 2005; 100:265–70.
160. Patten SF, Tomecki KJ. Wegener's granulomatosis: cutaneous and oral mucosal diseases. J Am Acad Dermatol 1993;1:710–8.
161. Allen CM, Camisa C, Salewskic C, et al. Wegener's granulomatosis: report of three cases with oral lesions. J Oral Maxillofac Surg 1991;49:294–8.
162. O'Devaney K, Ferlito A, Hunter BC, et al. Wegener's granulomatosis of the head and neck. Ann Otol Rhinol Laryngol 1998;1:439–45.
163. Erickson VR, Hwang PH. Wegener's granulomatosis: current trends in diagnosis and management. Curr Opin Otolaryngol Head Neck Surg 2007;15(3):170–6.
164. Steward C, Cohen D, Bhattacharyya I, et al. Oral manifestations of Wegener's granulomatosis: a report of three cases and a literature review. J Am Dent Assoc 2007;138:338–48.
165. Fessel WJ. Systemic lupus erythematosus in the community; incidence, prevalence outcome and first symptoms, the high prevalence in black women. Arch Intern Med 1974;134:1027–35.
166. Denchenko N, Satia JA, Antony MS. Epidemiology of systemic lupus erythematosus: a comparison of worldwide diseases burden. Lupus 2006;15:308–18.
167. Gill JM, Quisel AM, Rocca PV, et al. Diagnosis of systemic lupus erythematosus. Am Fam Physician 2003;68:2179–86.
168. Masi AT, Kaslow RA. Sex effects in systemic lupus erythematosus: a clue to pathogenesis. Arthritis Rheum 1978;21:480–4.

169. Lahita RG. Over view of lupus erythematosus. Clin Dermatol 1993;10:389–92.
170. Cervera R, Khamashta MA, Fout J. Morbidity and mortality in systemic lupus erythematosus during a 5 year period. Medicine (Baltimore) 1999;78:167–75.
171. De Rossi SS, Glick M. Lupus erythematosus. Considerations for dentistry. J Am Dent Assoc 1998;129:330–9.
172. Velthuis PJ, Kater L, Baart de la Faille H. Direct immunofluorescence pattern in clinically healthy skin of patients with collagen diseases. Clin Dermatol 1993;10: 423–30.
173. Mok CC, Lau CS. Pathogenesis of systemic lupus erythematosus. J Clin Pathol 2003;56:481–90.
174. Fox RI. Sjögren's syndrome: a review. Lancet 2005;366(9482):321–31.
175. Vitalic C, Bombardieri S, Moutosopoulos HM, et al. Primary criteria for the classification of Sjögren's syndrome. Results of a prospective concerted action supported by the European community. Arthritis Rheum 1993;36(3):340–7.
176. Al-Hashimi I, Khuder S, Haghighat N, et al. Frequency and predictive value of the clinical manifestations in sjogren's syndrome. J Oral Pathol Med 2001; 30(1):1–6.
177. Fox PC. Auto immune diseases and sjogren's syndrome : an auto immune exocrinopathy. Ann N Y Acad Sci 2007;1098:15–21.
178. Pedersen AM, Reibel J, Nauntofte B. Primary Sjogren's syndrome (pSS): subjective symptoms and salivary findings. J Oral Pathol Med 1999;28:303–11.
179. Mohoney EJ, Spiegel JH. Sjogren's diseases. Otolaryngol Clin North Am 2003; 36(4):733–45.
180. Wakamastsu TH, Sato EA, Matsumoto Y, et al. Conjunctiva in vivo confocal scanning laser microscopy in patients with Sjogren's syndrome. Invest Opthalmol Vis Sci 2010;51(1):144–50.
181. Vitalic C, Tavoni A, Simi U, et al. Parotid sialography and minor salivary gland biopsy in the diagnosis of sjogren's syndrome. A comparative study of 84 patients. J Rheumatol 1998;15(2):262–7.
182. Rout J. Radiographic diagnosis of Sjogren's syndrome. Sjogren's Today 2009; 24(4):1–3. Available at: www.bssa.uk.net/live/documents/20a.pdf. Accessed July 9, 2015.
183. Takagi Y, Sumi M, Sumi T, et al. MR microscopy of the parotid glands in patients with Sjogren's syndrome: quantitative MR diagnostic criteria. AJNR Am J Neuroradiol 2005;26:1207–14.
184. Greenberg MS, Glick M, Ship JA. Burket's oral medicine. 11th edition. Hamilton (Canada): BC Decker Inc; 2008.
185. Cocuroccia B, Gubinelhi E, Annessi G, et al. Persistant unilateral orbital and eyelid edema as a manifestations of Melkerson – Rosenthal syndrome. J Eur Acad Dermatol Venereol 2005;19(1):107–11.
186. Dodi I, Verri R, Brevi B, et al. A mono symptomatic Melkersson–Rosenthal syndrome is an 8 years old boy. Acta Biomed 2006;77(1):20–3.
187. Nally FF. Melkersson–Rosenthal syndrome. Report of two cases. Oral Surg Oral Med Oral Pathol 1970;29:694–703.
188. Zecha JJ, Van Dijk L, Hadders HN. Cheilitis granulomatosa (Melkersson Rosenthal syndrome). Oral Surg Oral Med Oral Pathol 1976;42:454.
189. Winnie R, Deluke DM. Melkersson Rosenthal syndrome: a review of the literature and case report. Int J Oral Maxillofac Surg 1992;21:115–7.

Systemic Diseases and Conditions Affecting Jaws

Arthur S. Kuperstein, DDS[a], Thomas R. Berardi, DDS[b], Mel Mupparapu, DMD, MDS[c],*

KEYWORDS

- Radiopacity • Radiolucency • Mixed lesion • Ill-defined border • Effaced-border
- Localized lesion • Generalized lesion • Root resorption

KEY POINTS

- Perform a detailed medical history and physical examination for each patient.
- Understand the potential osseous changes that may be caused by an underlying medical problem.
- Understand normal radiographic anatomy.
- Identify and describe any osseous changes noted on radiographic imagery of the patient.
- Develop a differential diagnosis and treatment plan.

This article is written to highlight and focus on patients with medical conditions seeking dental treatment. History and physical examination findings combined with laboratory and imaging findings lead the clinician to understand the burden of the underlying systemic condition and its effect on the impending dental treatment. It is the responsibility of the dental practitioner to be aware of these systemic conditions, diagnose and appropriately refer to a specialist when needed, and more commonly, manage them as dental patients. Any pertinent data must be used in conjunction with the radiographic investigation or other imaging modality to arrive at a clinical diagnosis. The systemic conditions that are covered range from endocrine abnormalities and developmental conditions to malignancies that have skeletal manifestations. Some of the systemic conditions that may affect the dental treatment or outcomes are described elsewhere in this issue.

[a] Oral Medicine Clinical Services, University of Pennsylvania School of Dental Medicine, 240 South 40th Street, Philadelphia, PA 19104, USA; [b] Oral Medicine, University of Pennsylvania School of Dental Medicine, 240 South 40th Street, Philadelphia, PA 19104, USA; [c] Oral and Maxillofacial Radiology, University of Pennsylvania School of Dental Medicine, 240 South 40th Street, Suite 214, Philadelphia, PA 19104, USA
* Corresponding author.
E-mail address: mmd@dental.upenn.edu

Dent Clin N Am 60 (2016) 235–264
http://dx.doi.org/10.1016/j.cden.2015.08.008
0011-8532/16/$ – see front matter © 2016 Elsevier Inc. All rights reserved.

dental.theclinics.com

SICKLE CELL ANEMIA
Introduction

Sickle cell disease (SCD) comes from a specific form of anemia that is the result of homozygosity for the mutation that causes sickling of hemoglobin (HbS). Sickle cell anemia also has been referred to as HbSS, SS disease, and hemoglobin S. In the heterozygous populations that have only one sickle gene and one normal adult hemoglobin gene, the condition is referred to as sickle cell trait or HBAS. Other forms of sickle disease includes sickle cell hemoglobin c (HbSC), sickle beta plus-thalassemia (HbS/β^+), and sickle beta zero-thalassemia (HbS/β^0) According to the Centers for Disease Control and Prevention[1] (CDC data) that looked into the data from 44 states representing 88% of population, the prevalence of SCD was approximately 73 per 1000 births among African American individuals and 7 per 1000 among Hispanic American individuals. The overall rate was approximately 15 per 1000 live births in the United States.

Summary of Clinical Features

Anemia, infection, and vaso-occlusion are the most common reasons for the complications related to SCD, episodes of pain in the chest, back, abdomen, or extremities. Multiple areas are often involved simultaneously. The acute chest syndrome leading to respiratory insufficiency will have the cardinal features of fever, pleuritic chest pain, referred abdominal pain, cough, lung infiltrates, and hypoxia. Patients with SCD now survive into their fifth or sixth decades in the industrialized countries.[2,3]

Radiographic Features

The vaso-occlusion leads to bone infarcts, osteomyelitis, orbital wall infarction, and subperiosteal hemorrhage. Chronic anemia leads to internal carotid artery stenosis and extramedullary hematopoiesis. The infections lead to osteomyelitis and regional lymphadenopathy. Bone involvement is the most common clinical feature of SCD, mainly the long bones and to a lesser extent the maxillofacial area, due to the small number of marrow spaces within these bones. In the head and neck, the most frequently reported location is the orbital wall, followed by the mandible and skull base. There are both acute and chronic phases of bone involvement; in the acute phase, vaso-occlusive crisis and osteomyelitis are notable, whereas in the chronic phase, bone marrow hyperplasia, osteoporosis, and iron deposition in the marrow due to repeated transfusions may be noted.[4] Avascular necrosis of the bone is a major problem in the long bones, especially the hip, although it is not a common occurrence within the jaws.

Imaging Protocols

Bone infarction leading to change in the trabecular pattern may be a radiographic sign noted in patients with SCD. MRI is a much more sensitive imaging technique over computed tomography (CT) for these changes.

Imaging Findings/Pathology

Radiographically, cortical defects, adjacent soft tissue fluid collection that communicates with the medullary compartment through cortical defects, and ill-defined bone marrow enhancement are indicative of osteomyelitis.[5] A panoramic radiograph (Fig. 1) of a 34-year-old woman with compensated SCD, who presented to the oral medicine admissions clinic with severe abdominal distension and vasculitis affecting the lower extremities showed inconsistent trabecular changes, enlarged bone marrow spaces, especially in the lower anterior region, and some cortical defects. Hypercementosis of some teeth was noted as an incidental finding.

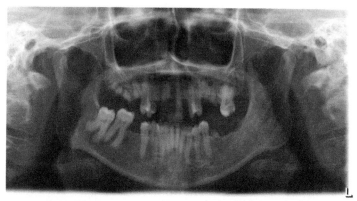

Fig. 1. Panoramic radiograph showing trabecular and cortical changes in a patient with SCD. Note the enlarged bone marrow spaces in the symphysis region.

Differential Diagnosis

- Sickle cell anemia
- Thalassemia
- Spherocytosis
- Elliptocytosis
- Iron deficiency anemia

Summary

It is important to remember that a reduction of the number of trabeculae, a generalized rarefaction accompanied by some thinning of the mandibular cortical plates, may be indicative of SCD.

END-STAGE RENAL DISEASE AND RENAL OSTEODYSTROPHY
Introduction

End-stage renal disease (ESRD) may cause a skeletal change known as renal osteodystrophy. The kidney disease results in decreased levels of 1,25-dihydroxy vitamin D, which is responsible for the active transport of calcium in the small bowel. These patients may present with hypocalcemia as a result of compromised calcium absorption and hyperphosphatemia resulting from reduction in renal phosphorus excretion. Secondary hyperparathyroidism may be a consequence of sustained serum calcium stimulating the parathyroid glands to produce parathyroid hormone (PTH).[6]

Imaging Findings/Pathology

The radiographic features of renal osteodystrophy are quite variable. Some changes of the skeleton resemble those changes observed in rickets, and other changes are consistent with hyperparathyroidism, including generalized loss of bone density and thinning of bony cortices (**Fig. 2**). There may be occasional findings of brown tumors, similar to those seen in primary hyperthyroidism. The occasional size increase of the mandible is due to enlargement of the cancellous bone component that has a dense granular trabecular pattern. In renal osteodystrophy, the density of the mandible and maxilla may be less than normal and intermittently may be greater than normal. Manifestations include a decrease or an increase in the number of internal trabeculae, and the trabecular bone pattern may be granular. The cortical boundaries may be thinner

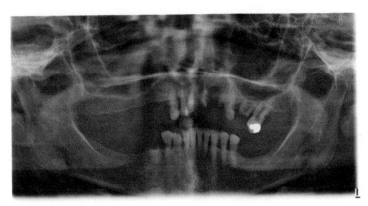

Fig. 2. Panoramic radiograph of a patient with secondary ESRD. Patient has multiple myeloma and osteoporosis who is receiving chemotherapy.

or less noticeable. It is important to note that these bone changes may persist after a successful renal transplant because of hyperplasia of the parathyroid glands, resulting in a continued elevation of PTH. The lamina dura may be absent or not as noticeable on occasion.[7]

Differential Diagnosis

- Osteomalacia and renal osteodystrophy
- Osteoporosis
- Multiple myeloma
- Osteomalacia and renal osteodystrophy
- Sickle cell anemia

Summary

Loss of calcium and vitamin D promotes demineralization of the skeleton (referred to as renal osteodystrophy). Risk of fractures increases with prolonged and uncontrolled secondary hyperparathyroidism and results in increased complications that result from fractures. Bone densitometry can be used to detect reduced bone density and monitor its response to treatment. Prevention or reversal of this complication can be achieved through regulation of parathyroid hormone, vitamin D, and calcium levels.

When treating an patient with ESRD or those on hemodialysis, expect to observe a generalized bony rarefaction when interpreting intraoral and extraoral images of the head and neck. Also, you should relate these finding to recent dialysis blood draws for osteodystrophic panels, as well as complete metabolic panels.[8]

HYPERPARATHYROIDISM

Hyperparathyroidism is an endocrine abnormality in which there is an excess of circulating PTH. An excess of serum PTH increases bone remodeling in preference of osteoclastic resorption, which mobilizes calcium from the skeleton. In addition, PTH increases renal tubular reabsorption of calcium and renal production of the active vitamin D metabolite 1,25(OH)2D. The net result of these functions is in an increase in serum calcium levels. Primary hyperparathyroidism usually results from a benign tumor[8–10] (adenoma) of 1 of the 4 parathyroid glands, resulting in the production of excess PTH. Infrequently, some individuals may have hyperplastic parathyroid glands that secrete excess PTH. The combination of hypercalcemia and an elevated serum level of PTH is diagnostic of primary hyperparathyroidism.

Secondary hyperparathyroidism results from an increase in the production of PTH in response to hypocalcemia. The underlying hypocalcemia may result from an inadequate dietary intake or poor intestinal absorption of vitamin D or from deficient metabolism of vitamin D in the liver or kidney.[11] This condition produces clinical and radiographic effects similar to those of primary hyperparathyroidism. PTH is produced and secreted by the parathyroid glands, whose activity is controlled by the free (ionized) serum calcium level. Increased PTH secretion results in a condition called hyperparathyroidism. Hyperparathyroidism is divided into primary, secondary, and tertiary types. Primary hyperparathyroidism is characterized by elevated PTH secretion. This is a result of an abnormality in one or more of the parathyroid glands. Adenomas are the main cause in approximately 85% of primary hyperparathyroidism cases. Most cases of primary hyperparathyroidism are identified by the presence of hypercalcemia and hypophosphatemia on routine multipanel serum analysis. Secondary hyperparathyroidism is caused by hypocalcemia or vitamin D deficiency acting as a stimulus for excessive PTH production. Chronic renal failure is the main cause of secondary hyperparathyroidism. It results in hypocalcemia and the parathyroid glands hyperactivity to compensate for this low serum calcium level.[12]

Radiographic Features

The principal radiographic change is calcification of the basal ganglia. On skull radiographs, this calcification appears flocculent and paired within the cerebral hemispheres on the posteroanterior (PA) view. Radiographic examination of the jaws may reveal dental enamel hypoplasia, external root resorption, delayed eruption, or root. The important radiographic presentation of hyperparathyroidism in the dental radiographs is the loss of lamina dura (**Fig. 3**), ground glass appearance of the bone, thinning of the mandibular cortex, and, in established cases, gives the appearance of "floating teeth" within the bone due to generalized loss of lamina dura. Intracranial calcifications noted

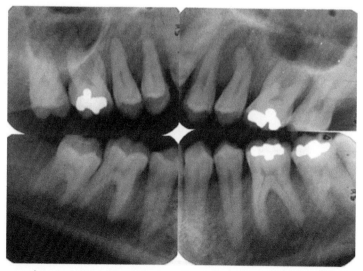

Fig. 3. Intraoral periapical molar views of a patient with primary hyperparathyroidism. Note the loss of lamina dura around the teeth.

in a patient with exuberant hyperparathyroidism secondary to long-standing ESRD are shown. Note the generalized thickening of skull vault (**Figs. 4–6**).

Differential Diagnosis

The following can be considered in the differential diagnosis:

- Hyperparathyroidism
- Central giant cell granuloma
- Fibro-osseous lesion

Summary

Panoramic radiographs, CT scans, ultrasonography, and parathyroid scintigraphy with 99m Tc were all useful radiographic methods for the correct diagnosis if serum analysis is suggestive of underlying disease.

OSTEOPOROSIS
Introduction

Osteoporosis is a systemic skeletal disease characterized by low bone mass and microarchitectural deterioration of bone tissue, with a subsequent increase in bone fragility and susceptibility to fracture.[13,14] Osteoporosis is identified internationally, affecting mostly old and middle-aged women.[15,16] An imbalance occurs in bone resorption and formation. Decrease in bone formation results in changes in trabecular architecture, the volume of trabecular bone, and the size and thickness of individual trabeculae. Osteoporosis occurs with the aging process of bone and can be considered a variation of normal (primary osteoporosis). By the third decade of life, there is a gradual and progressive decline, occurring at the rate of approximately 8% per decade in women and 3% per decade in men. The loss of bone mass with age is so gradual that it is virtually imperceptible until it reaches significant proportions. Secondary osteoporosis may result from nutritional deficiencies, hormonal imbalance, inactivity, or corticosteroid or heparin therapy.

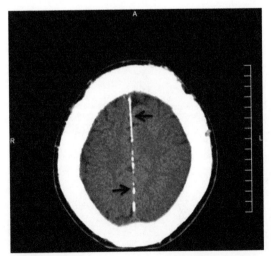

Fig. 4. Axial CT in soft tissue windows showing calcified falx cerebri (*arrows*) in a patient with hyperparathyroidism secondary to ESRD. Note the thickened cranial vault.

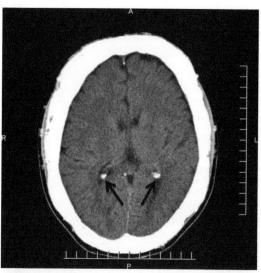

Fig. 5. Axial CT in soft tissue windows showing bilateral choroid plexus calcification (*arrows*). Note the thickened cranial vault.

Imaging Findings/Pathology

Osteoporosis results in an overall reduction in the density of bone (**Fig. 7**). This reduction may be observed in the jaws by using the unaltered density of teeth as a comparison. There may be evidence of a reduced density and thinning of cortical boundaries, such as the inferior mandibular cortex (**Fig. 8**). Reduction in the volume of cancellous bone is more difficult to assess, although new techniques to analyze the trabecular pattern in intraoral images are being developed. Reduction in the number of

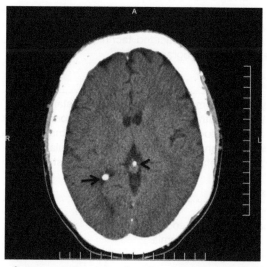

Fig. 6. Axial CT in soft tissue windows showing choroid plexus calcification (*arrow*) and pineal calcification (*arrowhead*) in the same patient as in **Figs. 4** and **5**. Note the thickened cranial vault.

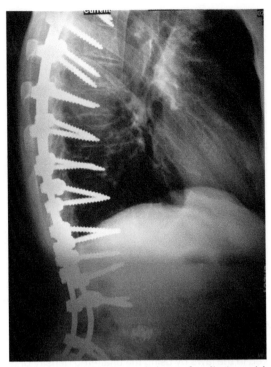

Fig. 7. Lateral thoraco-lumbar spinal radiograph (part of scoliotic study) showing the hardware used to correct the scoliotic deformity in this 70-year-old woman with significant osteoporosis.

trabeculae is least evident in the alveolar process, possibly because of the constant stress applied to this region of bone by the teeth. On occasion, the lamina dura may appear thinner than normal. In other regions of the mandible, a reduction in the number of trabeculae may be evident. Accurate assessment of bone mass loss is difficult, but may be done with sophisticated techniques, such as dual-energy photon absorption or quantitative CT programs.

Diagnostic Criteria

Dual-energy X-ray absorptiometry is considered the standard for measurement of bone density; the World Health Organization considers bone mineral density measurements diagnostic for osteoporosis.[15,17] Certain features may be observed on a panoramic image. A constellation of thinning of the mandibular cortex, external oblique ridges, and generalized rarefaction might represent an osteoporotic patient.

Differential Diagnosis

- Hyperparathyroidism
- Osteomalacia and renal osteodystrophy
- Homocystinuria/homocysteinemia
- Multiple myeloma
- Paget disease
- Sickle cell anemia
- Scurvy

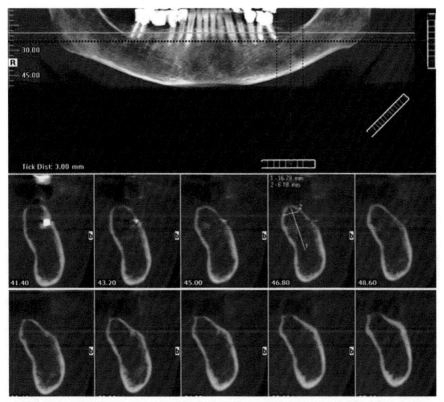

Fig. 8. CBCT orthogonal views from the mandibular left molar region showing thinned cortices and sparse trabeculation within in a patient with osteoporosis seeking dental implants.

Summary

We in the dental profession have the opportunity to use intraoral and extraoral imaging technology inherent to our field of patient care to identify osteoporotic changes in the maxillofacial skeleton that may influence patient care.[17] Of utmost importance is the current use of nitrogen-bearing bisphosphonate drugs that carry with them the potential for antiresorptive osteonecrotic jaw disease.

CUSHING SYNDROME

Cushing syndrome is caused by the clinical manifestation of pathologic hypercortisolism. These excess glucocorticoids can be from increased endogenous production or prolonged exposure to exogenous use of glucocorticoid products.[18–23] Although endogenous Cushing syndrome is a rare disease, drug-related or exogenous Cushing syndrome from glucocorticoid products is commonly seen in clinical practice. This section focuses on iatrogenic, or drug-related, Cushing syndrome.

Drugs that have been reported to result in hypercortisolism are glucocorticoids, megestrol acetate, and herbal preparations that contain glucocorticoids.

Individuals with Cushing syndrome can develop moon facies, facial plethora, supraclavicular fat pads, buffalo hump, truncal obesity, and purple striae.

Individuals often experience proximal muscle weakness, easy bruising, weight gain, hirsutism, and pediatric growth retardation. Hypertension, osteopenia, diabetes mellitus, and impaired immune function also may occur.[21,22] Additionally, subclinical hypercortisolism may be more common than is generally recognized in patients with osteoporosis in whom secondary causes of osteoporosis have been excluded.[23]

Imaging Findings/Pathology

Cushing syndrome, which cannot be differentiated radiologically from that of the natural form of the disease, has been frequently described. It is liable to occur with a cortisone or cortisone-equivalent dosage of 50 to 100 mg a day over periods varying from 6 months to 3 years. Osteoporosis, fractures, and joint degenerations may be observed in the absence of the fully developed picture of Cushing syndrome. Such changes may occur after much shorter periods of steroid therapy.[23]

TEMPOROMANDIBULAR JOINT DISEASES OF SYSTEMIC ORIGIN

The research diagnostic criteria that are universally accepted for the diagnosis of temporomandibular disorder (TMD) are quite stringent in their categorization of clinical and radiographic findings.[24] Only those cases of osteoarthritis in which there is clear-cut deformation of the condyles due to subcortical cyst, surface erosions, osteophytosis, or generalize sclerosis were classified into the category C (the most severe form), the other 2 categories, A and B, being less severely involved and imaging findings are within normal limits. These patients constitute a large majority of the patient population in which the abnormality is mostly soft tissue or disk-related in origin for which standard radiography is of no use. A magnetic resonance examination of the joints might show the changes related to the disk and whether or not it is displaced.

The imaging of the temporomandibular joint (TMJ) may be indicated based on the patient's signs and symptoms and examination findings. Clinical examination finding suggestive of joint restriction or progressive trismus should alert the clinician of an impending TMD, and extraoral imaging is indicated in such situations (**Fig. 9**). On the other hand, incidental findings may be observed on panoramic, cone beam CT (CBCT), and lateral and PA cephalometric and skull views acquired during the examination for other procedures. This patient population may be treated with drugs such

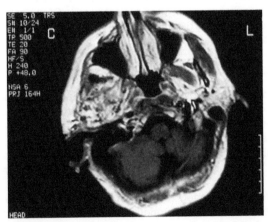

Fig. 9. Axial open MR (T1-weighted) image showing significant destruction of right TMJ due to synovial chondromatosis.

as corticosteroids, which of course may also contribute to osteoporotic changes in the bone, and antineoplastic drugs, such as methotrexate, which have the potential of causing severe bone marrow suppression.

TEMPOROMANDIBULAR JOINT DEGENERATIVE JOINT DISEASE
Introduction

There are a number of arthritides: osteoarthritis (OA) with the sequelae of biologic and mechanical events may destabilize the joint.[24] Degenerative joint disease (DJD), often a synonym of OA, is considered noninflammatory in nature. Joint deterioration is characterized by loss of articular cartilage and bone erosion. The proliferative component is characterized by new bone formation at the articular surface and in the subchondral region. Usually a variable combination of deterioration and proliferation occurs, but occasionally one aspect predominates; deterioration is more common in acute disease, and proliferation predominates in chronic disease[25,26]; rheumatoid arthritis (RA) is treated in the next section.

Imaging Findings/Pathology

Osseous changes in DJD are more accurately depicted in CT images, but gross osseous changes may be evident in MRI studies, particularly in T1-weighted images. When the patient is in maximal intercuspation, the joint space may be narrow or absent, which often correlates with an internal derangement and frequently with a perforation of the disk or posterior attachment, resulting in bone-to-bone contact of the joint components. Signs of previous remodeling, such as flattening and subchondral sclerosis, may be evident, although degenerative changes may obscure these findings. Loss of cortex or erosions of the articulating surfaces of the condyle or temporal component (or both) are characteristic of this disease (**Fig. 10**). In some cases, small, round, radiolucent areas with irregular margins surrounded by a varying area of increased density are visible deep to the articulating surfaces. The term, "Ely cyst" or subchondral bone cysts has been used to describe them, but they are not true cysts; they are areas of degeneration that contain fibrous tissue, granulation tissue, and osteoid (**Fig. 11**). Later in the course of the disease, bony proliferation occurs at the periphery of the articulating surface, increasing the articulating surface area. This new bone is called an osteophyte, which typically appears on the anterosuperior surface of the condyle, the lateral aspect of the temporal component, or both. Osteophytes also may form on the lateral, medial, and posterosuperior aspects of the condyle. In severe cases, osteophyte formation originating in the glenoid fossa extends from the articular eminence to almost encase the condylar head. Osteophytes may break off and lie free within the joint space, and these must be differentiated

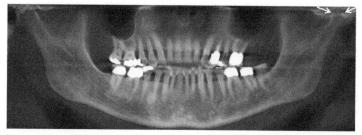

Fig. 10. Panoramic reconstruction of CBCT showing flattening of left condylar head as well as loss of joint space in relation to the left TMJ (*arrows*).

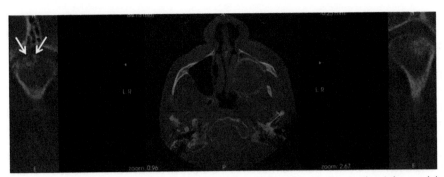

Fig. 11. CBCT coronal TMJ views showing a subchondral cyst in relation to the right condyle (*arrows*).

from other conditions that cause joint space radiopacity. In severe DJD, the glenoid fossa may appear grossly enlarged because of erosion of the posterior slope of the articular eminence, and the condyle may be markedly diminished in size and altered in shape because of destruction and erosion of the condylar head. This in turn may allow the condylar head to move forward and superiorly into an abnormal anterior position that may result in an anterior open bite.[26]

Differential Diagnosis

- Subchondral sclerosis
- Osteophyte formation (proliferative component)
- Extensive erosions: degenerative component
- RA
- Osteoma or osteochondroma

TEMPOROMANDIBULAR JOINT RHEUMATOID ARTHRITIS
Introduction

RA is a diverse group of systemic disorders that manifests mainly as synovial membrane inflammation in numerous joints. RA is a chronic inflammatory condition affecting approximately 1% of the population, making it the most common inflammatory arthritis seen by physicians.[26] It primarily affects the small joints of the hands and feet and if not treated aggressively may lead to diminished quality of life, need for joint replacement surgery, and mortality.[26] RA is a clinical diagnosis with laboratory and radiographic tests helping to confirm the diagnosis and providing useful prognostic information. The TMJ becomes involved in approximately half of affected patients (**Fig. 12**). The characteristic radiographic findings are a result of villous synovitis, which leads to formation of synovial granulomatous tissue (pannus) that grows into fibrocartilage and bone, releasing enzymes that destroy articular surfaces and underlying bone.[27]

Imaging Findings/Pathology

The initial changes may be generalized osteopenia (decreased density) of the condyle and temporal component. The pannus may destroy the disk, resulting in diminished width of the joint space. Bone erosions by the pannus most often involve the articular eminence and the anterior aspect of the condylar head, which permits anterosuperior positioning of the condyle when the teeth are in maximal intercuspation and results in an anterior open bite. Erosion of the anterior and posterior condylar surfaces at the attachment of the synovial lining may result in a "sharpened pencil" appearance of

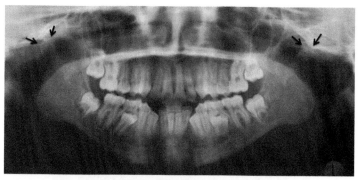

Fig. 12. Panoramic radiograph showing typical features of RA in a young patient. TMJ is affected bilaterally. *Arrows* indicates the condyles.

the condyle. Erosive changes may be so severe that the entire condylar head is destroyed, with only the neck remaining as the articulating surface. Similarly, the articular eminence may be destroyed to the extent that a concavity replaces the normally convex eminence. Joint destruction eventually leads to secondary DJD. Subchondral sclerosis and flattening of articulating surfaces may occur, as well as subchondral "cyst" and osteophyte formation. Fibrous ankylosis or, in rare cases, osseous ankylosis, may occur; reduced mobility is related to the duration and severity of the disease.[28]

Differential Diagnosis

The American College of Rheumatology/European League Against Rheumatism collaborative initiative has created and published guidelines for establishing diagnostic criteria.[26]

- Severe DJD
- Systemic lupus erythematosus
- Osteopenia and severe erosions of the articular eminence, are more characteristic of RA
- Psoriatic arthritis

Summary

Subtle or no changes in the radiographic image of the TMJ may not correlate with a symptomatic presentation of the patient. Conversely, a severely degenerated condyle, as viewed on a radiograph, may be asymptomatic. Therefore, thorough clinical evaluation must be used with imaging in a patient workup.

PAGET DISEASE
Introduction

Paget disease (osteitis deformans) was described by Sir James Paget in 1877. It is a chronic skeletal disorder characterized by abnormal and excessive remodeling of bone.[29] The disease typically appears in the population beginning in the fourth decade.[29]

Imaging Findings/Pathology

The progression of Paget disease (**Fig. 13**) has been described as consisting of 3 phases that may be coexistent. The affected areas have an amorphous shape. Other

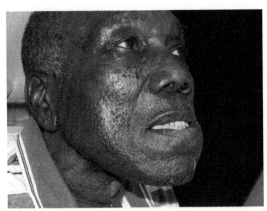

Fig. 13. Facial profile of an 80-year-old patient with Paget disease. Note the mandibular prognathism. (*Courtesy of* Dr Maano Milles, Rutgers School of Dental Medicine, Newark, NJ.)

common radiographic features may be observed, such as a ground glass appearance in the second phase (**Fig. 14**) to a cotton wool appearance blending into the third phase.

	Phase 1	Phase 2	Phase 3
Bone changes	Osteolytic	Mixed osteolytic and osteoblastic	Sclerotic
Radiographic findings	Radiolucent	Mixed radiolucent and radiopaque	Radiopaque

Diagnostic Criteria

The disease is typically found in the fourth to sixth decades. Bony expansion is a constant finding.

Differential Diagnosis

- Paget disease
- Florid osseous dysplasia
- Fibrous dysplasia

Variants

Although sarcomatous change is rare, the clinician should be aware of unexpected bony changes observed on the patient's radiographs. The sarcomas arising from pagetic lesions tend to have poor prognosis. The 5-year survival rate averaged at approximately 10% for adults with this transformation, whereas the 5-year survival rate is approximately 70% to 80% in pediatric osteosarcomas.

What the Referring Dentist Needs to Know

The 2014 Endocrine Society Clinical Practice Guideline on Paget disease recommends among its management protocol the consideration of treatment with single-dose intravenous zolendronic acid as the treatment of choice,[30] seen as follows:

- Plain radiographs of the pertinent regions of the skeleton in patients with suspected Paget disease

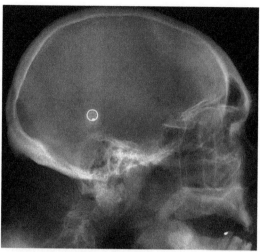

Fig. 14. Cropped lateral cephalometric radiograph of the patient in **Fig. 13** with established Paget disease showing typical changes associated with Paget. Note the generalized increased bone density, as well as thickening of the cortices. (*Courtesy of* Dr Maano Milles, Rutgers School of Dental Medicine, Newark, NJ.)

- A radionuclide bone scan to determine the extent of the disease if the diagnosis is confirmed
- Measurement of serum total alkaline phosphatase or, when warranted, a more specific marker of bone formation or bone resorption to assess the response to treatment or evolution of the disease in untreated patients
- Consider treatment with a bisphosphonate for most patients with active Paget disease who are at risk for future complications
- Consider a single 5-mg dose of intravenous zoledronate as the treatment of choice in patients who have no contraindication
- Consider measurement of a specific marker of bone formation and bone resorption in patients with monostotic disease who have a normal serum total alkaline phosphatase
- Consider serial radionuclide bone scans to determine the response to treatment if the markers are normal
- Bisphosphonate treatment may be effective in preventing or slowing the progress of hearing loss and osteoarthritis in joints adjacent to Paget disease and may reverse paraplegia associated with spinal Paget disease
- Consider treatment with a bisphosphonate before surgery on pagetic bone

This, of course, caries the potential risk of antiresorptive agent related osteonecrosis of the jaw associated with surgical procedures. These patients also may develop congestive heart failure as a consequence of having Paget disease and should be treated accordingly.

Summary

It is important to remember the diagnostic criteria of advanced age, total bone involvement, elevated alkaline phosphatase, bony expansion, and variable radiographic presentation in establishing and refining a working differential diagnosis for Paget disease. Consider the medical management of the disease and coordinate with any oral surgical procedures.[30]

Paget disease is a common skeletal disorder of middle-aged and elderly persons characterized by excessive and abnormal remodeling of bone. The disease varies considerably in severity and evolves through various phases of activity, followed by an inactive phase. The radiographic features of Paget disease are virtually diagnostic, including an initial osteolytic phase and a subsequent osteosclerotic phase. Bone enlargement with increased radiodensity (**Figs. 15** and **16**), accentuated trabecular pattern, and deformity is typical. Complications associated with Paget disease are pathologic fractures, neurologic symptoms, skeletal deformities, articular derangements, and secondary neoplasms. CT and MRI help delineate pagetic bone changes and have proven extremely useful in the diagnosis of sarcomatous transformation, which constitutes the most dreaded complication of the disease.[27]

HYPERPITUITARISM
Introduction

Hyperpituitarism, also known as *acromegaly*, is a sequela of hyperfunction of the anterior lobe of the pituitary gland, which escalates the production of growth hormone after the epiphyseal closure. This excess of growth hormone causes overgrowth of all tissues in the body still capable of growth. Gigantism is the term used with disease onset in children before epiphyseal closure. Active growth occurs in those bones in which the epiphyses have not united with the bone shafts. Those affected may ultimately

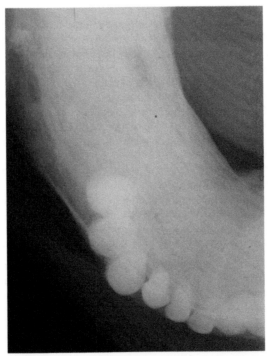

Fig. 15. Cropped mandibular floor of the mouth occlusal radiograph (right side) of the patient showing generalized increased bone density suggestive of Paget disease. (*Courtesy of* Dr Maano Milles, Rutgers School of Dental Medicine, Newark, NJ.)

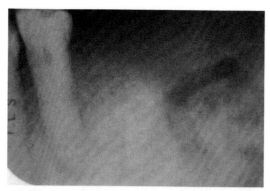

Fig. 16. Mandibular left premolar periapical radiograph showing loss of lamina dura and irregular, patchy dense bone suggestive of a multistage bone loss and bone gain (osteolytic and osteoblastic). (*Courtesy of* Dr Maano Milles, Rutgers School of Dental Medicine, Newark, NJ.)

attain heights of 7 to 8 feet or more, yet exhibit remarkably normal proportions.[28] Adult hyperpituitarism, called acromegaly, has an insidious clinical course, quite different from the clinical profile seen in the childhood disease. In adults, the clinical effects of a pituitary adenoma develop quite slowly because many types of tissues have lost the capacity for growth. This is true of much of the skeleton; however, an excess of growth hormone can stimulate the mandible and the phalanges of the hand. Mandibular condylar growth may be very prominent. Also, the supraorbital ridges and the underlying frontal sinus may be enlarged. Excess growth hormone in adults may also produce hypertrophy of some soft tissues.[31] The lips, tongue, nose, and soft tissues of the hands and feet typically overgrow in adults with acromegaly, sometimes to a great extent.

Imaging Findings/Pathology

The pituitary adenoma responsible for hyperpituitarism often produces enlargement (ballooning) of the sella turcica. It is important to note that in some examples the sella may not expand at all. Skull radiographs characteristically reveal enlargement of the paranasal sinuses (especially the frontal sinus). These air sinuses are more prominent in acromegaly than in pituitary giantism because sinus growth in giantism tends to be more in step with the generalized enlargement of the facial bones. Hyperpituitarism in adults also produces diffuse thickening of the outer table of the skull.[32–34]

Hyperpituitarism causes enlargement of the jaws, most notably the mandible. The increase in the length of the dental arches results in spacing of the teeth. In acromegaly, the angle between the ramus and body of the mandible may increase. This, in combination with enlargement of the tongue (macroglossia), may result in anterior angulation of the teeth and the development of an anterior open bite. The sign of incisor flaring is a helpful point of differentiation between acromegalic prognathism and inherited prognathism. In acromegaly the most profound growth occurs in the condyle and ramus, often resulting in a class III skeletal.

An example of acromegaly manifesting as excessive growth of the mandible results in a class III skeletal relationship of the jaws. Lateral skull view of a patient demonstrating the osseous changes and enlargement of the sella turcica is shown in **Fig. 17**. The thickness and height of the alveolar processes may also increase, and in some cases, hypercementosis is noted (**Fig. 18**). A CBCT with 3D reconstruction

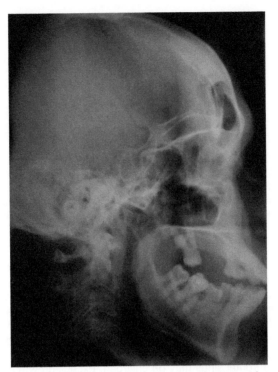

Fig. 17. Lateral cephalometric radiograph showing enlarged sella and frontal sinus. Note the steep mandibular angle and a class III malocclusion. (*From* Kashyap RR, Babu GS, Shetty SR. Dental patient with acromegaly: a case report. J Oral Sci 2011;53:135; with permission.)

is shown in **Fig. 19**. The midsagittal CBCT view demonstrates the anterior skeletal class III relationship (**Fig. 20**). Other skeletal changes that are noted in the sagittal view in are in relation to the sella (enlarged), cervical vertebrae (sclerosis, hypertrophy of the dens), and the clivus (sclerosis).

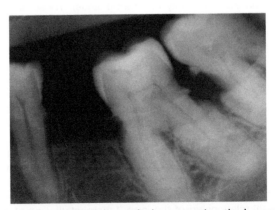

Fig. 18. Mandibular left molar PA radiograph demonstrating the hypercementosis of the roots of both the molars in the same patient as noted in **Fig. 17**. Missing apices are secondary to positioning error. (*From* Kashyap RR, Babu GS, Shetty SR. Dental patient with acromegaly: a case report. J Oral Sci 2011;53:135; with permission.)

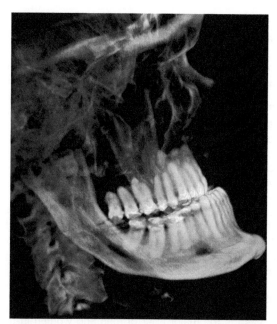

Fig. 19. A CBCT 3-dimensional reconstruction of a patient with hyperpituitarism showing the accentuated jaw growth leading to a class III profile. (*Courtesy of* Dr Mansur Ahmad, University of Minnesota School of Dentistry, Minneapolis, MN.)

The tooth crowns are usually normal in size, although the roots of posterior teeth often enlarge as a result of hypercementosis. This hypercementosis may be the result of functional and structural demands on teeth instead of a secondary hormonal effect. Super-eruption of the posterior teeth may occur in an attempt to compensate for the growth of the mandible.[35,36]

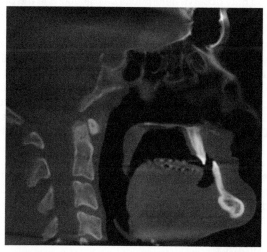

Fig. 20. Midsagittal CBCT view of the same patient noted in **Fig. 19** demonstrating the mandibular prognathism and enlarged sella. Note the calcification of pineal gland noted on this image intracranially. (*Courtesy of* Dr Mansur Ahmad, University of Minnesota School of Dentistry, Minneapolis, MN.)

Diagnostic Criteria

Diagnostic criteria include thickened cranial vault, enlarged sella (pituitary fossa), prominence of occipital protuberance, enlarged frontal sinus, mandibular prognathism and elongation, increase in gonial angle, enlarged supraorbital ridge, and increased thickness of calvaria.[34–36]

Differential Diagnosis

- Familial tall stature
- Exogenous obesity
- Cerebral gigantism
- Weaver syndrome
- McCune-Albright syndrome

Summary

The prognosis of hyperpituitarism has improved due to modern surgical and pharmacologic treatment strategies. Patients' survival, as well as their quality of life, has been improved by the diagnosis and treatment of comorbidities such as hypertension, diabetes, and sleep apnea.[37]

ATHEROSCLEROSIS

Cardiovascular disease is the major killer of men and women in the United States. Many studies cite findings of calcifications of the carotid artery on panoramic radiographs as being predictors of stroke[38–41]; however, even as early as 2005, researchers have been investigating the pathology of the plaques, and not necessarily the calcification, as a means to prevent ipsilateral and contralateral stroke. The extent of calcification has been found to be unassociated with stroke symptoms in their sample.

Imaging Findings/Pathology

During the examination of the panoramic radiograph and/or the CBCT (panoramic or full field) the clinician may observe amorphous calcifications in the posterior lateral region of the pharynx at the level of C3-C4. This level corresponds with a grouping of anatomic mineralized structures: thyroid cartilage, triticeous cartilage, and proximal great cornu of the hyoid bone. Additionally, the nonmineralized bifurcation of the common carotid artery is typically located in this area. On occasion, a calcified carotid artery atheroma may be observed in the visual field captured by the detector or in a CBCT/CT volume (**Fig. 21**). This pathologic structure may have significant cardiovascular implications, such as transient ischemic attack and stroke in certain patients at risk.[38–42] Consultation with their primary care physician, and perhaps a recommendation for a duplex Doppler ultrasound of the carotids should be considered.[41]

Summary

Even though there may be limited predictive value of stroke risk in identifying a calcified carotid artery atheroma (CCAA) on a panoramic radiograph or CBCT,[43] once the lesion is observed, the patient may be at risk[42] and therefore the primary care physician should be advised.

METASTATIC MALIGNANCY
Introduction

Metastatic tumors represent the establishment of new foci of malignant disease from a distant malignant tumor, usually by way of the blood vessels. An interesting feature of

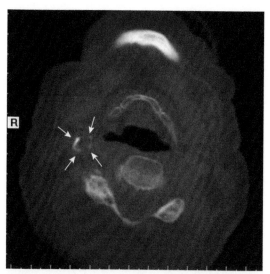

Fig. 21. Axial CBCT view at the level of hyoid bone shows calcified carotid atheroma on the right side (*arrows*).

these lesions is that metastatic lesions in the jaws usually arise from sites that are anatomically inferior to the clavicle. Metastatic lesions of the jaws usually occur when the distant primary lesion is already known, although on occasion the presence of a metastatic tumor may reveal the presence of a silent primary lesion. Jaw involvement accounts for less than 1% of metastatic malignancies found elsewhere, with most affecting the spine, pelvis, skull, ribs, and humerus. Most frequently, the tumor is a type of carcinoma; the most common primary sites are the breast, kidney, lung, colon and rectum, prostate, thyroid, stomach, melanoma, testes, bladder, ovary, and cervix. Metastatic carcinoma must be differentiated from the more common locally invading squamous carcinoma.

Metastatic disease is more common in patients in their fifth to seventh decades of life. Patients may complain of dental pain, numbness or paresthesia of the third branch of the trigeminal nerve, pathologic fracture of the jaw, or hemorrhage from the tumor site.[44,45]

Metastatic tumors do not possess any pathognomonic radiographic appearance. Radiographic appearances of metastatic lesions may range from no manifestation to lytic (**Fig. 22**) or opaque lesion with ill-defined margins (**Fig. 23**). Metastatic lesions from prostate nearly always form osteoblastic lesions in the bone. The metastatic lesions from lung, breast, or kidney are more often lytic in nature.

Imaging Findings/Pathology

The posterior areas of the jaws are more commonly affected with the mandible favored over the maxilla. The maxillary sinus may be the next most common site, followed by the anterior hard palate and mandibular condyle. Frequently, metastatic lesions of the mandible are bilateral. Also, lesions may be located in the periodontal ligament space (sometimes at the root apex), mimicking periapical and periodontal inflammatory disease, or in the papilla of a developing tooth.

Periphery and shape

Metastatic lesions may be moderately well demarcated but have no cortication or encapsulation at their tumor margins; they may also have ill-defined invasive margins.

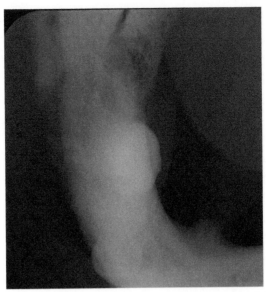

Fig. 22. Cropped mandibular floor of the mouth occlusal radiograph of right body showing expansion, and cortical and trabecular changes secondary to metastatic bone disease from prostate. A pathologic fracture was noted in this patient at the site.

The lesions are not usually round but polymorphous in shape. Both prostate and breast lesions may stimulate bone formation of the adjacent bone, which will be sclerotic. The tumor may begin as a few zones of osseous destruction separated by normal bone. After a time, these small areas coalesce into a larger, ill-defined mass and the jaw may become enlarged.

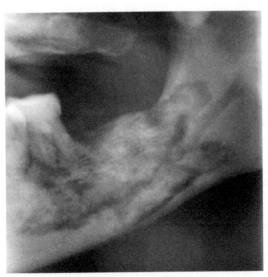

Fig. 23. Cropped panoramic radiograph of a 75-year-old man with metastatic lesion from prostate cancer. Note the pathologic fracture with diffuse lytic and dense areas suggestive of medication-related osteonecrosis of the jaw.

Internal structure

Lesions are generally radiolucent, in which case the internal structure is a combination of residual normal trabecular bone in association with areas of bone lysis. If sclerotic metastases are present (ie, prostate and breast), the normally ragged radiolucent area may appear as an area of patchy sclerosis, the result of new bone formation.[45] The origin of this new bone is not the tumor but stimulation of surrounding normal bone. If the tumor is seeded in multiple regions of the jaw, the result is a multifocal appearance (multiple small radiolucent lesions) with normal bone between the foci. Significant dissemination of metastatic tumor may give the jaws a general radiolucent appearance or even that of osteopenia.

Effects on surrounding structures

Metastatic carcinomas may stimulate a periosteal reaction that usually takes the form of a spiculated pattern (prostate and neuroblastoma, typical of malignancy), the lesion effaces the lamina dura and can cause an irregular increase in the width of the periodontal ligament space. If the tumor has seeded in the papilla of a developing tooth, the cortices of the crypt may be totally or partially destroyed. Teeth may seem to be floating in a soft tissue mass and may be in an altered position because of loss of bony support. Extraction sockets may fail to heal and may increase in size. Resorption of teeth is rare (sometimes associated with multiple myeloma and chondrosarcoma); this is more common in benign lesions. The cortical bone of adjacent structures, such as the neurovascular canal, sinus, and nasal fossa, is destroyed. On occasion the tumor breaches the outer cortical plate of the jaws and extends into surrounding soft tissues or presents as an intraoral mass.

Differential Diagnosis

In most cases, the patient will have a preexisting diagnosis. However, one must be ever conscious of changes from previous radiographic examination.

Summary

Consistent updates from oncologists, and considerations of dosing, fields of intensity-modulated radiation therapy (IMRT), and shielding have influence on dental treatment of these patients.

CHERUBISM

Originally published by A.W. Jones[45] in 1933, cherubism is a rare, inherited developmental anomaly causing bilateral enlargement of the jaws, giving the child a "cherubic" facial appearance.[46] It was originally named familial multilocular cystic disease of the jaws by Jones and later renamed as cherubism. It was also known by the name, "familial fibrous dysplasia" because the biopsy of the lesions published in the early literature (from the early twentieth century) consistently showed histologic features similar to fibrous dysplasia. Hence, it was thought to be a familial version of the disease. It is inherited as an autosomal dominant disorder of variable penetrance (100% in male individuals and 50%–70% in female individuals). The disease usually develops at 2 to 6 years of age and is characterized by painless bilateral swellings of the posterior mandible. Researchers have isolated the gene responsible for cherubism: chromosome 4p16.[46]

Radiographic Features

The lesions are always bilateral, multilocular in nature, with well-defined periphery. The condition may affect maxilla as well as mandible. The epicenter is typically the ramus or the maxillary tuberosity area. The lesions are well demarcated with corticated borders. Thin trabeculae or septae are noticed within the lesions. The lesions assume the "soap bubble" appearance. The lesion expands the cortices of the mandible. Maxillary lesions may expand into the maxillary sinus. Teeth are usually displaced anteriorly as the lesions expand. The lesions are filled with bone after the active phase ends, leading to the reduction in size (**Figs. 24–26**).

RADIATION AND CHEMOTHERAPEUTIC EFFECTS ON ORAL CAVITY

After irradiation of the head and neck, if the oral cavity is in the *line of fire*, there will be changes to the oral mucosa, tongue, teeth, and bone.[47,48]

Based on the literature reports, there is minimal tooth damage below 30 Gy (salivary gland threshold) and a significant damage at or above 60 Gy.[47] Changes to the salivary composition added with the increase in the amount of cariogenic bacteria leads to rapid decalcification of enamel. Radiation caries sets in on all available tooth surfaces, leading to progression of caries ultimately leading to breakdown of tooth structure (**Fig. 27**).

Irradiation also may induce disturbances in tooth formation. Various effects of radiation include microdontia, taurodontism, short or blunted roots, premature closure of apices, and arrested development of teeth have been noted.[47,48] The development of osteoradionecrosis is described in the article by Omolehinwa and Akintoye, elsewhere in this issue. Common side effects of chemotherapy include pain in gums and oral cavity, burning mouth, peeling of oral mucosa, change of taste, and infection. As immunity can be suppressed temporarily, chances of infection are high for these patients. Any focus of infection should be eliminated. It is recommended that fixed orthodontic appliance be removed before chemotherapy. Common side effects that are noted after any chemotherapy include fatigue, pain, oral ulcers secondary to mucositis, diarrhea, nausea, and vomiting.[48] Patients who are undergoing either chemotherapy or radiation therapy or both may need dental care either prophylactically or for interceptive purposes. The assessment of these patients has to be done with utmost care, taking into consideration the total dose received, status of bone marrow suppression, secondary infections, and nutritional status.

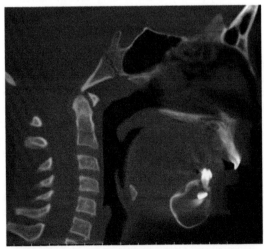

Fig. 24. Midsagittal CBCT image showing the expansion of anterior mandible in a case of cherubism. Note the beginnings of the expansile lesion in the maxilla. (*Courtesy of Dr Mansur Ahmad, University of Minnesota School of Dentistry, Minneapolis, MN.*)

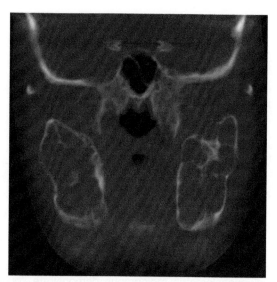

Fig. 25. Coronal CBCT section at the level of vertical ramus showing the bilateral expansile areas of the mandible that demonstrate smaller compartments in the same patient as seen in **Fig. 20**. (*Courtesy of* Dr Mansur Ahmad, University of Minnesota School of Dentistry, Minneapolis, MN.)

MULTIPLE MYELOMA

Multiple myeloma, a common malignancy of bone in adults, often presents with bone pain, especially lower back, Ben Jones proteinuria, tooth mobility (jaw involvement), parasthesia, oral ulceration, temporal arteritis, and macroglossa (due to deposition

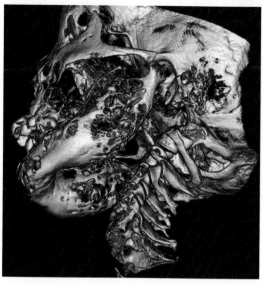

Fig. 26. CBCT 3-dimensional reconstruction of the patient noted in both **Figs. 24** and **25**. Note the bilateral expansion of the body and ramus of the mandible. (*Courtesy of* Dr Mansur Ahmad, University of Minnesota School of Dentistry, Minneapolis, MN.)

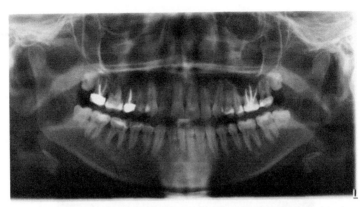

Fig. 27. Panoramic radiograph of a patient status post radiation therapy showing extensive proximal carious lesions.

of amyloid). In the United States, the lifetime risk of getting multiple myeloma is 1 in 143 (0.7%). Lateral cephalometric radiographs demonstrate "punched out" skull lesions that appear as distinct, round, or oval lucencies (**Fig. 28**).[49] Skull lesions may be present in approximately 45% of patients. Plain radiography appears to be better for the diagnosis of cortical bone lesions, their sequelae, and follow-up (**Fig. 29**).

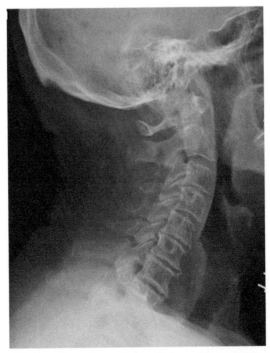

Fig. 28. C-Spine radiograph of a patient with multiple myeloma showing multiple punched out radiolucencies in the skull. Significant osteopenia is noted in the cervical vertebrae and evidence of DJD.

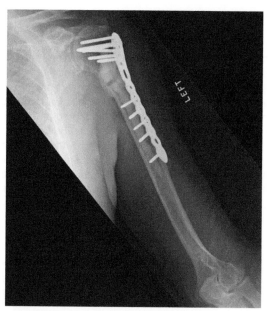

Fig. 29. Fractured neck of the humerus reduced via internal fixation in a patient with multiple myeloma. Note the significant callus formation at the fracture site.

CT is a very sensitive imaging modality in the detection of osteolytic lesions of multiple myeloma and has higher sensitivity than planar radiography when used to detect small cortical lesions. CT or CBCT features in multiple myeloma consist of punched out lytic lesions, expansile lesions with soft tissue masses, osteopenia, fractures, and, rarely, osteosclerosis. Although standard pulse sequences have been tried to image multiple myeloma lesions (T1-weighted, T2-weighted, T2*, short tau inversion recovery), the preferred technique now is diffusion-weighted imaging. Bone scintigraphy is of limited use in multiple myeloma. PET/CT is a very useful tool in the identification of active myeloma lesions (fluorodeoxyglucose positive) from that of monoclonal gammopathy of undermined significance (MGUS) or smouldering disease. MGUS is usually negative on PET/CT with neither diffuse marrow uptake nor focal disease in marrow sites. PET/CT has also been shown to be useful in evaluating response to therapy, especially when other imaging techniques like MRI or CT are inconclusive.

The diagnosis of multiple myeloma should be based on many tests. The following are some of the frequently recommended tests[50]:

1. The detection and evaluation of monoclonal component by serum and urine protein electrophoresis (24-hour urine specimen)
2. Quantification of immunoglobulin (Ig)G, IgA, and IgM immunoglobulins
3. Evaluation of bone marrow plasma cell infiltration via bone marrow biopsy
4. Evaluation of lytic bone lesions via skeletal survey to detect the plasmacytoma lesions and possible pathologic fractures
5. MRI if spinal cord compression is suspected
6. Serum calcium, serum creatinine, hemoglobin, and complete blood count

A common staging system (stages I, II, and III), known as the Durie-Salmon classification, is used to stage the disease based on the recommended tests. The international staging system has 3 groups, International Prognostic Index (IPI) Group I, IPI Group II, and the IPI Group III, based on the concentration of β_2M (Beta macroglobulin).[50]

Most patients with myeloma receiving antimyeloma therapy (chemotherapy), also receive bisphosphonates, regardless of whether or not they show evidence of bone disease radiographically. As bone disease is a common complication of multiple myeloma, bisphosphonates are given to slow down and prevent bone destruction. The most commonly prescribed bisphosphonates are zolendronic acid and pamidronate. Patients with multiple myeloma should be monitored for complications, such as kidney failure and osteonecrosis of the jaw. Renal function tests should be measured before each bisphosphonate infusion and patients with mild to moderate kidney impairment should receive reduced doses of bisphosphonates. Apart from chemotherapeutic agents and bisphosphonates, corticosteroids and immunomodulation agents are also given as part of the therapy. Solitary lesions, called plasmacytomas could be a problem, as the lesions may affect the vitality of teeth and necessitate endodontic therapy and minor oral surgery.

REFERENCES

1. Available at: www.cdc.gov/ncbddd/sicklecell/data.html. Accessed July 1, 2015.
2. Steinberg MH. Management of sickle cell disease. N Engl J Med 1999;340: 1021–30.
3. Platt OS, Brambilla DJ, Rosse WF, et al. Mortality in sickle cell disease: life expectancy and risk factors for early death. N Engl J Med 1994;330:1639–44.
4. Saito N, Nadgir RN, Flower EN, et al. Clinical and radiographic manifestations of sickle cell disease in the head and neck. Radiographics 2010;30:1021–34.
5. Ejindu VC, Hine AL, Mashayekhi M, et al. Musculoskeletal manifestations of sickle cell disease. Radiographics 2007;27(4):1005–21.
6. Moe S, Drüeke T, Cunningham J, et al, Kidney disease: improving global outcomes (KDIGO). Definition, evaluation, and classification of renal osteodystrophy: a position statement from kidney disease: improving global outcomes (KDIGO). Kidney Int 2006;69:1945–53.
7. White SC, Pharoah MJ. Oral radiology—principles and interpretation. 7th edition. Philadelphia: Elsevier. 2014.
8. Trunzo JA, McHenry CR, Schulak JA, et al. Effect of parathyroidectomy on anemia and erythropoietin dosing in end-stage renal disease patients with hyperparathyroidism. Surgery 2008;144:915–8.
9. Selvi F, Cakarer S, Tanakol R, et al. Brown tumour of the maxilla and mandible: a rare complication of tertiary hyperparathyroidism. Dentomaxillofac Radiol 2009; 38:53–8.
10. Kar DK, Gupta SK, Agarwal A, et al. Brown tumor of the palate and mandible in association with primary hyperparathyroidism. J Oral Maxillofac Surg 2001;59: 1352–4.
11. Altay C, Erdogan N, Eren E, et al. Computed tomography findings of an unusual maxillary sinus mass: brown tumor due to tertiary hyperparathyroidism. J Clin Imaging Sci 2013;3:55.
12. Praveen AH, Thriveni R. Maxillary and mandibular hyperparathyroidism. Natl J Maxillofac Surg 2012;3:51–4.
13. Consensus development conference: diagnosis, prophylaxis and treatment of osteoporosis. Am J Med 1993;94:646–50.
14. NIH consensus development panel on osteoporosis prevention, diagnosis, and therapy. Osteoporosis prevention, diagnosis, and therapy. JAMA 2001;285:785–95.

15. WHO Scientific Group on the Prevention and Management of Osteoporosis. Prevention and management of osteoporosis: report of a WHO scientific group. (WHO technical report series: 921). Geneva (Switzerland): WHO; 2000.

16. Harvey N, Dennison E, Cooper C. Osteoporosis: impact on health and economics. Nat Rev Rheumatol 2010;6:99–105.

17. White SC, Rudolph DJ. Alterations of the trabecular pattern of the jaws in patients with osteoporosis. Oral Surg Oral Med Oral Pathol Oral Radiol Endod 1999;88:628–35.

18. Rockall AG, Babar SA, Sohaib SA, et al. CT and MR imaging of the adrenal glands in ACTH dependent Cushing's syndrome. Radiographics 2004;24:435–52.

19. Friedlander AH. The physiology, medical management and oral implications of menopause. J Am Dent Assoc 2002;133:73–81.

20. Leibowitz G, Tsur A, Chayen SD, et al. Pre-clinical Cushing's syndrome: an unexpected frequent cause of poor glycaemic control in obese diabetic patients. Clin Endocrinol (Oxf) 1996;44:717–22.

21. Omura M, Saito J, Yamaguchi K, et al. Prospective study on the prevalence of secondary hypertension among hypertensive patients visiting a general outpatient clinic in Japan. Hypertens Res 2004;27:193–202.

22. Chiodini I, Mascia ML, Muscarella S, et al. Subclinical hypercortisolism among outpatients referred for osteoporosis. Ann Intern Med 2007;147:541–8.

23. Murray RO. Radiological bone changes in Cushing's syndrome and steroid therapy. Br J Radiol 1960;33(385):1–19.

24. Ahmad M, Hollander L, Anderson Q, et al. Research diagnostic criteria for temporomandibular joint disorders (RDC/TMD) development of image analysis criteria and examiner reliability for image analysis. Oral Surg Oral Med Oral Pathol Oral Radiol Endod 2009;107:844–60.

25. Pincus T, Sokka T. How can the risk of long-term consequences of rheumatoid arthritis be reduced? Best Pract Res Clin Rheumatol 2001;15:139–70.

26. Aletaha D, Neogi T, Silman AJ, et al. 2010 Rheumatoid arthritis classification criteria: an American College of Rheumatology/European League Against Rheumatism collaborative initiative. Arthritis Rheum 2010;62:2569–81.

27. Siris ES, Lyles KW, Singer FR, et al. Medical management of Paget's disease of bone: indications for treatment and review of current therapies. J Bone Miner Res 2006;21(Suppl 2):P94–8.

28. Melmed S. Medical progress: acromegaly. N Engl J Med 2006;355:2558–73.

29. Hamdy R. Paget's disease of the bone. Clin Geriatr Med 1994;10:719–35.

30. [Guideline] Singer FR, Bone HG 3rd, Hosking DJ, et al. Paget's disease of bone: an Endocrine Society clinical practice guideline. J Clin Endocrinol Metab 2014;99(12):4408–22.

31. Daly AF, Rixhon M, Adam C, et al. High prevalence of pituitary adenomas: a cross-sectional study in the province of Liege, Belgium. J Clin Endocrinol Metab 2006;91:4769–75.

32. Holdaway IM, Rajasoorya C. Epidemiology of acromegaly. Pituitary 1999;2:29–41.

33. Kashyap RR, Babu GS, Shetty SR. Dental patient with acromegaly; a case report. J Oral Sci 2011;53:133–6.

34. Chew F. Radiologic manifestations in the musculoskeletal system of miscellaneous endocrine disorders. Radiol Clin North Am 1991;29(1):139.

35. Resnick D. Bone and joint disorders. 4th edition. vol. 3. Philadelphia: W.B. Saunders Company. 2004.

36. Katznelson L, Atkinson JL, Cook DM, et al. American Association of Clinical Endocrinologists medical guidelines for clinical practice for the diagnosis and treatment of acromegaly-2011 update. Endocr Pract 2011;17:1–44.

37. Melmed S, Casanueva FF, Cavagnini F, et al. Guidelines for acromegaly management. J Clin Endocrinol Metab 2002;87:4054–8.

38. Stary HC. Natural history and histological classification of atherosclerotic lesions: an update. Arterioscler Thromb Vasc Biol 2000;20:1177–8.

39. Fatahzadeh M, Glick M. Stroke: epidemiology, classification, risk factors, complications, diagnosis, prevention, and medical and management. Oral Surg Oral Med Oral Pathol Oral Radiol Endod 2006;02:80–91.

40. Cohen SN, Friedlander AH, Jolly DA, et al. Carotid calcification on panoramic radiographs: an important marker for vascular risk. Oral Surg Oral Med Oral Pathol Oral Radiol Endod 2002;94(4):510–4.

41. Nederkoorn PJ, van der Graaf Y, Hunink MG. Duplex ultrasound and magnetic resonance angiography compared with digital subtraction angiography in carotid artery stenosis: a systematic review. Stroke 2003;34:1324–32.

42. Friedlander AH, Garret NR, Norman DC. The prevalence of calcified carotid artery atheromas on the panoramic radiography of patients with type 2 diabetes mellitus. J Am Dent Assoc 2002;133:1516–23.

43. Mupparapu M, Kim IH. Calcified carotid artery atheroma and stroke: a systematic review. J Am Dent Assoc 2007;138(4):483–92.

44. Kumar GS, Manjunatha BS. Metastatic tumors to the jaws and oral cavity. J Oral Maxillofac Pathol 2013;17:71–5.

45. Worth HM. Principles and practice of oral radiologic interpretation. Chicago: Year Book Medical Publishers Inc; 1963.

46. Tiziani V, Reichenberger E, Buzzo CS, et al. The gene for cherubism maps to chromosome 4p16. Am J Hum Genet 1999;65(1):158–66.

47. Walker MP, Wichman B, Cheng AL, et al. Impact of radiotherapy dose on dentition breakdown in head and neck cancer patients. Pract Radiat Oncol 2011;1:142–8.

48. Otmani N. Oral and maxillofacial side effects of radiation therapy on children. J Can Dent Assoc 2007;73:257–61.

49. Koenig LJ. Diagnostic imaging: oral and maxillofacial. 1st edition. Salt Lake City, Utah: Amirsys; 2012.

50. Harousseau JL, Dreyling M. Multiple myeloma: ESMO clinical recommendations for diagnosis, treatment and follow-up. Ann Oncol 2009;20(Suppl 4):iv97–9.

Chemical and Radiation-Associated Jaw Lesions

Temitope T. Omolehinwa, BDS, Sunday O. Akintoye, BDS, DDS, MS*

KEYWORDS

- Osteoradionecrosis • Medication-related osteonecrosis • Chemical • Radiation
- Recreational drug • Damage • Diseases • Necrosis

KEY POINTS

- The role of radiographic imaging in diagnosis of osteonecrotic lesions cannot be overemphasized.
- Treatment options for jaw osteonecrosis include the use of local and systemic antibiotics, pain medications, debriding, sequestrectomy, hyperbaric oxygen treatment, and use of the antioxidants, tocopherol and Pentoxifylline. Surgical resection is usually a last resort, when all other forms of therapy fail.
- The effects on the quality of life in patients with jaw osteonecrosis, makes it an important area of research, especially to researchers interested in bone and tissue engineering.

INTRODUCTION

Bone is a unique connective tissue because it is functionally dynamic, consisting of different cells that continuously interact together. Unlike other connective tissues within the body, bone is physiologically mineralized. There is also an abundance of osteoprogenitor cells that reside within the bone microenvironment that can be activated to form different cell types.[1] The ability of bone to constantly remodel plays a vital role in the maintenance of mineral homeostasis, as old bone is removed by the activities of osteoclasts and new bone matrix is deposited by osteoblasts. Essentially, external and internal insults from radiation, drugs, or other chemical insults can induce a pathologic process that disrupts the bone microenvironment, turnover, and homeostasis. The outcome is dysregulation of the bone healing process that can potentially lead to loss of bone tissue, as in osteonecrosis.

This work was supported in part by the grants K22CA169089 and R21DE022826 (awarded to S.O. Akintoye) by United States Department of Health and Human Services/National Institutes of Health, Bethesda, MD.

Department of Oral Medicine, University of Pennsylvania School of Dental Medicine, Robert Schattner Center Room 211, 240 South 40th Street, Philadelphia, PA 19104, USA
* Corresponding author.
E-mail address: akintoye@dental.upenn.edu

Osteonecrosis is characterized by tissue dehiscence, chronic bone devitalization, hypocellularity, and osteolysis. The term osteonecrosis is often used interchangeably with ischemic necrosis, avascular necrosis, or aseptic necrosis, but there are different types of osteonecrosis. Depending on the etiologic agent, osteonecrosis can occur in any bone including the orofacial, appendicular, and axial bones. Osteonecrosis may or may not be associated with exposed bone with delayed healing. Specifically, the femoral head and mandible are highly susceptible to osteonecrosis. In the orofacial region, jaw osteonecrosis can lead to significant loss of bone tissue, tooth loss, and facial disfigurement. The unfortunate outcomes are significant morbidity, debility, and diminished quality of life.[2] The high susceptibility of the femoral bone to osteonecrosis is associated with a variety of factors that include alcohol abuse and steroid therapy. However, jaw osteonecrosis is much more associated with complications of radiation therapy, and long-term therapy with bone antiresorptives used to control skeletal events of cancer metastasis and osteoporosis.[3,4] In a randomized controlled study that assessed 792 cases of osteonecrosis in general, 76% of the cases occurred in the hip, and 4.4% occurred in the jaw mainly as a result of bisphosphonate therapies. The remaining cases were associated with the wrist, knee, foot, or ankle.[5] Several pathophysiologic theories have been proposed for osteonecrosis based on correlations of clinical signs with histologic and radiologic analyses. Although many of these theories have not been conclusively established, radiographic imaging has played a major role in the diagnosis, management, and follow-up assessment of osteonecrosis. Even more importantly is the increasing use of the combination of functional imaging with planar images to fully understand the metabolic changes that lead to osteonecrosis.[6]

TYPES OF OSTEONECROSIS
Osteoradionecrosis

Osteoradionecrosis (ORN) of the jaw is defined as nonhealing bony exposure and necrosis that starts with a breach in the oral mucosa, and persists for at least 3 months, in a patient who has undergone previous radiation therapy. The necrosis, however, must be evidently different from a recurrent, vestigial, or metastatic tumor.[7,8] This definition, however, does not include cases of ORN in which the oral mucosa is intact, but osteonecrotic changes can be observed by diagnostic imaging.[9] ORN is a chronic condition that can last for months or even years after the initial radiation therapy. The incidence of ORN can range from 2.6% to 22.0%[10] and it develops when the radiation dose exceeds 50 Gy. Specifically, radiation doses between 50 and 70 Gy have been implicated in the etiology of ORN.[11] Within the orofacial complex, the mandible is commonly affected because the mandible is usually in the line of radiation delivery and it is believed that the mandible is less vascularized than the maxilla.[12,13] Radiation also affects teeth secondarily, due to pronounced xerostomia noted in patients receiving radiation therapy (**Fig. 1**). The extensive carious lesions can be readily noted on bitewing radiographs, as demonstrated in **Figs. 2** and **3**.

Pathogenesis

Osteoradionecrosis was first described in 1926.[14] It was not until 1970 that a triad of radiation, trauma, and infection was proposed as the mechanistic process in ORN. However, this theory was later replaced in 1983 by another proposal that radiation causes development of hypoxic-hypocellular-hypovascular tissue (3H theory),[15] when it was reported that microorganisms do not play any causative but rather a contaminant role in ORN. It was also reported that trauma mainly creates a portal of entry for microorganisms to invade the radiation-suppressed bone. The 3H theory

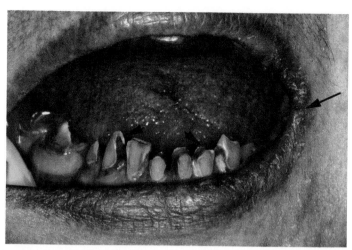

Fig. 1. Intraoral photograph of a patient who received radiation therapy for oral cancer. Note the several complications of radiation therapy that include extensive caries involving multiple surfaces as well as the incisal edges (*arrowheads*). The chalky white appearance of teeth is characteristic of radiation caries. Also note the angular cheilitis due to radiation-induced xerostomia (*arrow*).

of ORN takes into account that several tissues from exterior to interior are damaged by radiation, ranging from the skin or mucosa to periosteum, bone, and finally endothelium within the bone marrow compartment.[16] So the combination of tissue fibrosis, vascular and cellular damage induces a hypoxic environment within the radiated tissue.[16] The 3H theory was quickly followed by development of hyperbaric oxygen (HBO) therapy protocols to prevent and treat ORN, but this had only modest effectiveness, and HBO therapy is limited because it is contraindicated in patients with metastatic cancer.[3,4,17]

The radiation-induced fibroatrophic process is another mechanism associated with radiation damage more commonly to the superficial structures. This is associated with the activity of reactive oxygen species that cause damage to fibroblasts, endothelium,

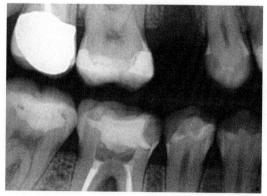

Fig. 2. Right premolar bitewing radiograph of a patient who received radiation therapy for head and neck cancer. Note the extensive carious lesions and failing restorations.

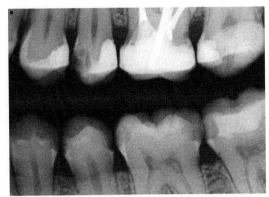

Fig. 3. Left premolar bitewing of the same patient as in **Fig. 2** with evidence of extensive dental caries due to a combination of decreased salivation and increased biofilm.

and bone cells, eventually causing tissue and bone necrosis (**Fig. 4**). However, the direct application of this theory to deep-seated radiation damage within the bone is yet to be conclusively clarified.[16] Another proposed pathophysiologic hypothesis is that ORN can be precipitated by a combination of dysregulated turnover, osteoclast

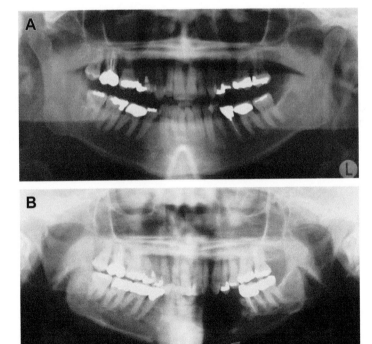

Fig. 4. Osteoradionecrosis of the mandible. This patient received radiation therapy for head and neck cancer. The panoramic radiographs before radiation therapy (*A*) show intact and well-corticated outline of the mandible. However, the patient developed left mandibular osteoradionecrosis (*B, red arrow*) after undergoing postirradiation extraction of the left mandibular premolars.

depletion, local tissue injury, and infection.[11] As all these theories do not conclusively define the pathophysiological process of ORN, more research is still needed to further our understanding of ORN pathogenesis.

Risk factors and classification

Several risk factors predispose to ORN; these include poor oral health, smoking, alcohol abuse, and most importantly, type and dose of radiation. Brachytherapy and radiation doses greater than 50 Gy have been associated with higher incidence of ORN. Additionally, any surgical manipulations of the irradiated area, including dental extractions, pose a significant risk. Several different classifications of ORN have been proposed, but one recently proposed combines clinical description, presence or absence of symptoms, and the treatment option for each of the different stages of ORN (**Table 1**).[9]

Clinical presentation

Patients with ORN usually present with pain that is typically neuropathic in nature. Also swelling may be accompanied by fever depending on the extent of the inflammatory process. Follow-up clinical evaluation may reveal tissue breakdown and bone necrosis that may be associated with paresthesia/anesthesia. If untreated, ORN especially in the mandible may result in pathologic fracture. Definitive diagnosis of ORN is a combination of clinical, radiologic, and histologic evaluations.

Medication-Related Osteonecrosis of the Jaws

Medication-related osteonecrosis of the jaw (MRONJ) is a more recent class of jaw osteonecrosis first described in 2003 in patients taking nitrogen-containing bisphosphonates (nBPs).[18] It is defined as exposed bone in the intraoral cavity persisting for 8 weeks or more, in patients who have previously undergone, or are currently undergoing treatment with antiresorptives and/or antiangiogenic agents and with no

Table 1
Classification of osteoradionecrosis

Stage	Length of Affected Bone/ Associated Structures (Damaged/Exposed)	Presence/Absence of Symptoms	Treatment
1	<2.5 cm	Asymptomatic.	Medication treatment only.
2	>2.5 cm	Asymptomatic. Includes pathologic fracture and/or involvement of inferior dental nerve.	Medication treatment only; except for presence of dental sepsis and loose/ necrotic bone.
3	>2.5 cm	Symptomatic. No other features of bone necrosis. However, symptoms persist despite medication treatment.	Debridement of loose/ necrotic bone. Local pedicle flap.
4	>2.5 cm	Symptomatic. Pathologic fracture. Involvement of inferior alveolar nerve and/or orocutaneous fistula.	Reconstruction with free flap, if patient's overall health allows.

Adapted from Lyons A, Osher J, Warner E, et al. Osteoradionecrosis: a review of current concepts in defining the extent of the disease and a new classification proposal. Br J Oral Maxillofac Surg 2014;52(5):394; with permission.

previous history of radiation therapy to the jaw. This excludes primary or metastatic cancer within the jaw region.[18] However, this definition does not take into account the nonexposed bone variant of the disease process, which makes up about a third of all cases of MRONJ cases.[19]

The nBPs, especially the intravenous nBPs, such as zoledronic acid, were the first group of drugs initially associated with MRONJ. The high efficacy of intravenous nBPs, such as zoledronic acid and pamidronate, to control altered bone remodeling make them highly favored for the treatment of skeletal events of cancer metastasis, Paget disease, osteogenesis imperfecta, and hyperparathyroid jaw tumors, so it is understandable that nBPs were the first to be associated with osteonecrosis exclusive to the jaws. Other medications also have been implicated in MRONJ; these include another antiresorptive drug, denosumab, which acts as an inhibitor of receptor activator for NFκB ligand (RANKL), and antiangiogenic drugs like bevacizumab, an inhibitor of vascular endothelial growth factor, and sunitinib, a tyrosine kinase inhibitor.

Because of the vast array of medications associated with osteonecrosis of the jaw (ONJ), the nomenclature for this disorder has evolved over the years from ONJ, bisphosphonate osteonecrosis (BON), bisphosphonate-related osteonecrosis of the jaw (BRONJ), and anti-resorptive osteonecrosis of the jaw (ARONJ) to the more recent MRONJ.[20] The incidence of MRONJ in patients taking intravenous nBPs ranges from 0% to 27.5%,[19,20] and denosumab 1.7%.[19] The relative risks of MRONJ occurring in patients taking intravenous nBPs, denosumab, or bevacizumab are 0.7% to 6.7%, 0.7% to 1.9%, and 0.2% respectively.[20] MRONJ affects the mandible and maxilla at a ratio of 2:1,[21] because the mandible is partly associated with a single vascular supply from the inferior alveolar artery compared with the superior, inferior, and middle arteries in the maxilla. Severe cases of MRONJ in the mandible can lead to pathologic fracture, whereas in the maxilla it can result in oroantral fistulation.

Pathogenesis

The pathophysiology of MRONJ is still unclear, but different investigators have proposed several theories.[22,23] These include a decrease in bone turnover, presence of infection (especially *Actinomyces* species), inhibition of angiogenesis, and a dysregulation or dysfunction of innate and acquired immunity.[24] The infection theory is based on the premise that a "complex biofilm" is present on the surface of exposed necrotic bone.[25] Definitive elucidation of MRONJ pathogenesis is hampered because the offending drugs have different mechanisms of action (**Table 2**) and nonoral bones are spared by MRONJ. The role of bone mesenchymal stem cells (MSCs) also cannot be overlooked, considering that jaw MSCs are phenotypically and functionally different from those of axial and appendicular bones[1] and they are disproportionately more sensitive to both zoledronic acid and pamidronate, both of which are strongly associated with MRONJ.[26]

Risk factors and classification

The local risk factors that may predispose to MRONJ include trauma, overall poor dental health, presence of tori or bony exostosis, and invasive dental procedures, such as dental extractions and periodontal treatment. In addition, the systemic risk factors include diabetes, smoking, alcohol, and an ongoing immunosuppressive therapy.[28]

Clinical presentation

Patients with MRONJ have variable clinical presentation depending on the clinical course of the disease. This can vary from nonexposed bone to extensive bone loss and pathologic fracture (**Fig. 5**). Therefore, a staging algorithm has been proposed to aid not only in the diagnosis but also management of MRONJ (**Table 3**). A detailed

Table 2
Implicated drugs in medication-related osteonecrosis of the jaw and their mechanisms of action

	Zoledronic Acid	Denosumab	Bevacizumab
Half-life	Binds to bone: longer half-life	Does not bind to bone: short half-life (approximately 28 d)	Does not bind to bone: short half-life (approximately 20 d)
Mechanism	Apoptosis of osteoclasts	Prevents formation of osteoclasts	Inhibits angiogenesis
Target pathways/ transcription proteins	Inhibits farnesyl pyrophosphate through mevalonate pathway	Inhibits receptor activator of nuclear factor kappa-B ligand	Inhibits tyrosine kinase by binding to vascular endothelial growth factor
Effects on immune system	No effect on immune system	Tendency to cause immunosuppression by action on B and T cells	Has effects on the immune system
Clearance	Clearance through kidneys: nephrotoxic (up to 12 y)	Clearance through immunoglobulin pathway in reticuloendothelial system (within 6 mo)	Clearance by pinocytosis with binding to neonatal Fc receptor[27]

history, clinical examination, and carefully selected radiographic imaging will aid in the diagnosis of MRONJ (**Figs. 6** and **7**).

Recreational Drug–Induced Osteonecrosis

Chronic use of recreational or illicit drugs, such as cocaine, amphetamine, and methamphetamine, are established independent risk factors for osteonecrosis, termed recreational drug–induced osteonecrosis (RDIO).[29–32] It is more common in the maxilla.[29]

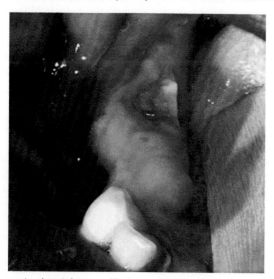

Fig. 5. Exposed bone in the right mandibular posterior region in a patient with MRONJ. (*Courtesy of* Arthur Kuperstein, DDS, and Mel Mupparapu, DMD, University of Pennsylvania School of Dental Medicine, Philadelphia, PA.)

Table 3	
Clinical staging of medication-related osteonecrosis of the jaw	
Clinical Staging	**Presentation**
Stage 0	Nonspecific odontogenic symptoms in patients with a history of antiresorptive treatments.
Stage 1	Asymptomatic bony exposure.
Stage 2	Bony exposure, pain, and infection, well contained in the dentoalveolar area.
Stage 3	Stage 2 disease symptoms extending beyond the alveolar area. Includes pathologic fractures, oroantral communication, maxillary sinusitis, sinuses, and fistula.

Adapted from Ruggiero SL, Dodson TB, Fantasia J, et al. American Association of Oral and Maxillofacial Surgeons position paper on medication-related osteonecrosis of the jaw—2014 update. J Oral Maxillofac Surg 2014;72(10):1938; with permission.

The incidence of RDIO is unknown because many addicts do not seek medical care. Additionally, most illicit drug addicts are also heavy smokers and may be abusing alcohol or other prescription drugs, which also heightens their predisposition to osteonecrosis.[31] The pathogenesis of RDIO is multifactorial. Although several recreational drugs have been implicated, cocaine in particular induces vascular constriction that results in local ischemia of the adjacent soft and hard tissues.[33] It has been proposed that the combined effect of chemical irritation from additives to the recreational drug, trauma, and superimposed microbial infection accentuate the necrotic process that leads to bone destruction.[32] Therefore, excessive bone destruction caused by nasal inhalation or snorting of a recreational drug like cocaine initially starts as ulceration of mucosal tissue that progressively leads to osteocartilaginous necrosis. If uncontrolled, the nasal septum and palate become perforated, consequently leading to oronasal and oroantral fistulations.[30,34] Specifically, cocaine-induced midline destructive lesion (CIMDL) has been used to describe extensive destruction caused by cocaine addiction to the oronasal structures, including the hard palate.[32] This extensive osteonecrosis of the bony structures is one of the hallmarks used to identify CIMDL in the assessment of human skeletal remains by medical examiners and forensic scientists. If the addicted individual seeks treatment early, which often does not happen, RDIO can be controlled before extensive bone destruction occurs by discontinuation of the offending recreational drug.

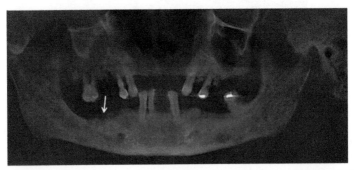

Fig. 6. Panoramic reconstruction of the mandible and maxilla CBCT image of a patient with MRONJ (*arrow* points to the area of osteonecrosis). (*Courtesy of* Arthur Kuperstein, DDS, Mel Mupparapu, DMD, University of Pennsylvania School of Dental Medicine, Philadelphia, PA.)

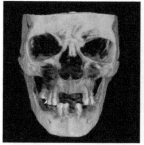 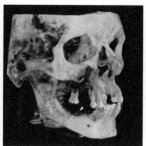 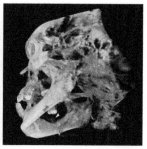

Fig. 7. Same patient as in **Figs. 5** and **6**. CBCT 3-dimensional reconstruction of the facial skeleton showing the separated osteonecrotic alveolar portion of the mandible (*arrowheads*). (*Courtesy of* Arthur Kuperstein, DDS, and Mel Mupparapu, DMD, University of Pennsylvania School of Dental Medicine, Philadelphia, PA.)

Steroid-Induced Osteonecrosis

Steroid-induced osteonecrosis, also referred to as aseptic, ischemic, or avascular necrosis, develops as a result of long-term administration of corticosteroids. It is more common in the appendicular bones, such as the femur or humerus rather than the jaw[35,36] and it is not induced by trauma or external insults, so it is a form of atraumatic osteonecrosis. Corticosteroids affect multiple organs and systems, have immunosuppressive effects, and can disrupt bone homeostasis.[36] Long-term use of corticosteroids of more than 20 mg per day can result in osteopenia and eventually osteoporosis. To further complicate the situation, the patient may need to be placed on bisphosphonate therapy to control dysregulated bone remodeling, consequently resulting in the development of medication-induced osteonecrosis of the jaw. Smoking, alcohol abuse, and comorbid conditions, such as osteoporosis and systemic lupus erythematosus, predispose patients to steroid-induced osteonecrosis.[37]

HISTOLOGIC FEATURES OF OSTEONECROSIS

Definitive diagnosis of osteonecrosis is based on clinical, histologic, and radiological findings. Histologically, vascular damage with hyperemia, inflammatory cells, and osteoclastic activity are often seen at the early stages of osteonecrosis. Thereafter, osteonecrosis displays regions of acellular marrow with loss of hematopoietic cells, adipocytic infiltration suggestive of fatty marrow, and some regions of patchy calcifications within the marrow components due to osteoclastic activity. The bone is also hypocellular with regions of empty lacunae devoid of osteocytic nuclei. There may be attempts at healing demonstrated by reparative granulation tissue and some degree of new osteoid deposition. Histologic features of osteonecrosis are similar in the oral and nonoral bone and are independent of the bone type.

RADIOLOGIC FEATURES OF OSTEONECROSIS

Radiologic features of osteonecrosis must be correlated with histologic findings. A good starting point for diagnosis of osteonecrosis is the use of plain film and panoramic radiography (see **Figs. 2–4**), cone beam computerized tomography (CBCT) (see **Figs. 6** and **7**), and conventional CT. Plain film radiographs will display mixed radiolucent and radiopaque trabecular pattern. Depending on the cause of the osteonecrosis, there could be regions of osteolysis and sclerosis. Similarly, CT will display altered trabeculation, cortical thinning, and sclerosis. Unfortunately, there needs to be approximately 30% to 50% loss of bone mineral content for a bone lesion to be better defined in a panoramic radiograph or CT.[6]

Other limits of panoramic radiograph and CT are that some of the radiographic features are not specific to osteonecrosis; also, these imaging modalities cannot differentiate necrotic bone from metastatic lesion, especially in oncology patients in whom this may be a concern.[38] Bone scintigraphy or bone scan provides better information about the metabolic activities and pathophysiological changes in osteonecrosis much earlier than panoramic radiographs, as osteonecrosis will display high uptake of 99mTc-methylene diphosphonate in a bone scan. But a major diagnostic challenge of using bone scintigraphy to diagnose osteonecrosis is its high signal sensitivity and low specificity, as many dental disorders can present as osteonecrosis in a bone scan.

The additional use of the combinations of fluorodeoxyglucose/positron emission tomography (FDG/PET) and single photon emission computed tomography (SPECT)/CT combination have also been shown to improve diagnostic accuracy because they provide functional and anatomic coregistration of the extent of the osteonecrosis.[32,39-41] MRI can display osteonecrosis as decreased marrow signal intensity on T1-weighted images and increased signal intensity on T2-weighted images. Interestingly, studies using osteonecrosis of the hip samples have also shown that MRI findings correlate well with histologic features of osteonecrosis.[42] As MRI displays excellent visualization of soft tissues, it may be useful in the diagnosis of osteonecrosis in the mandibular condyle and around the temporomandibular joint complex where it may be clinically impracticable to obtain biopsy samples.

SUMMARY

The role of radiographic imaging in diagnosis of osteonecrotic lesions cannot be overemphasized. However, there are limitations in the use of radiologic imaging only as the standard of diagnosis without correlating the findings with other aspects of diagnosis: clinical presentation and histologic findings. This is because most types of jaw osteonecrosis have similar radiographic presentations and cannot be differentiated from other diseases affecting the jaw bone; for example, osteomyelitis and periapical lesions.

Treatment options for jaw osteonecrosis include the use of local and systemic antibiotics, pain medications, debriding, sequestrectomy, hyperbaric oxygen treatment, and use of the antioxidants, tocopherol and Pentoxifylline.[28] Surgical resection is usually a last resort, when all other forms of therapy fail.

The effects on the quality of life in patients with jaw osteonecrosis make it an important area of research, especially to those interested in bone and tissue engineering. An interesting area of ongoing research right now is the possible role of MSCs in possible reconstruction of the defect caused by jaw osteonecrosis and the use of pharmacologic compounds; for example, antisclerostin antibody in the prevention of the osteonecrotic process especially in patients with MRONJ.[43-46]

REFERENCES

1. Akintoye SO, Lam T, Shi S, et al. Skeletal site-specific characterization of orofacial and iliac crest human bone marrow stromal cells in same individuals. Bone 2006; 38(6):758–68.
2. Edwards BK, Ward E, Kohler BA, et al. Annual report to the nation on the status of cancer, 1975-2006, featuring colorectal cancer trends and impact of interventions (risk factors, screening, and treatment) to reduce future rates. Cancer 2010; 116(3):544–73.

3. Aapro M, Saad F, Costa L. Optimizing clinical benefits of bisphosphonates in cancer patients with bone metastases. Oncologist 2010;15(11):1147–58.

4. Mauri D, Valachis A, Polyzos NP, et al. Does adjuvant bisphosphonate in early breast cancer modify the natural course of the disease? A meta-analysis of randomized controlled trials. J Natl Compr Canc Netw 2010;8(3):279–86.

5. Cooper C, Steinbuch M, Stevenson R, et al. The epidemiology of osteonecrosis: findings from the GPRD and THIN databases in the UK. Osteoporos Int 2010; 21(4):569–77.

6. Bedogni A, Fedele S, Bedogni G, et al. Staging of osteonecrosis of the jaw requires computed tomography for accurate definition of the extent of bony disease. Br J Oral Maxillofac Surg 2014;52(7):603–8.

7. Madrid C, Abarca M, Bouferrache K. Osteoradionecrosis: an update. Oral Oncol 2010;46(6):471–4.

8. Pitak-Arnnop P, Sader R, Dhanuthai K, et al. Management of osteoradionecrosis of the jaws: an analysis of evidence. Eur J Surg Oncol 2008;34(10):1123–34.

9. Lyons A, Osher J, Warner E, et al. Osteoradionecrosis: a review of current concepts in defining the extent of the disease and a new classification proposal. Br J Oral Maxillofac Surg 2014;52(5):392–5.

10. D'Souza J, Lowe D, Rogers SN. Changing trends and the role of medical management on the outcome of patients treated for osteoradionecrosis of the mandible: experience from a regional head and neck unit. Br J Oral Maxillofac Surg 2014;52(4):356–62.

11. McCaul JA. Pharmacologic modalities in the treatment of osteoradionecrosis of the jaw. Oral Maxillofac Surg Clin North Am 2014;26(2):247–52.

12. Parliament M, Alidrisi M, Munroe M, et al. Implications of radiation dosimetry of the mandible in patients with carcinomas of the oral cavity and nasopharynx treated with intensity modulated radiation therapy. Int J Oral Maxillofac Surg 2005;34(2):114–21.

13. Salama JK, Vokes EE, Chmura SJ, et al. Long-term outcome of concurrent chemotherapy and reirradiation for recurrent and second primary head-and-neck squamous cell carcinoma. Int J Radiat Oncol Biol Phys 2006;64(2): 382–91.

14. Phemister DB. Radium necrosis of bone. Am J Roentgenol 1926;16:340.

15. Marx RE. Osteoradionecrosis: a new concept of its pathophysiology. J Oral Maxillofac Surg 1983;41(5):283–8.

16. Delanian S, Lefaix JL. The radiation-induced fibroatrophic process: therapeutic perspective via the antioxidant pathway. Radiother Oncol 2004;73(2):119–31.

17. Marx RE. A new concept in the treatment of osteoradionecrosis. J Oral Maxillofac Surg 1983;41(6):351–7.

18. Ruggiero SL, Mehrotra B, Rosenberg TJ, et al. Osteonecrosis of the jaws associated with the use of bisphosphonates: a review of 63 cases. J Oral Maxillofac Surg 2004;62(5):527–34.

19. Campisi G, Fedele S, Fusco V, et al. Epidemiology, clinical manifestations, risk reduction and treatment strategies of jaw osteonecrosis in cancer patients exposed to antiresorptive agents. Future Oncol 2014;10(2):257–75.

20. Ruggiero SL, Dodson TB, Fantasia J, et al. American Association of Oral and Maxillofacial Surgeons position paper on medication-related osteonecrosis of the jaw—2014 update. J Oral Maxillofac Surg 2014;72(10):1938–56.

21. Franco-Pretto E, Pacheco M, Moreno A, et al. Bisphosphonate-induced osteonecrosis of the jaws: clinical, imaging, and histopathology findings. Oral Surg Oral Med Oral Pathol Oral Radiol 2014;118(4):408–17.

22. Landesberg R, Woo V, Cremers S, et al. Potential pathophysiological mechanisms in osteonecrosis of the jaw. Ann N Y Acad Sci 2011;1218:62–79.

23. Sarin J, DeRossi SS, Akintoye SO. Updates on bisphosphonates and potential pathobiology of bisphosphonate-induced jaw osteonecrosis. Oral Dis 2008; 14(3):277–85.

24. Li D, Gromov K, Proulx ST, et al. Effects of antiresorptive agents on osteomyelitis: novel insights into the pathogenesis of osteonecrosis of the jaw. Ann N Y Acad Sci 2010;1192:84–94.

25. Katsarelis H, Shah NP, Dhariwal DK, et al. Infection and medication-related osteonecrosis of the jaw. J Dent Res 2015;94(4):534–9.

26. Stefanik D, Sarin J, Lam T, et al. Disparate osteogenic response of mandible and iliac crest bone marrow stromal cells to pamidronate. Oral Dis 2008;14(5): 465–71.

27. Kazazi-Hyseni F, Beijnen JH, Schellens JH. Bevacizumab. Oncologist 2010;15(8): 819–25.

28. Epstein MS, Wicknick FW, Epstein JB, et al. Management of bisphosphonate-associated osteonecrosis: pentoxifylline and tocopherol in addition to antimicrobial therapy. An initial case series. Oral Surg Oral Med Oral Pathol Oral Radiol Endod 2010;110(5):593–6.

29. Rustemeyer J, Melenberg A, Junker K, et al. Osteonecrosis of the maxilla related to long-standing methamphetamine abuse: a possible new aspect in the etiology of osteonecrosis of the jaw. Oral Maxillofac Surg 2014;18(2):237–41.

30. Seyer BA, Grist W, Muller S. Aggressive destructive midfacial lesion from cocaine abuse. Oral Surg Oral Med Oral Pathol Oral Radiol Endod 2002; 94(4):465–70.

31. Ziraldo L, O'Connor MB, Blake SP, et al. Osteonecrosis following alcohol, cocaine, and steroid use. Subst Abus 2011;32(3):170–3.

32. Rubin K. The manifestation of cocaine-induced midline destructive lesion in bone tissue and its identification in human skeletal remains. Forensic Sci Int 2013; 231(1–3):408.e1–11.

33. Nastro Siniscalchi E, Gabriele G, Cascone P. Palatal fistula resulting from cocaine abuse: a case report. Eur Rev Med Pharmacol Sci 2012;16(2):280–2.

34. Goodger NM, Wang J, Pogrel MA. Palatal and nasal necrosis resulting from cocaine misuse. Br Dent J 2005;198(6):333–4.

35. Chiu CT, Chiang WF, Chuang CY, et al. Resolution of oral bisphosphonate and steroid-related osteonecrosis of the jaw–a serial case analysis. J Oral Maxillofac Surg 2010;68(5):1055–63.

36. Powell C, Chang C, Gershwin ME. Current concepts on the pathogenesis and natural history of steroid-induced osteonecrosis. Clin Rev Allergy Immunol 2011;41(1):102–13.

37. Nowak DA, Yeung J. Steroid-induced osteonecrosis in dermatology: a review. J Cutan Med Surg 2015;19(4):358–60.

38. Gander T, Obwegeser JA, Zemann W, et al. Malignancy mimicking bisphosphonate-associated osteonecrosis of the jaw: a case series and literature review. Oral Surg Oral Med Oral Pathol Oral Radiol 2014;117(1):32–6.

39. Fleisher KE, Raad RA, Rakheja R, et al. Fluorodeoxyglucose positron emission tomography with computed tomography detects greater metabolic changes that are not represented by plain radiography for patients with osteonecrosis of the jaw. J Oral Maxillofac Surg 2014;72(10):1957–65.

40. Lapa C, Linz C, Bluemel C, et al. Three-phase bone scintigraphy for imaging osteoradionecrosis of the jaw. Clin Nucl Med 2014;39(1):21–5.

41. Dore F, Filippi L, Biasotto M, et al. Bone scintigraphy and SPECT/CT of bisphosphonate-induced osteonecrosis of the jaw. J Nucl Med 2009;50(1):30–5.
42. Larheim TA, Westesson PL, Hicks DG, et al. Osteonecrosis of the temporomandibular joint: correlation of magnetic resonance imaging and histology. J Oral Maxillofac Surg 1999;57(8):888–98 [discussion: 899].
43. Xu J, Zheng Z, Fang D, et al. Mesenchymal stromal cell-based treatment of jaw osteoradionecrosis in swine. Cell Transplant 2012;21(8):1679–86.
44. Damek-Poprawa M, Stefanik D, Levin LM, et al. Human bone marrow stromal cells display variable anatomic site-dependent response and recovery from irradiation. Arch Oral Biol 2010;55(5):358–64.
45. Chandra A, Lin T, Tribble MB, et al. PTH1-34 alleviates radiotherapy-induced local bone loss by improving osteoblast and osteocyte survival. Bone 2014;67:33–40.
46. Fessel J. There are many potential medical therapies for atraumatic osteonecrosis. Rheumatology (Oxford) 2013;52(2):235–41.

Index

Note: Page numbers of article titles are in **boldface** type.

A

Actinomycosis, 200–201
Adenoid cystic carcinoma, 148–150
Adenomatoid odontogenic tumors, 134, 135
Ameloblastic fibro-odontoma, 134
Ameloblastoma, 132, 133
Amelogenesis imperfecta, 50–51
Aneurysmal bone cyst, 138
Anthrax, 202–203
Aspergillosis, 208–209, 210
Atherosclerosis, 254, 255
Autoimmune and vascular diseases, 222–225

B

Bifid condyle, 120, 121
Bitewing radiograph, premolar, 3, 4
Blastomycosis, 205–206
Bone cyst, aneurysmal, 138
    simple, 127
Brucellosis, 203
Burkitt lymphoma, 153

C

Cementoblastoma, 133, 134
    benign, 177–178, 181, 182
Cementum, defects of, 54
Cephalometric radiograph, lateral, 13
Chemotherapy, effects on oral cavity, 258
Cherubism, 257–258, 259
Cholesterol granulomas, 215–216
Chondromatosis, synovial, 114–116
Chondrosarcomas, 151
Cleidocranial dysplasia, 62–64
Cocaine-induced granulomas, 216–217
Computed tomography, multidetector/multislice, for oral and maxillofacial imaging, 18–22
Condylar aplasia, 61, 119–120
Condylar hyperplasia, 59–61
Condylar hypoplasia, 61, 119–120
Coronoid process hyperplasia, 61–62
Craniosynostosis, 64

Dent Clin N Am 60 (2016) 279–285
http://dx.doi.org/10.1016/S0011-8532(15)00129-9
0011-8532/16/$ – see front matter © 2016 Elsevier Inc. All rights reserved.

dental.theclinics.com

Crohn disease, 221–222
Crozon syndrome, 64–67
Cryptococcosis, 209
Cushing syndrome, 243–244
Cysts. See specific cysts.

D

Degenerative joint disease, 109
    radiodiagnostic criteria in, 109–114
Dens evaginatus, 48–49
Dens invaginatus, 47–48
Dental implant patient, radiographic evaluation of, 99–103
Dentigerous cysts, 126, 128
Dentin, defect of, 51–53
Dentine dysplasia, 53
Dentinogenesis imperfecta, 51–53
Developmental diseases, 226
Down syndrome, 74–81
Drugs, osteonecrosis related to, 269–270, 271
    recreational, osteonecrosis induced by, 271–272

E

Ectodermal dysplasia, 71–72, 73
Ehlers-Danlos syndromes, 72–74, 75–76, 77, 78
Enamel, defect of, 50–51
Enamel pearls, 49
Epithelial odontogenic tumor, calcifying, 133
Ewing sarcoma, 151, 152
Exostosis, and tori, 54
    buccal and palatal, 56–57

F

Fibro-odontoma, ameloblastic, 134
Fibro-osseous lesions, 189–191
Fibroma, ossifying, cemento-ossifying or cementifying, 137–138
Fibrosarcoma, 151
Fibrous dysplasia, craniofacial, 183–192
    monostotic, 178–181, 182–186
    polystotic, 181–182, 186, 187
Foreign body, infections due to, 215–218
    oral reaction to, 215
Frontal bone, skull lesions within, 13
Fungal infections, 205–211

G

Gardner syndrome, 82–86
Ghost teeth, 53–54

Giant cell granuloma, central, 136–137, 138
Gorlin syndrome, 81–82, 83, 84
Gout, 217–218
Granulomatous diseases, of jaws, **195–234**

H

Hansen disease, 197–198, 199, 200
Hemifacial atrophy, 58–59
Hemihyperplasia, facial, 57
Histiocytosis X, 218–219
Histoplasmosis, 205
Hypercementosis, 54
Hyperparathyroidism, 238–240
Hyperpituitarism, 250–254
Hypodontia/anodontia, 41

I

Infections, caused by trauma, 213
    of jaws, 195–205
Infectious arthritis, 114

J

Jaws, benign fibro-osseous lesions of, **167–193**
    benign lesions of, **125–141**
    chemical and radiation-associated lesions of, **265–277**
    cysticlike lesions of, salient imaging of, 137
    developmental disorders affecting, **39–90**
    granulomatous diseases of, **195–234**
        and etiologic agents, 196
    MRI of, 157–158
    osseous dysplasia in, 168–192
    radiographic examination of, 156
        imaging modalities in, 156–157
        imaging protocols for, 156
    systemic diseases and conditions affecting, **235–264**
Jwas, genetic conditions affecting, 62–86

K

Klebsiella rhinoslerosis infection, 201–202

L

Leishmaniasis, 211
Leprosy, 197–198, 199, 200
Lethal midline granulomas, 220–221
Leukemia, 153, 154

M

Macrodontia, 39–40
Magnetic resonance imaging, of jaws, 157–158
Malignant tumor-gingival carcinoma, mandibular, 158, 159
Mandibular body, oblique radiography of, 12
Mandibular condyle, hyperplasia of, 120, 121
Mandibulofacial dysostosis, 67–69, 70
McCune Albright syndrome, 186
Melkersson-Rosenthal syndrome, 226
Metastatic tumors, 254–257
Microdontia, 40–41
Microsomia, hemifacial, 69–71, 72
Multiple myeloma, 153, 259–262
Myiasis, 211–212, 213
Myxoma, odontogenic, 133, 134

N

Nasopalatine duct/incisive canal cysts, 127, 128
Neoplastic diseases, 218–221
Nevoid basal cell carcinoma syndrome, 81–82, 83, 84
Non-Hodgkin lymphoma, 153
Nonodontogenic cysts, 127–129
Nonodontogenic tumors, benign, 135–136
        neural, 135

O

Odontodysplasia, regional, 53–54
Odontogenic cysts, 126, 127
Odontogenic myxoma, 133, 134
Odontogenic tumors, adenomatoid, 134, 135
    benign, 129–134
    epithelial calcifying, 133
    keratocystic, 129, 132
Odontoma, 132, 133
Oral and maxillofacial imaging, **1–37**
    extraoral, 7
    findings and pathology of, 5
    for differential diagnosis, 6
    kilovoltage peak rule for, 5
    quality of, factors affecting, 3–4, 5
    skull radiographs for, 7–12
    technique of, and normal anatomy, 2
    why, where, how, and when to image, 2
Orofacial pain, temporomandibular joint disorders and, **105–124**
Orofacial region, malignant tumors in, classification of, 146–155
        clinical examination of, 145
        diagnostic imaging of, **143–165**
        differential disgnosis of, 162–163

management of, 161, 162
oral cancer screening in, 145
radiographic appearance of, 160–161
viruses associated with, 144
Osseous dysplasia, florid, 173–177, 180
focal, 172–173, 175–179
of jaws, 168–192
periapical, 169–172, 173, 174, 175
Osteitis deformans, 247–250, 251
Osteoarthrosis, 109–114
Osteodystrophy, renal, 237–238
Osteoma, 136
Osteonecrosis, histologic features of, 273
medication-related, 269–270, 271
radiologic features of, 267, 268, 273–274
recreational drug-induced, 271–272
steroid-induced, 273
types of, 266–273
Osteoporosis, 240–243
Osteoradionecrosis, 266–269
Osteosarcoma, 151, 152

P

Paget disease, 247–250
Pantomyography, oral and maxillofacial, 16–18
Papillon-Lefèvre syndrome, 74, 79
Parasitic infections, 211–213
Parry-Romberg syndrome, 58–59
Periodontal cysts, lateral, 126
Periodontal patient, radiologic assessment of, **91–104**
Periodontics, cone beam computed tomography in, 97–99
conventional radiography in, 92–97
film and sensor characteristics for, 92
options and selection criteria for, 92–97
Phycomycosis, 206–207
Polymorphic reticulosis, 220–221
Pyogenic granulomas, 213–215

R

Radiation, effects on oral cavity, 258, 259
Radicular (periapical) cysts, 126, 128
Radiography, extraoral, cone beam computed tomography in, noncontrast, 22–26
linear and complex motion tomography, 14–22
MRI, for oral and maxillofacial imaging, 26
PET scanning, for oral and maxillofacial imaging, 28–29
intraoral, 2–7
imaging protocols for, 2–5
Radioisotope imaging, for oral and maxillofacial imaging, 31–32
Radiosialography, for oral and maxillofacial imaging, 32–34

Renal disease, end-stage, 237–238
Renal osteodystrophy, 237–238
Reticulosis, polymorphic, 220–221
Rheumatoid arthritis, 113–114, 246–247
Rhinosporidiosis, 210–211

S

Salivary gland depression, lingual, 138, 139
Sarcoidosis, 221, 222
Sarcomas, 151
Scintigraphy, for oral and maxillofacial imaging, 31, 32
Septic arthritis, 114
Sialendoscopy, for oral and maxillofacial imaging, 34
Sialography, for oral and maxillofacial imaging, 32–34
Sialometaplasia, necrotizing, 219–220
Sickle cell anemia, 236–237
Simple bone cyst, 127
Sjögren syndrome, 224–225
Squamous cell carcinoma, 147–150
Steroids, osteonecrosis induced by, 273
Synovial chondromatosis, 114–116
Syphillis, 203–205
Systemic lupus erythematosus, 223–224

T

Taurodontism, 46–47
Teeth, concrescence of, 44–46
    dilaceration of, 49–50
    fusion of, 42–43, 44
    germination of, 43–44, 45
    number of, developmental defects of, 41–42
    shape of, developmental defects of, 42
    size of, developmental defects of, 39–40
    supernumerary, 41–42
Temporomandibular joint complex, fracture of, 116
Temporomandibular joint(s), akylosis of, 118
    development disturbances of, 118–119
    disc displacement in, 107–108
    diseases of, degenerative, 245–246
        of systemic origin, 244–245
        rheumatoid arthritis, 246–247
    dislocation of condyles of, 116–117
    disorders of, and orofacial pain, **105–124**
        taxonomy of, 105, 106
    hypomobility of, 118
    inflammatory disturbances of, 108
    loose bodies, 114–116
    MRI of, 109, 110
    traumatic disturbances of, 116–118

Tomography, linear and complex motion, for oral and maxillofacial imaging, 14–22
Tori, exostosis and, 54
Torus mandibularis, 55–56
Torus maxillaris, 56–57
Torus palatinus, 54–55
Toxoplasmosis, 212–213
Treacher Collins syndrome, 67–69, 70
Tuberculosis, 195–197

U

Ultrasound, for oral and maxillofacial imaging, 29–31

W

Wegener granulomatosis, 222–223

Moving?

Make sure your subscription moves with you!

To notify us of your new address, find your **Clinics Account Number** (located on your mailing label above your name), and contact customer service at:

Email: journalscustomerservice-usa@elsevier.com

800-654-2452 (subscribers in the U.S. & Canada)
314-447-8871 (subscribers outside of the U.S. & Canada)

Fax number: 314-447-8029

Elsevier Health Sciences Division
Subscription Customer Service
3251 Riverport Lane
Maryland Heights, MO 63043

*To ensure uninterrupted delivery of your subscription, please notify us at least 4 weeks in advance of move.

Printed and bound by CPI Group (UK) Ltd, Croydon, CR0 4YY

07/10/2024

01040499-0012